EUGENICS, H1
AND HUM

What is the history of the British eugenics movement? Why should it be of interest to how scientists work today?

This outstanding study follows the history of the eugenics movements from its roots to its heyday as the source of a science of human genetics. The primary contributions of the book are fourfold. First, it points to nineteenth-century social reform as contributing to the later eugenics movement. Second, it is based upon important archival material newly available to researchers. This material gives the reader an insight into the inner councils of the Society that could not have been obtained by relying upon published sources alone. Third, it treats the statistical methods involved in human genetics historically, in a way that allows the reader to follow their development and tie them to their context within the eugenics movement. Previous treatment of eugenics has not tended to view it as a science whose methods required serious consideration. Fourth, it provides a historical introduction to the current problems connected with the huge international projects for the mapping of the human genome. New methods developed in the 1980s have created new interest in pinpointing the genes for diseases such as Huntington's chorea. With this scientific success there has come a renewal of interest in, and fears of, eugenics in both Europe and America.

Comprehensive and compelling, this book will be of interest to historians of medicine and science, sociologists, social historians, psychologists and human geneticists.

Scholarly and penetrating, Pauline Mazumdar's study of eugenics is a major contribution not only to the sociology of science, but to our understanding of the complex relation between science, ideology and class.
Bryan S. Turner, Professor in Sociology, *University of Essex*

Pauline M.H. Mazumdar is Associate Professor in the History of Medicine, Toronto University.

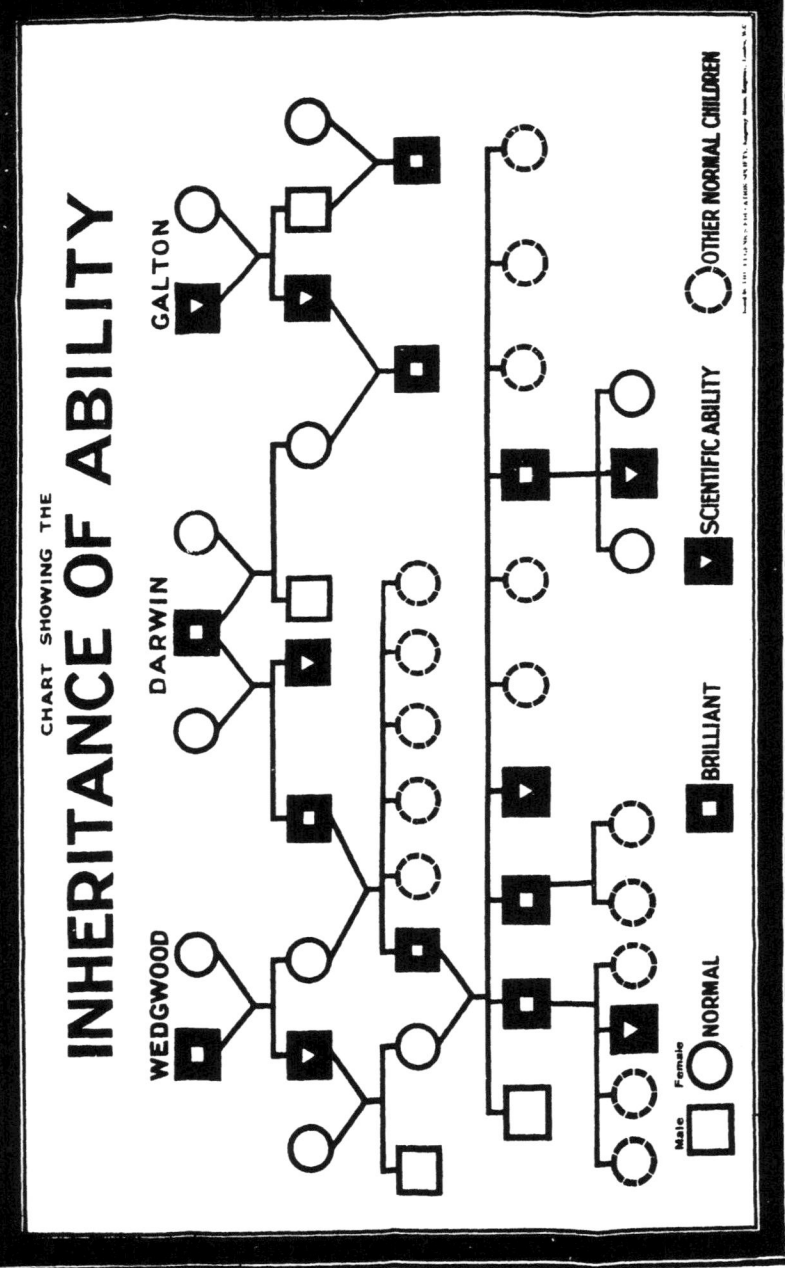

Frontispiece Pedigree of the Wedgwood–Darwin–Galton family, the model family of the eugenics movement

EUGENICS, HUMAN GENETICS AND HUMAN FAILINGS

The Eugenics Society, its sources and its critics in Britain

Pauline M.H. Mazumdar

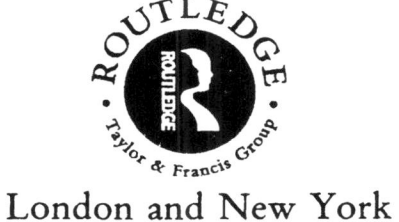

London and New York

First published 1992
by Routledge
2 park Square, Milton Park, Abingdon, Oxon, OX14 4RN

Simultaneously published in the USA and Canada
by Routledge
a division of Routledge, Chapman and Hall, Inc.
711 Third Avenue, New York, NY 10017

Reprinted 1998, 2001 (twice)

Routledge is an imprint of the Taylor & Francis Group

First issued in paperback 2011

© 1992 Pauline M. H. Mazumdar

Typeset by J&L Composition Ltd, Filey, North Yorkshire

British Library Cataloguing in Publication Data
Mazumdar, Pauline M.H.
Eugenics, human genetics and human failings: the Eugenics
Society, its sources and critics in Britain.
1. Great Britain. Eugenics, history
I. Title
363.920941

Library of Congress Cataloging in Publication Data
also available

ISBN13: 978-0-415-04424-0 (hbk)
ISBN13: 978-0-415-51481-1 (pbk)

CONTENTS

ILLUSTRATIONS

PLATES

TABLES

PREFACE

The most obvious debt I incurred in writing this book has been to the Eugenics Society itself.

I first became interested in the Society through the work of the statistician R.A. Fisher on the genetics of the blood groups; it was this that led me to investigate the background to the setting up of the blood grouping unit at the Galton Laboratory in 1935. When I contacted the Society in 1976, the Secretary, Ms Eileen Walters, made me welcome at its library and offices, and gave me access to many documents that were not public property in any way. I was later elected to a Fellowship of the Society. No one at the Society has seen this text, however. I hope that when they do, they will not feel that their kindness was a mistake. In those days, one felt a certain amount of awkwardness and hesitation in asking to see private materials, in spite of Ms Walters' politeness. It is otherwise nowadays, when the Society's papers are beautifully catalogued and easily accessible at the Wellcome Institute. Working in the Society's library at 69 Eccleston Square, too, is no longer an experience that the historian can have: in 1989, the library was transferred to the Wellcome, and the Society itself has changed its name to the Galton Institute.

Besides the Society, many others have helped me in this work. I should particularly mention Ms Julia Sheppard, Archivist at the Wellcome, and Mrs Dorothy Hanks at the National Library of Medicine, Bethesda, MD, who made my summers at the library a pleasure for many years, until her retirement in 1987. She has been greatly missed. Several colleagues read my slowly evolving manuscript and made helpful comments: they include Bruce Sinclair, Charles Rosenberg,

Daniel Kevles and Bernard Norton, a deeply admired friend who is now dead.

I should also acknowledge the inspiration generated by the lively discussions at the Eugenics Seminar that we organised in 1985 at the Institute for the History and Philosophy of Science and Technology, University of Toronto. Among the participants, Gordon McOuat and Cyril Greenland were of special significance in helping me to straighten out my thoughts on several problems.

Funding for my work came at the beginning and the end: at the beginning, from the Wellcome Institute, which very generously funded my early work on R.A. Fisher, and at the end, from the Hannah Institute for the History of Medicine, Toronto, which paid for several long stays in London, as well as from a Leave Fellowship of the Social Sciences and Humanities Research Council of Canada.

Finally, I must thank my husband, Dipak, both for additional insights into the economic problems of the urban poor, and for putting up so patiently with all kinds of aggro as this work slowly reached its conclusion.

INTRODUCTION

This book is an account of the eugenics movement in Britain. It is centred mainly on the Eugenics Society, founded in 1907 as the Eugenics Education Society, with the purpose of promoting, to paraphrase Francis Galton, those agencies under social control which might improve the human race. As this definition shows, its interests lay both in human biology *and* in social problems. Its members were mainly either biological or social scientists, with a proportion of social activists who were not scientists, but who found its social goals important enough to devote themselves to the Society and the eugenics movement.

The eugenists, and, as I shall argue, their successors the human geneticists, worked within a well-defined and quite recognisable problematic. A *problematic* has been defined as a field of concepts which organises a particular science by making it possible to ask some kinds of questions and suppressing others.[1] It determines the choice of problems which are to seem significant. In the case of the science of eugenics as it developed in Britain, a central part in the problematic was played by social class, which made itself felt not only in the narrow social group which actually joined the Eugenics Society, but in the Society's programme of investigation and advocacy.

This part of the eugenic problematic reaches far back into the nineteenth century, to the efforts of the reforming middle class to improve the lives of their inferiors in the classes below them. It was established well before the appearance of the hereditarianism associated with Francis Galton, but it was this Galtonian element which provided the particular solution to the problem of the pauper class that distinguished the Society from its sister societies of the middle-class activist network, and it was

1

this element that was critical in bringing the Society into existence. Seen from this point of view, the eugenics movement in Britain has a long pre-history that links it to the currents of nineteenth-century legislative reform.

There were several of these reforming movements, all typically focused on the urban poor, but generally led by members of the middle class. They were the response of the middle class to the growth of an industrial proletariat and a sub-proletariat that was known at various times as the residuum, the pauper class, the social problem group, and sometimes as the dangerous class. They include the legislative attempt to control pauperism by means of the New Poor Law of 1834, the drive to provide a suitable education for the working classes, and the temperance movement, as well as the sanitary movement, which was directed towards improving urban conditions, and to minimising the losses to industry caused by the high death rate of the urban poor. The tradition of middle-class meliorism, together with the new ideas about heredity introduced by Charles Darwin and his cousin Francis Galton, and the Malthusian concept of the dangerous fertility of the poor, provided the elements that came together at the beginning of the twentieth century to form the eugenics movement.

It is this background in Victorian social reform that gives the British eugenics movement its peculiar national colouring. The Eugenics Education Society was organised to press for legislative remedies for what it saw as the fundamental cause of pauperism. The concern with the pauper class was central to the Society's programme from the start, and was to remain so until the political part of its programme came to an end about sixty years later. The Society was not, however, the only group that could trace its ancestry back to the nineteenth-century meliorists. That part of the problematic was shared by a number of sister societies of the middle-class activist network. Each one of them had its own specific suggestion for the means to be employed in the manipulation of their common object, the urban poor.

The eugenist problematic that was formed from these elements consisted of a group of interrelated claims concerning the nature of the pauper class. As a class, it was defined by its dependence upon the Poor Law, but the eugenists saw it in biological or hereditarian terms as a breeding isolate at the margin of the human race, rather than an administrative

2

category. The physical unfitness of this class had been clear for many years, at least since 1842, when the sanitary reformer Edwin Chadwick had shown the working class as a whole to have a higher death rate than other classes of society, and what was true of the working class was true *a fortiori* of its social inferiors, the so-called residuum or pauper class. Chadwick, and before him T.R. Malthus, had pointed out that a high death rate usually went with a high birth rate, so it was no surprise when the lowest class was found to have the highest fertility. The assumed inheritance of their negative moral as well as physical qualities made it seem to the members of the Eugenics Education Society that if the prolific breeding of this class were not controlled, pauperism and its associated undesirable qualities must necessarily keep on increasing until the direction of evolution of the human race was reversed. To persuade an audience of the obvious truth of this principle of negative eugenics, the Society's lecturers made good use of the pedigrees of pauper families, which showed in a chilling manner how pauperism was passed on. It was to discussion and persuasion, backed up by these telling case studies, that the Society looked for the passage of the legislative remedies for which they agitated. As a scientific method of persuasion, the pedigree worked perfectly. There was also a positive eugenics, devoted to encouraging the reproduction of the eugenically valuable or prudential classes, as Malthus had called them. It may have been this aspect of the eugenics movement that attracted so many educated women to the Society, but it generally had less emphasis in practice than the negative side.

The eugenics movement as a whole was an international one, an aspect that has been well brought out by Daniel Kevles in his recent book, *In the Name of Eugenics*.[2] From its beginning in Britain, eugenics spread to many other countries, and although it had features that could be found in all or almost all of the countries in which it flourished, in each country it took on local colouring that distinguished it from the parallel movements elsewhere. In each country, the eugenists' *Wunschbild*, their ideal type, and its negative image, were determined by national background and historical context. In Britain, it was the casual labourers or pauper class whose low intelligence and high fertility were dangerous to society, as it had been throughout the nineteenth century. The feeble-minded were taken to be the epitome of this class. In the United States, the undesirables with the high birth rate who provided the source of feeble-mindedness and crime, and who filled up the asylums and the prisons, were the immigrants from Southern Europe. In Germany, it was the psychotics and psychopaths who were the main target of eugenic research, though when sterilisation laws came with National Socialism, the feeble-minded were on the list too. There was no suggestion in Germany that danger to the race was associated with class.

This book, then, does not aim at being a general history of a world-wide movement. It tries, first, to characterise the British movement, based largely on the unpublished papers of the Eugenics Society. It is this archival material, rather than the published writings of its supporters, that have made it possible to reconstruct the inner life of the Society. In particular, the Society's archives have brought to light the central importance of the long-running Pauper Pedigree Project, a project whose published results are only the tip of an iceberg of organisation, effort and discussion that lasted for several decades. It is this material that has enabled me to offer a historical explanation for the Society's thinking. It shows how the problematic that had originated during the nineteenth century persisted within the investigative science of human genetics as well as in the sociology and social psychiatry that were directly linked to the movement. This problematic, whose diverse features were united by a concern with social class biologically defined, disintegrated as a movement with the diminution of class feeling that followed the end of the Second World War.

A second theme of the book is the development of scientific methodology and its relationship to the ideological needs of those who used it. The earliest method adopted was the pedigree. It was the Eugenics Society's preferred tool for both investigation and propaganda, in Britain as it was generally throughout Europe and America in the years before the First World War. But although the Society used the American standardised pedigree as its model, the British group did not use it in the way it was used in America, to claim that a trait was inherited as a Mendelian unit character. Instead, they saw a pedigree as a straightforward demonstration that like engendered like, with no specific theory of inheritance implied. As long as there was no need to try to answer the question of the relative parts played by heredity and environment in the creation of pauperism, pedigree construction worked very well as a general technique for both investigation and demonstration. During the twenties, however, discussions within the Society show that this perfect match between ideology and method became strained. Demands from within the Society, rather than from any outside opponents, for research rather than demonstration, for statistical treatment, for controls, and above all, for investigation of the effects of environment, made the simple pedigree seem inadequate.

The new mathematical methods which irrupted suddenly upon the scene in 1930, in the hands of the new breed of aggressively outspoken left-wing critics of eugenics, appeared to their advocates to be able to fulfil all these demands and more: they would make it possible to distinguish scientifically not only between the effects of heredity and environment, but also between the simply biological and what was social and human, and between 'value-free science' and class prejudice.

These new mathematical techniques had been developed in Germany, within the German eugenics movement, but in Britain they were introduced by the *contras*, in the hope of purifying their science of the ideological accretions attached to human genetics through the eugenist problematic. I have discussed elsewhere the development of the mathematical models that constituted German *Vererbungsmathematik* or mathematical Mendelism, and its successor, *empirische Erbprognose*.[3] The transfer of German mathematical Mendelism to Britain placed it for the most part in a new and different context, that of an attack on a highly local form of main-line eugenics. The method of empirical prognosis, on the other hand, essentially retained its old context in the new setting: it began as a justification for eugenic sterilisation, and that was how it was used in Britain too.

The final part of the book deals with the persistence of the eugenist problematic, with its insistence on class as an inherited factor. The problematic retained its organising power through the thirties in the face of the powerful critique of the eugenists' class position that came from the geneticists of the left, a critique that was linked to the upgrading and mathematisation of the methods of human genetics in Britain. Throughout the decade, as I shall show, it was eugenics that determined the type of question to which the new methods were applied, even by the Society's critics.

5

After the end of the Second World War, the links between human genetics and class began to dissolve, the eugenic problematic broke up, and the eugenics movement in its original form came slowly to an end. The possible reasons for this are discussed in the concluding section of the book. I suggest that the decline of the eugenics movement in Britain is one aspect of the post-war change in *mentalité* that some contemporary sociologists saw as the 'end of ideology' – the perceived growth of egalitarianism that followed the establishment of the Welfare State and the final break-up of the Poor Law. The movement in its original form did not long survive the disappearance of the pauper class as an administrative category.

These linked themes describe a network of connections that together form a problematic. Each modifies the others: ideology is formed in the long term through the interaction of social groups that, in the case discussed, precedes by decades the movement in question. Scientific procedures and mathematical methods are chosen for their ability to answer the questions posed by ideological needs. The methods themselves may be utilised in more than one context, each of which contributes something to their growth in complexity, through the ways in which they are applied and criticised by the scientific community that uses them. In a new setting, imported swords may become ploughshares, and ploughshares, swords, without losing their sharp edge. In spite of this mobility, however, they are not value-free in any given setting.

The British eugenics movement, with its long social history, its strong ideological commitment, and its use of distinctive scientific and technical methods, is an ideal subject for an examination of the interaction of these elements.

1

THE EUGENICS
EDUCATION SOCIETY
The tradition, the setting
and the programme

The Eugenics Education Society was founded in 1907, a result of the enthusiasm and organising drive of Sybil Gotto, then aged twenty-one and recently widowed.[1] She was already interested in social problems, but it was Francis Galton's books that inspired her to act. According to Lady Theodore Chambers, who worked with her on the Society's council in those early days, Sybil Gotto 'had the vision to see the effect eugenics would have once Galton's teaching permeated the mind of mankind no matter to what race they belonged. ... She was a born organizer with an almost tireless energy which infected and stimulated all those who came in contact with her'.[2]

Her first contact was through the Sociological Society. Its Secretary, James W. Slaughter, was excited by her idea, and introduced her to Montague Crackanthorpe, a lawyer friend of Galton's. Crackanthorpe in turn became interested and introduced her to Galton himself. Together they set to work to form a society founded upon Galton's definition of eugenics as 'the study of all agencies under social control which can improve or impair the racial quality of future generations'.[3]

Eugenics was to apply an understanding of the laws of biology to the laws that determined the lives and environments of the subjects of the realm, to immigration and emigration, to marriage and prostitution, to the quality and quantity of the human race. In particular, British eugenics was to concentrate on applying the laws of inheritance to the social problems of poverty and pauperism. The Committee of the Moral Education League was next approached, and a provisional committee including some of their members was set up in 1907. Georgina Chambers remembered, forty years later, that 'Mrs Gotto was the moving spirit which inspired them all; the idea of educating the public on such broad and varied lines filled all with what might almost be called a religious zeal. The success of the movement without any thought of self dominated all those who joined.'[4]

The Eugenics Education Society was the only group to concentrate its attention solely on human biology and 'racial responsibility'; but, as Georgina Chambers pointed out, most of its members were also active in a variety of other social and environmental concerns, and there were many invitations to expound their aims before other similar groups. Before long, Sybil Gotto's energetic organising had brought together a society with 341 members, and the eugenics movement in Britain had begun to move.[5]

Every historian who has read the public statements of the British eugenists has recognised that as a movement they spoke on behalf of the educated middle class; their position is as obvious to us as it was to the movement's founders. The rollicking spirit in which men like the Dean of St Paul's damned the lower classes leaves no doubt as to the special position of eugenics as an expression of the aggressively outspoken class-consciousness of these early enthusiasts.

The Australian historian Lyndsay Farrall, writing in 1970, was the first to analyse the membership of the Eugenics Education Society from the point of view of a class and its interests. His counts showed that nearly 80 per cent of the early membership was eminent enough to be included in the *Dictionary of National Biography*. Most of them were university people, and two-thirds of these were biological or social scientists. There were a few only who were medical or physical scientists and fewer still from the humanities, although medical men were better represented on the Council of the Society.[6] Farrall called them middle-class radicals, a phrase which has been used to describe the middle-class leaders of reform movements from the days of Henry Brougham and his Whig friends.[7]

Donald MacKenzie brought out another implication of Farrall's membership counts. He suggested that it was the interests of the more modern and more scientific professions that were served by eugenics, rather than those of the older traditional professions such as law and the Church.[8]

However, there were many exceptions among the movement's

early leaders. The first president of the Society was a lawyer, Galton's friend Montague Crackanthorpe, and one of the most outspoken of the early members was the Reverend William R. Inge, later Dean of St Paul's. The Society's founder, Sybil Gotto, belonged to no profession but was interested in social questions generally. MacKenzie went on to suggest that less science-oriented members of the same group of people might join the Fabian Society instead of the Eugenics Society.[9]

Within the 'modern professions', G.R. Searle picks out a still smaller group, those whose professions were based on the biological sciences: the biologists, the statisticians and the medical men, especially if their speciality involved diseases thought to be inherited. Searle finds very few members of what he calls the environmental professions, local government officials, civil servants and social workers. Middle-class opinion, he feels, tended to group itself not so much along traditional versus modern lines, but on whether the biological sciences were actually part of one's job or not.[10] However, although there was quite a number of doctors among the Society's members, eugenics was not supported by the British Medical Association, nor did it ever become part of the medical curriculum.

Each of these generalisations follows Farrall's in being based on the membership of the Eugenics Education Society alone. But the Eugenics Education Society was just one of a network of organisations representing a common front of social activists who might be doctors, teachers or social workers, or simply ladies interested in social problems. Many were active in more than one society; social activism did not confine itself to a single remedy, though a given society might be specialised in its interests. The same person might join the Eugenics Education Society, the Moral Education League, the Charity Organisation Society, the National Association for the Care and Protection of the Feeble Minded, or the Society for the Study of Inebriety. All these organisations shared members, interests and programmes with one another. With the exception of the Eugenics Education Society, all of them were formed before 1900: the Charity Organisation Society in 1869, the Society for the Study of Inebriety in 1884, the National Association for the Care and Protecion of the Feeble Minded in 1896, the Moral Education League in 1898. The Eugenics Education Society itself was founded in 1907. It had particularly close links with the Moral

Education League, but it drew members from all the older groups. Environmentalism had not yet become the dividing issue. Their common appeal was to the 'educated class', and their common goal the control of pauperism and the management of the class they called the residuum.

The history of middle-class efforts to deal with this difficult group goes far back into the nineteenth century, long before the appearance of the eugenics movement. These themes, the causes of pauperism and the problem of the residuum, were to constitute the core of eugenic thinking in Britain. They were already being discussed by the social activists of the 1850s, a cross-section of whose concerns can be discovered in the programmes of the National Association for the Promotion of Social Science, a group founded in 1857.[11]

The purpose of the Social Science Association, as it was called for short, was to bring together people actively interested in social reform, who were working in five different areas: jurisprudence and amendment of the law, education, punishment and reformation, public health and social economy. This last was intended to cover 'social questions related to Capital, Labour and Production', under which it grouped together economic science and statistics, population, labour and capital, the condition of the working class, including the problem of intemperance, and workhouse management.[12]

The first President of the Social Science Association was Lord Brougham, the Whig reformer and the original middle-class radical, by then an old man. He was well known for his interest in education, particularly working-class education.[13] In the 1820s he had formed and led the Mechanics Institute movement and the Society for the Diffusion of Useful Knowledge, and he had been active in organising the University of London when it was founded in 1826.[14]

The problems of the causes and control of crime and pauperism were the Association's central interests. Social science adopted a point of view and a method of empirical investigation that was very close to that of sanitary science. It linked statistics on crime, education and sanitation into a complex whole enthusiastically discussed by middle-class reformers as a basis for legislative changes that were intended to lead to the moral and physical improvement of the lower class. The Association's *Handbook* of 1857 stated its aims in these words:

while statistics reveal that crime is not the necessary atten-
dant upon poverty or low wages, they show that it is found
most abundant [sic] in closely crowded houses, in ill-
drained localities, while the morals of the poor quickly
manifest an improvement when sanitary reform has been
carried out in their dwellings. ... The religious condition
of the people, the education of their children, the wretched
sanitary state of crowded neighbourhoods, the connexion
of intemperance with crime, have all been tested and
proved by statistical science.[15]

The sanitary movement seems to have been the model for the
Association's methods, as the British Association for the Advancement of Science had been for its initial formation. The Public
Health Section was supported by most of the movers of the
sanitary movement. At various times, it heard papers from
Edwin Chadwick, author of the famous Sanitary Report of 1842
and from his two main informants on the sanitary condition of
the working class in England, Dr Southwood Smith and Sir
James Kay-Shuttleworth, the first Secretary of the Committee of
Privy Council on Education.[16] Chadwick and Kay-Shuttleworth
had also been the movers behind the Poor Law Amendment Act
of 1834, that had abolished outdoor relief for the poor, and had
established the principle of less eligibility.[17]

A focus on problems connected with the urban poor was
typical of all sections of the Social Science Association. At its first
Annual Meeting in 1857 the Education Section of the Association listened to a few papers on middle-class education, but like
the section on crime control, its major interest was the education
of the working class, and particularly in the extension of
education to the sub-proletariat through the Ragged Schools,
the Industrial Schools and the Reformatories.[18]

The best-known authority on the education of this class was
Mary Carpenter, who had devoted herself to the Ragged School
movement, and to the organisation of reformatories for the
education of the 'children of the perishing and dangerous
classes'.[19] Mary Carpenter spoke at the first two meetings of the
Association, on Reformatories and on Ragged and Industrial
Schools.[20] She argued passionately that the education of this
kind of child should concentrate on moral training rather than
intellectual instruction, and that it should include industrial

discipline.[21] Papers on this borderland between education, discipline and punishment, or education, that is, as it applied to the 'dangerous classes', were to be a common feature of Association meetings of the future.

The working class did not, it seems, make the members of the Association feel particularly welcome when they appeared at the door with advice on hygiene and educational enlightenment. As one of the Association's speakers said:

> All who have had to deal with working men have encountered similar manifestations of suspiciousness, Why should they be, as a class, so suspicious? ... By looking back a little ... we may detect causes ... that have produced a set of traditional notions concerning the relations between the different classes of society, that are calculated to render the bulk of the poorer classes very suspicious of political interference that comes or seems to come from those who are socially above them. It is still held as an hereditary article of popular faith that the leading effect of political and social effort on the part of the rich is to keep the people down and to secure to themselves the perpetual maintenance of their own existing advantages.[22]

The stated aim of the society was not, of course, to 'keep the people down'. But the connection between pauperism, crime, intemperance and lack of sanitation in streets and houses was perfectly clear to the meliorists. To 'promote the comfort, the health and the morals of the sunken masses of the people by a sanitary reformation' was also the way to make the streets safer for their betters.[23] As we have often been warned, historians should be careful not to use the concept of social control too facilely.[24] But the list of social evils which were to be ameliorated, and the coerciveness of the suggested remedies, certainly sound more like a programme of control than one of comfort, in common with much of the Victorian reformers' rhetoric.

It was generally held that one of the root causes of both pauperism and crime was drink:

> City missionaries regard it as the most powerful obstacle to their labours among the sunken masses of the people. Poor-Law Guardians ascribe to it the majority of cases of pauperism. Our judges and prison governors declare that

12

it occasions most criminal offences. Medical men ... find it the most prolific source of disease. Governors of lunatic asylums refer the insanity of many of their unhappy patients to its dire influence.[25]

A speaker at the 1860 meeting of the Social Science Association argued that dipsomania was often hereditary, and that it affected children, particularly if the parents had suffered from repeated delirium tremens. He suggested that the dipsomaniac or insane drunkard should be subject to voluntary or involuntary commitment to an institution.[26] The temperance advocates demanded legislation to control dipsomaniacs, and to confine them, either voluntarily or involuntarily, in institutions.[27] These were the remedies that were to appeal strongly to the eugenists at a later date. Fifty years on, with the Royal Commission on the Care and Control of the Feeble Minded of 1908, advocates of the care and control, who made up a substantial part of the eugenics movement, were making the same hereditarian claims, and demanding the same kind of legislation to control the spread of feeble-mindedness. A pattern of demand for legislation that would control people who constituted a social problem by putting them into closed homes was already established by the middle of the nineteenth century. The tense relationship between the middle and upper classes and the casual poor in nineteenth-century London has been brilliantly treated by Gareth Stedman Jones in his *Outcast London*. The separation of classes in the town had led, so the upper classes felt, to the 'demoralisation' of the poor and to their increasing pauperisation. Thrift and self-respect were ebbing away from the poor as they began to depend more and more on impersonal charity handed out by agencies to whom they felt no sense of personal responsibility. The Settlement movement and the Charity Organisation Society were attempts to bring the classes back into contact and to stop indiscriminate charity. The casual poor were to be led back to thrift, work and self-respect by the example and the supervision of their betters. As Stedman Jones put it, the Victorian social critics of the 1860s and 1870s saw casual labour not as an economic problem, but as a problem of pauperism and demoralisation.[28] In the 1880s the emphasis changed from demoralisation to degeneration, as the growth of social Darwinism added a biological side to the picture of the casual poor.[29]

Paupers were not only morally weak, they were also visibly physically degenerate, as a result of the conditions of town life. It was this group of small, thin, sickly-looking men and women, the unfit, who bred the most freely, and would gradually outbreed the fit members of society who supported them. The problem of the residuum became even more pressing following the employment crisis of the 1880s. The riots of February 1886 in London showed convincingly that the casual poor were a real threat to the propertied classes.[30]

The Charity Organisation Society had always insisted on distinguishing those in temporary difficulties, who deserved charitable help, from the permanent casual poor who were to be left to the Poor Law. Fear of the rioting mob of the 1880s laid even more stress on this distinction. There were proposals for more coercive solutions to the problem, such as the suggestion of 'voluntary' labour camps for segregating the degenerate residuum from the respectable working class. These dangerous degenerates would then be removed from the towns into the country, where they would be subjected to healthy farm labour and firm discipline. The state would take over from charity in providing this more permanent solution to the perennial problem. This kind of proposal had already been carried out in the field of education, where the adult labour camp had its parallel in the reformatory school.

The problem of the urban poor was one of the main foci of the nineteenth-century meliorist tradition. Beginning with the Poor Law Amendment Act of 1834, the sanitary and the temperance movements and their forum for discussion, the Social Science Association, all concentrated their attention on the causes of pauperism. They had in common a middle-class membership which interested itself in the amelioration of the conditions of life of the very poor, in the cleaning up of their environment, their bodies and their morals.

In the early part of the century, the Eugenics Education Society, as it was called at first, was one of a network of societies of progressive activists, each interested in a different aspect of the problem of urban poverty. Since this chapter describes a network, it is a little difficult to know in what order to discuss the different groups and their interests, which were all interlocking and overlapping. I shall start with the Charity Organisation Society, formed in 1869, since it provides a kind of master-plan

14

for the rest; I shall try to sketch a position in which the Charity Organisation Society's views on individualism, character and poverty are repeated with varying emphasis by each of several different organisations, and I shall show that the Eugenics Society, or the Eugenics Education Society, as it was from its foundation in 1907 until 1926, was one among many, holding its own variant of the common viewpoint, and pushing its own solution of the common problem, the problem of the urban poor.

In a deeply class-divided society, these groups represent the attempts of the middle and upper middle class, the urban bourgeoisie, to try to understand the poor, to explain their lives by one set or another of natural laws, and to account for the huge gulf which separated the lives of the working class from their own (see Figure 1.1). Each group had its own explanation and its plan for making working-class society more like the orderly, moral, healthy and ambitious society in which the bourgeois reformers themselves lived. Beatrice Webb, herself a bourgeois reformer, says that

> The origin of the ferment is to be discovered in a new consciousness of sin among men of intellect and men of property. ... The consciousness of sin was a collective or class consciousness; a growing uneasiness, amounting to a conviction, that the industrial organisation, which had yielded rent, interest and profits on a stupendous scale, had failed to provide a decent livelihood and tolerable conditions for a majority of the inhabitants of Great Britain.[31]

Yet it was very seldom that the industrial organisation was in fact blamed for the failure, and the consciousness that is most striking in much of the writing of these middle-class enthusiasts for reform is of superiority, rather than sin. It is a consciousness that shows itself rather plainly in the insistence of the Charity Organisation Society, for example, on giving charitable help only to those who, like the members of the Society, have the strength of character, and the will, to help themselves.

Bernard Bosanquet, Professor of Moral Philosophy at St Andrew's University in Aberdeen, was on the Administrative Committee of the Charity Organisation Society from 1890.[32] In

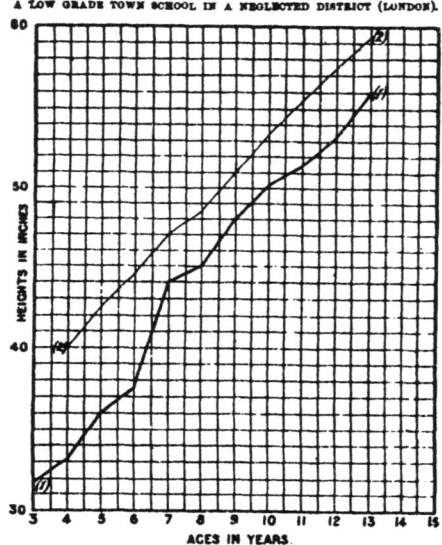

A LOW GRADE TOWN SCHOOL IN A NEGLECTED DISTRICT (LONDON).

(1) *Lambeth.* Johanna Street Board School.
(2) *Honeywell Road* (Standard). *Note.*—Irregular growth and severe retardation of a very grave nature.

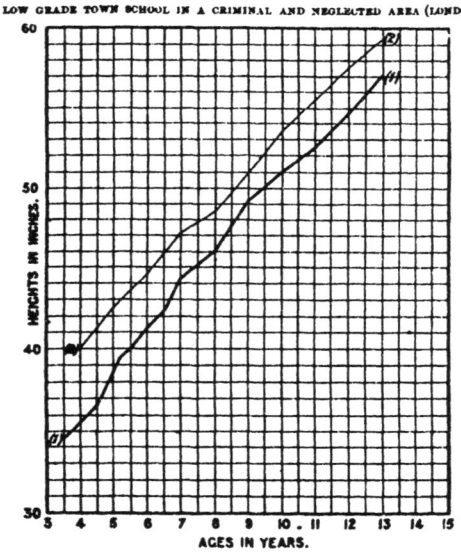

A LOW GRADE TOWN SCHOOL IN A CRIMINAL AND NEGLECTED AREA (LONDON).

(1). *Notting Hill.* St. Clement's Road Board School.
(2) *Honeywell Road* (Standard). *Note.* -Conspicuous retardation in growth, only less than Johanna Street.

Figure 1.1 Curves showing the retarded growth of the lower-class
schoolchild compared to children from middle-class homes
Source: Fitzroy Report (1904) n. 140

the introduction to a series of essays by members of his Society, entitled *Aspects of the Social Problem*, he said:

> The writers [the authors of the essays] have seen and felt as well as reflected that the individual member of society is above all things a character and a will, and that society as a whole is a structure in which will and character 'are the blocks with which we build.' Among the influences which operate upon the will they of course take note of some that are due to material or economic condition ... but in watching the social process, life by life and generation by generation, the skilled observer becomes aware that circumstances are modifiable by character, and so far as character is a name for human action, by character alone.[33]

Helen Dendy, a Charity Organisation Society activist who married Professor Bosanquet in 1895, contributed several of the essays to his collection. One of these, 'The Industrial Residuum', was reprinted from *The Economic Journal* of December 1895. In it, she distinguished the 'true industrials', the genuinely self-supporting wage earners, from a residuum, who differ from the former, and from the ideal economic man, in having no foresight or self-control, who live only in the present and who every day merely repeat the mistakes and follies of the day before. 'To fully realise the facts', she says, 'it is necessary to live among these people, to see them day after day, watch their extraordinary freaks, and feel the burden of their total irresponsibility.' The absence of economic virtue is accompanied by a low order of intellect and a degradation of the natural affections to something little better than animal instincts.[34]

The people to whom she is referring are those who filled the many economic niches in what is now called the 'informal sector' of the urban industrial scene. Her examples of this degraded group are the oil man, the coal man, the wood man, the coke man and the coster, whose commodities, unlike those of the milk men, do not *necessitate* their being brought round from house to house:

> The whole method of retail industry differs from that pursued in the higher classes of the community. ... It is a difference of the imaginative faculty which well illustrates the disposition of the Residuum; for the educated person

anticipating her needs, the sight of the store's list is sufficient to provoke a purchase but for the uneducated person, the sight and touch of the commodities themselves is found to be necessary.[35]

Other examples of this class are the girl who cleans steps, the old woman who minds babies, the knocker-up and the charwoman. The charwoman is 'a typical instance of the development and results of partial employment. Under any satisfactory arrangement a household will find within its own internal economy sufficient labour power to carry on its necessary and normal work', and should not need to engage casual labour.

Helen Dendy's difficulty is transparent: she cannot understand how people could live like this. She belongs to the 11 per cent of Londoners who kept servants, according to Charles Booth's survey, rather than to the 30 per cent who lived below subsistence level.[36] She was one of the most active of the Charity Organisation Society's workers, writing and lecturing, and setting up training courses in the case-work methods of the Society. The counterpart to the Society's insistence on individual responsibility in theory was the investigation of each case in practice, before relief could be permitted. Help could be authorised only in cases that were 'helpable', whose need was short term, and not for those whose utter helplessness showed them to be without the necessary strength of character. These, the residuum whom she discusses in the essay quoted above, were to be left to the Poor Law and the workhouse; they were the paupers whose lives were so incomprehensibly different that no charity could help them.

Helen Dendy's distinction of the residuum from the 'true industrials' parallels the traditional distinction between the so-called labour aristocracy the small unionised urban proletariat, and the rest of the working class.[37] As the labour historian Hobsbawm pointed out, the organised labour movement excluded the 'half-world of misery which emerges from ... Charles Booth's survey'.[38] Hobsbawm feels that unionisation helped to produce the distinction between these two groups of workers.

The members of the unionised labour aristocracy often shared Helen Dendy's sense of superiority to the struggling mass of the very poor. Hobsbawm quotes the evidence of a carpenter to the 1895 Royal Commission on the Aged Poor. This man was

President of a Sick Society, secretary of a Trade Society and a Birmingham City Councillor. He divides the working class into three groups: the first were those skilled men who were too prosperous ever to need assistance; the second were those who, although they honestly tried to do well, did not manage to hold their own towards the end of their lives, due to lack of intelligence, or education or moral strength and courage. The third group, the true paupers, were 'the produce of the street corner; loafers I should call them'.

Hobsbawm's suggestion is that the labour aristocracy shared the individualist attitudes and the interests of the employers. It was not until 1889 that the newer large general unions began to include the unskilled and extended to them the bargaining power of organisation.[39]

Present-day economists have described a two-tier structure of this kind in urban labour markets from the late nineteenth century onwards. A superior, industrialised sector earns wages in large, formal concerns, such as factories, and a mixed informal sector earns irregularly in small family or individual enterprises, or in the street, outside the industrial-capitalist system. This dual structure is found at present in both highly industrialised countries such as the United States and developing ones such as India and West Africa. Economists have mainly followed a tradition of regarding the informal sector as surplus labour.[40] The workers in this sector have usually been found to have some kind of disability: they were either very young, or old, or limited in education, or not the primary earners, or were new entrants to the labour market, passing through the informal sector on their way to regular industrial employment.[41] These findings do not support Hobsbawm's suggestion, that the two-sector labour market is a product of unionisation: it has in fact been found to exist in the absence of trade unions.

It has usually been agreed by both economists and historians that the members of the informal sector have all been sufferers from some kind of crippling disadvantage in the urban labour market. However, two recent writers on West Africa have taken a radically different view. They suggest that the informal sector exists on the small-scale provision of inexpensive goods and services for the wage-labouring aristocracy, and in the case they looked at, they felt that this sector was more vigorous and was growing more rapidly than the traditional proletariat.[42]

It seems likely that both types of worker, the provider of services to the regular wage-earner and also the disadvantaged man, or very often woman, find a place in the informal sector of the work force. Helen Dendy, in describing the people she saw around her in a London street in 1893 as a residuum of paupers, was lumping them all together from the point of view of her class. To her, and to the members of the Charity Organisation Society, as to Hobsbawm's witness before the 1895 Commission on the Aged Poor, their position was due to a defect of character, a moral defect which made it useless to try to help them out of their pitiable condition. They were to be abandoned to the Poor Law and the workhouse.

In 1909, the Royal Commission on the Poor Laws reported its findings in the form of two separate conclusions, a Majority and a Minority Report. It was signed by fourteen of the eighteen members of the Commission, of whom six were members of the Society. They included C.S. Loch, the Secretary, and Helen Dendy.[43] The list of causes of urban pauperism cited by the Majority from the statement of a Poor Law Relieving Officer at Leeds is significant of the determination to see urban poverty as due to different kinds of individual pathology, rather than to an overall economic situation enveloping a whole class:

> The most important causes of pauperism are a) old age b) the early marriage of persons dependent on casual labour. Large families are the rule. .... c) Imprisonment for criminal offences is a large factor in pauperism d) venereal disease also contributes largely. .... Its ramifications are appalling. e) Intemperance is another contribution, and in this I find females to be the worst offenders. Many men are perforce paupers by the intemperance of their wives. f) Indiscriminate relief by private persons and religious bodies also contribute to pauperism, and cases have occurred where relief has been in the first instance given in this manner and the recipients eventually become confirmed paupers. g) Cases are not wanting to show that pauperism is hereditary – two generations being quite common, and third generations generally occur.[44]

As Beatrice Webb said, it was the Charity Organisation Society's position that the category of pauper should be kept quite separate from the normal population. Unlike paupers, normal people saved for their old age, prudently married late and had small families, committed no crimes, were not promiscuous or intemperate, did not accept 'indiscriminate relief' and came from healthy stock.[45] Some other causes of destitution had been suggested to the Poor Law Commissioners, but these, the Commissioners stated, they did not propose either to endorse or controvert. They were listed as (1) capitalism (four witnesses); (2) free trade (one witness); (3) the system of land tenure (one witness).[46] Beatrice Webb's very partisan description in her diary of one of the Poor Law Commission's sessions pictures the man behind these statements:

> May 22nd [1906]. C.S. Loch completely lost his temper yesterday at my cross-examination of Lockwood. ... Loch got white with rage, and protested against my questions as misleading statements of economic doctrine. ... What makes him angry is that the enquiry is drifting straight into the [economic] causes of destitution instead of being restricted to the narrower question of *granted destitution is inevitable, how can we best prevent pauperism?*[47]

The casting of the Charity Organisation Society as the enemy, the isolated representative of *démodé* individualism in an age of growing collectivism, is perhaps a result of the vigour and volume of the writing of Sidney and Beatrice Webb and the Fabian Society, and particularly their 'Campaign for the Break-Up of the Poor Law' and for the establishment of a state-guaranteed 'national minimum of civilised life' for all its citizens.[48] This campaign was organised by the Webbs following the publication of the dissenting Minority Report of the Royal Commission on the Poor Law.[49]

However, in many ways the Charity Organisation Society continued to represent an important part of middle-class opinion. Its list of the causes of poverty was assented to by a number of the other middle-class reformist societies active then and later. Societies interested in feeble-mindedness, in temperance, in the large families of the poor and in hereditary pauperism – all the causes cited by the Majority Report – were all concerned to show that the poor were pathologically different from the rest of the population. These groups shared both interests and members with one another; many people were active in two or more of the societies. Their multilateral connections make it extremely difficult to describe the situation with any kind of clarity: the societies must be taken as a complex whole, a tissue of strands of thought and feeling of the highly educated professional middle class of the period, both men and women.

The Eugenics Education Society was one of these groups.[50] Very early in its existence the Eugenics Education Society arranged lectures on both the Reports of the Royal Commission on the Poor Laws, by C.S. Loch for the Majority and by Sidney Webb for the Minority.[51] However, the Society was not in complete sympathy with either of them. Its presidential address for 1910 deals with the two Reports. Montague Crackanthorpe, KC, second President of the Society, presents them, as he puts it, as if he were the impartial chairman of a Quarter Sessions Court. His summing up seems to lean a little towards the Minority Report, which had claimed to 'prevent destitution before destitution sets in'. But the methods the Minority proposed were all inadequate to a eugenist. They consisted of 'searching out' neglected children, cases of preventable and curable disease, and people who were failing economically, and giving them support through state agencies. It was not the socialist nature of this solution that Crackanthorpe found objectionable. For the eugenist, these were not primary causes of destitution. Behind them all lay defects either inherited or transmitted *in utero*.[52] Neither the Majority nor the Minority faced the question of the biological basis of destitution – as a lesion of the germ cell which Auguste Forel, professor of psychiatry in Zürich, had called *Blastophthoria*, said Crackanthorpe.[53]

In 1896, eleven years before the foundation of the Eugenics Society, Mary Dendy and Mrs Hume Pinsent founded the National Association for the Care and Protection of the Feeble Minded (its title varies slightly).[54] Mrs Pinsent was Chairman of the Special Schools Subcommittee of the Birmingham Education Committee, and Mary Dendy Honorary Secretary of the Lancashire and Cheshire Association for the Permanent Care of the Feeble Minded, as well as the founder of the permanent care institution at Sandlebridge near Birmingham. These active workers were devoted to the idea of seeking out children of low intelligence in the schools, and transferring them to a closed institution, namely the Sandlebridge Homes, where they would be segregated for life from normal society. Both ladies joined the Eugenics Education Society within a year or two of its foundation. The National Association for the Care and Protection of the Feeble Minded was well represented on the Royal Commission on the Care and Control of the Feeble Minded of 1908. W.H. Dickenson, MP, Chairman of the National Association for Promoting the Welfare of the Feeble Minded, was a Commissioner along with Mrs Hume Pinsent. One of their colleagues on the Commission was C.S. Loch, Secretary of the Charity Organisation Society.

The Report of the Royal Commission on the Care and Control of the Feeble Minded reappeared in 1909 in the form of a popular summary, prepared, according to its Preface, by a joint committee of members of the Eugenics Education Society and the National Association.[55] It was introduced by Sir Edward Fry of the well-known philanthropic family, who commended the feeble-minded as objects of charity whose numbers would not be increased by generosity to them. As Professor Pigou, the economist, also pointed out, the 1834 Poor Law principle of ineligibility, the principle that relief must be less pleasant than poverty, does not apply to them. Their numbers would be diminished rather than increased by taking them into institutions, where they would be unable to breed, and would no longer swell the pauper class with their feeble-minded progeny.[56]

The Eugenics Education Society was from the first interested, like the Charity Organisation Society, in the causes of pauperism. But where the Charity Organisation Society saw the lack of character of the residuum as the underlying cause of all their problems – their intemperance, their venereal disease, their irresponsible fertility and their economic difficulties – the Eugenics Education Society felt that inherited defect in turn underlay the lack of character, and that control of the excessive fertility of these people would get to the root of the matter. The fertility control method that they preferred was that of compulsory detention in state institutions: campaigns for the detention of inebriates, of those with venereal disease and of the feeble-minded were all carried on vigorously in the Society's first few years.

In 1910 the Cambridge Association for the Care of the Feeble Minded wrote to the Council of the Eugenics Society to suggest that the two societies cooperate in pressuring the government to put the Royal Commission's recommendations into effect, with a

23

bill for the compulsory segregation of the feeble-minded.[57] The Executive Committee of the Eugenics Society appointed James Slaughter and Dr A.F. Tredgold, author of the standard text-book on mental deficiency, as its representatives.[58] Together with the National Association's Medical Committee, they drafted a 'Short Bill' for compulsory detention, but when the Home Secretary promised to make a government move in the matter, the Medical Committee withdrew its bill in favour of the government one.[59] The Parliamentary Committee of the Society then arranged to send letters to all members of Parliament and members of Boards of Guardians asking for their support, and to hold a non-party meeting at the House of Commons to explain the Bill to Members.[60] This Bill was at first defeated in committee, and dropped. The Society then arranged to send a letter to every Board of Guardians and 'nearly' every Education Committee in the country, asking them to pass a resolution urging the government to reintroduce the Bill, and to send a copy of it to both the Home Secretary and the local Member of Parliament. As we shall see below, this was a campaign strategy that the Society had learned from one of its forerunners, the Moral Education League. Five hundred of the addressees wrote back to the Society, although they had not been specifically asked to, saying that they had done as they had been asked.

On 1 April 1914, the Mental Deficiency Act came into force. The Society felt that some of the credit for the passage of the Act should be theirs. It was, they said, 'the only piece of English social law extant in which the influence of heredity has been treated as a practical factor in determining its provisions'.[61]

The Moral Education League, the Eugenics Society's direct forerunner, was founded in 1898.[62] Its object was to provide ethical and character training for schoolchildren, independent of religion. Its slogan was 'character is everything'. The League developed a Syllabus of Moral Instruction for Elementary Schools (1902), and a Secondary Syllabus (1913), and it organised a Moral Instruction Circle made up of schoolteachers, whose method was to give a sample or demonstration lesson to a small group of children, who were then to discuss it among themselves. The League sent circulars to every Local Education Committee in England and Wales, as well as to 7,000 individual members of the Committees. It approached the Board of Education with a 'very influentially signed Memorial', and persuaded the Board to recommend moral education in the Code of the Board of Education of 1906. In the election of 1906, all candidates were contacted by the League, and a Parliamentary Committee was set up to keep the subject before Parliament. In 1908, the League joined with the International Union of Ethical Societies to stage the First International Congress on Moral Education.[63] The list of authorities and other bodies at the Congress includes forty-five British and many European education authorities. Besides the Ethical groups, such as the famous South Place Ethical Society, representatives were sent by the Charity Organisation Society; by teachers' organisations such as the Association of Headmistresses and the Headmasters' Conference, the National Union of Teachers, the Association for the Education of Women, and the Parents' National Educational Union; by temperance groups such as the Society for the Study of Inebriety and the National Temperance League; by the Positivist Society and the Rationalist Press Association; and by religious organisations such as the British and Foreign Unitarian Association, the Society of Friends and the Theosophical Society; and by the Sociological Society, among many others.[64]

The central problem debated at the Congress was the 'Relation of Religious to Moral Education', the 'possibility of finding any meaning or relevance in the ordinary religious ideas that could be acknowledged by teachers and educationists who were in touch with the modern spirit'. Professor J.H. Muirhead of Birmingham University presented two points of view on this question: the one he calls positivist, which emphasised the connection of conduct with social, industrial, civic and political well-being; the other, the religious, which in his view stood not for any particular religion, but for 'the indefeasible claim for the inwardness of morality', part of the 'witness of consciousness', rather than the belief in a supernatural being. Muirhead synthetically combined these positions by suggesting that the new religious thought would appropriate with gratitude the noble teachings of Positivism. There would be no duties to God which were not also duties to ourselves and our fellow men. Religion so defined gave conduct a deeper significance by connecting its laws with the general purposes of the universe.[65]

The Moral Education League is a model of the social activism of the turn of the century. Its members were the socially responsible, advanced thinkers of their day, progressives who actively worked for the programmes in which they believed. By 1914, they had an international organisation with about 1,000 members, and with branches in several countries, notably in India.[66] They knew how to press claims on the political process in England, and how to lobby Members of Parliament and local Boards of Education. They succesfully managed to have their programmes accepted both at the central government and the local school level. The League's members seem to have almost all been connected with the teaching profession. At the Moral Education Congress, it was remarked that the audience showed no imbalance between the sexes. The participation of large numbers of educated women was a feature of socio-political activism at this time. It has been noticed in several different societies, including both the Fabians and the eugenists.[67] As long ago as the 1850s, at the Social Science Association's meetings, there had been a few women on the programme. Mary Carpenter, speaking on schools for the 'Ragged and Dangerous Classes', had been one of the first women to address a scientific meeting. At the Moral Education Congress, very many of the speakers were women, and many of them were leaders in the teaching profession, in teacher training and in women's education. They included Alice Ravenhill of King's College London Women's Department, Sara Burnstall of the Manchester School for Girls, the didactic writer Mrs Humphrey Ward, Alice Woods of the Maria Grey Training College in London and Professor Millicent MacKenzie of the University College of Cardiff. There were also at least two woman physicians, one of them Dr Ettie Sayer, and Mrs Bridges Adams, who spoke for the Social Democratic Federation and the Gas Workers' Trade Union. There were many other English women speakers whose affiliation was not mentioned, as well as European women who represented institutions abroad.

The membership, as in the other societies, was probably solidly middle class: teaching was a middle-class activity. But the writing and speeches of the Moral Educationists shows less class specialisation than, say, the writing of the Charity Organisation Society. Their concerns cover the type of schools that made up the Headmasters' Conference, the elite private schools, that is, as well as the state elementary schools that came under the Board of Education. Professor J.S. MacKenzie, President of the League, rejected the idea that the League's type of moral discipline had anything to do with economic success in an industrial world. He felt that the growth of 'moral ideas' might well make people less rather than more fit to carry on commercial life. 'It must be true to some extent of every real moral awakening', he wrote, 'that its immediate effect is to bring us not peace but a sword.'[68] Along with the lack of concentration on a particular class, the social control aspect of education is at a minimum here. Unlike the Social Science Association, the League seems to have been more interested in promoting moral leadership among the upper class than industrial discipline among the lower. Little time at the 1908 Congress was given to the familiar problems of penal education, hooliganism and the education of defectives, although these things were mentioned. A presentation on eugenics, however, by James Slaughter, Secretary of the Sociological Society, seems to have been received with general sympathy. The 'new moral principle and driving force supplied by the new chapter in ethics, based on a knowledge of man's nature and the conditions of his descent' was acclaimed, according to the Report, by 'such diverse elements as young Oxford men, foreign university professors, secondary and elementary teachers.' One of the few dissidents present was a woman doctor, perhaps Dr Marion Hunter, who disagreed with the claim that a Science of Eugenics was needed to provide teachers with better human material. There was plenty of good material, she said. The present social system, not the material, was the source of evil.[69] There was one other outstanding presentation by a eugenist at the Moral Education Congress: that too was by a woman doctor. Dr Ettie Sayer's lecture, illustrated with 'limelight pictures' on morally defective children, was reported as 'arousing the keenest interest'. The press was particularly interested in both Slaughter's and Sayer's contributions.[70] Dr Sayer's was head-lined in the *Daily Mail*:

A WOMAN DOCTOR'S REMEDIES
As to real moral degenerates ... If diagnosed as so actively antisocial and morally indirigible as to be unfit ever to live among a pure, honest, unselfish and public-spirited people, they should be classified and shipped off to various un-inhabited isles.[71]

It seems that although both of these items on the programme were rather different in tone from the rest of the Congress, they still received a fair amount of assent from the audience. Progressive educationists were primarily committed to using the methods of their own profession, but the appeal to natural law was quite acceptable to them. It was not incompatible with the positivist ethic. The suggestion made by Sir Francis Galton that eugenics might become the basis of a scientific religion would have sounded quite reasonable to a positivist of the school of Auguste Comte.[72]

The formation of the Eugenics Education Society followed closely the traditional pattern of social activism among the upper middle class. Its prime mover was the young widow Sybil Gotto, daughter of Admiral Sir Cecil Burney.[73] According to Lady Chambers, later her colleague on the Society's Council, Sybil Gotto's talent for organising people, and her enthusiasm for the cause of eugenics, were the prime movers in the foundation of the Society.[74] Sybil Gotto was already involved in many social problems when she came across Sir Francis Galton's work on eugenics, and decided to focus her energies on eugenical reform. She had the contacts needed, and she knew how to go about matters. Her first step was to go to the Sociological Society. This group of scientific meliorists had been formed in 1904, and it had heard papers on eugenics from Galton himself in 1904 and 1905.[75] As Lyndsay Farrall noted, the 1904 paper was followed by a discussion, and many of the discussants later became members of Sybil Gotto's new group.[76] But before that opportunity arose, the Sociological Society itself had heard several more papers on the 'biological foundations of sociology'.[77] These papers argue for a science-based sociology that chimes well with the positivistic ethics adopted by the progressive educators of the Moral Education League.

Sybil Gotto's contact at the Sociological Society was the Secretary, James Slaughter, the same who was to speak on eugenics at the Moral Education Congress of the following year.[78] Slaughter introduced her to his colleague Montague Crackanthorpe, KC, a friend of Sir Francis, and Crackanthorpe took her to Galton himself to put before him her idea of forming a Society to educate the public in eugenics.[79] Galton responded to her enthusiasm, and before long they had interested more of their friends, including Lady Emily Lutyens, wife of Sir Edwin Lutyens, the distinguished architect.

The group then approached the Committee of the Moral

Education League, of which Lady Emily was a member, and a proposal, presumably written by Sybil Gotto, was laid before the League's membership at a meeting at Caxton Hall on 15 November 1907. Sybil Gotto proposed to them that 'an organisation of parents and teachers for the study of Natural Laws' might be 'grafted onto your existing committee'. She emphasised the relationship of the new organisation to existing societies and associations: 'The ground has been so ably prepared during the last 25 years, by the devoted work of individuals, societies and this committee, that the time seems ripe for a banding together of all existing sympathisers in a recognised association.' She felt that the formation of a recognised association might help to interest some medical men, whose authority and support were important to her plan.

The aims of the new society were to be three: firstly, to break down the 'present conspiracy of silence that envelops the subject of birth and parenthood' in children's education; secondly, to raise public opinion on questions of morality; and thirdly, to 'strengthen public opinion against unhealthy marriages, and a wilful propagation of an unhealthy and suffering race'.[80]

An early agenda shows that the Moral Education League was at first asked to reconstitute itself as the Eugenic and Moral Education League, but it was decided that the League should continue as a separate entity alongside its offshoot, the new Eugenics Education Society.[81] One member of the League, Dr Marion Hunter, had objected to the amalgamation.[82] But the two groups had many members and many interests in common. The Society's early lectures were often on moral-education subjects: 'Mental Integrity and How to Attain It', for example, or 'Moral Education' itself.[83] The Society's Subcommittee on Education arranged discussions on the position of eugenics in education.[84]

The Education Committee had decided as a matter of policy to concentrate on girls' schools, and had contacted Mrs Woodhouse of the Girls' Public Day School Trust for advice.[85] Later, in the first year of its life, the Committee prepared a circular letter and a pamphlet by Alice Ravenhill of King's College, who was an active member of both the Eugenics Education Society and the Moral Education League. The pamphlet gave a statement of the Society's views on eugenics in education, and it was sent out to the headmistresses of girls' schools proposing an education conference.[86] It was Alice Ravenhill, too, who suggested that the Society should send a representative to the Moral Education Congress.[87] Slaughter's talk and a display on eugenics in the literature room at the Congress were the result. It is clear that the new Society was following up on both the contacts and the policies of its parent group, the Moral Education League.

The Society's first political act was a legacy from another parent group, the Society for the Study of Inebriety.[88] Sir James Crichton-Browne, FRS, first President of the Eugenics Education Society, was also Vice-President of the Society for the Study of Inebriety; that Society's Honorary Secretary, T.N. Kelynack, MD, was a member of the Eugenics Society also, and so were several of the Society for the Study of Inebriety's Council: G. Archdall Reid, who was a surgeon who wrote on heredity, the neuro-pathologist F.W. Mott, the Surgeon-General Evatt, and W.C. Sullivan, MD.[89] Archdall Reid and Mott were among those who had heard Galton's paper at the Sociological Society in 1904, and Archdall Reid himself had also talked to the Sociologists on the 'biological foundations of sociology' in 1906.[90] The Society for the Study of Inebriety was a mostly medical group. It was founded in 1884 but it had had a precursor, the Society for Promoting Legislation for the Control and Cure of Habitual Drunkards, which was started in 1876. The newer version united the medical and legal aspects of alcoholism. At its inauguration, Lord Shaftesbury, famous for his patronage of social reforms, said that he hoped the new Society would join with others in the amelioration of slum housing and sanitation, as well as alcoholism. But the Society does not seem to have taken that direction: its interests stayed with legislation on alcoholism and research into its pathology.

Both these tendencies were expressed in the inaugural lectures that followed Shaftesbury's. The physiologist William B. Carpenter, whose sister Mary Carpenter had been active in the Social Science Association, spoke on the inheritance of the alcoholic constitution. The craving for alcohol was a physical problem, he said. The Society's first President, Norman Kerr, took a similar line. The inebriate constitution was inherited, but it was not in itself harmful if the individual did not drink. The Society should try to protect those who were hereditarily at risk of succumbing to the desire for drink, and to help those who had succumbed to climb back to normal life. Kerr called for homes for inebriates where they could be cared for and controlled, and for legislation to support them.[91] In 1899, the Society set up a committee to examine the problem of heredity and inebriety. Archdall Reid, W.C. Sullivan and Sir Victor Horsley were among its members. They agreed with Kerr's position that the craving was constitutional and heritable, but they were not sure that alcohol was a cause of degeneration. Sullivan, however, refused to sign this report. He felt that alcoholism *was* an important cause of germ cell injury and degeneration. It is rather surprising that the committee took this stand; Sullivan's position was the more common. Alcohol was very often seen as a so-called race-poison, a cause of damage to the germ cells and of degeneration.[92] Frederick Mott, who was Director of the Laboratory and Pathologist to the London County Asylums, was a proponent of that point of view. For Mott, alcoholism was among the stresses of town life, a 'powerful coefficient' along with sexual excess, celibacy and competitive examinations, that went to produce the neurasthenias, the prelude to neurosis and insanity in a stock.[93] Mott also believed in the 'law of anticipation', which he found predicted by the French writer on degeneration, Benedict-Augustin Morel, whom he frequently quoted. Morel had said that transmission of the tainted constitution produced earlier and more severe forms of degenerative neurasthenia with each affected generation, ending in imbecility and idiocy, and the dying-out of the degenerative family.[94]

The Society for the Study of Inebriety had its own organ, the *British Journal of Inebriety*, which mainly carried papers on the pathology of alcoholism. Archdall Reid contributed one on 'Human Evolution and Alcohol' in which he argued that alcohol was quite safe for races that had evolved along with it, but that it eliminated the savage and inferior races that could not deal with it.[95] Mott wrote on alcohol and insanity.[96] There was even an occasional article on pauperism and inebriety, a subject which would have interested both the Charity Organisation Society and the Social Science Association of the nineteenth century, as much as the eugenists and inebriologists of the twentieth (see above, note 27).[97]

The first public act of the new Eugenics Education Society was to pass a resolution proposed by Dr Saleeby, who also belonged to the Sociological Society, deploring the closing of the homes for inebriate women in the London area, setting 'some hundreds of chronic inebriate women ... adrift in London, with an inevitable detrimental result to the race'.[98] Copies of the resolution were sent to the Home Secretary and to the London County Council, and a correspondence took place which was published by *The Times*. Eventually the Home Office appointed a Departmental Committee of Enquiry. The Society was invited to submit a brief answering questions in writing and a subcommittee was set up to do it. A Bill was drafted on the segregation of inebriates which embodied most of the Society's recommendations. The Society recorded it proudly in one of their recruiting pamphlets, though to their great disappointment it was dropped by Parliament in 1913.[99] The Inebriates Act of 1898 already gave Local Authorities the power of detaining chronic inebriates.

Venereal disease was another of the causes of pauperism emphasised by the Commissioners of the Majority Report of 1909. One of the physicians whose evidence was quoted in the Report makes the connection between the disease and the amorality of the slum dwellers:

> I am convinced that the greater majority of children born in the poorest districts (slum) are tainted with syphilis. ... They are mostly feeble in body and mind, possess no inhibitory power, and readily give way to the vices by which they are surrounded. It is from this class that paupers and criminals are made, and that prisons and workhouses are filled.
>
> We recommend, therefore, that subject to certain safeguards against abuse, the Public Assistance Authorities should have the power to detain cases of venereal disease.[100]

The Eugenics Education Society was engaged here too. Since the subject was so sensitive, there was little public activity at first. The Medical Committee of the Society 'followed the line of policy proposed by the President' and 'urged the consideration of the subject on medical bodies, but refrained from definite publication on behalf of the Society'.[101]

In July 1912, the Eugenics Education Society was represented on a deputation to the President of the Local Government Board, to present a memorial urging the implementation of the recommendations of the Majority Report that those suffering from venereal disease should be detained in Poor Law institutions. The members of the deputation included Sir James Crichton-Browne, Sir Victor Horsley, the well-known surgeon, Frederick (later Sir Frederick) Mott and the Reverend E. de M. Rudolf, all four of whom were also members of the Society for the Study of Inebriety, and C.S. Loch, Secretary of the Charity Organisation Society and one of the signatories of the Majority Report. They were told that there was no hope of legislation giving powers of detention.[102]

It was not until the beginning of the 1914–18 war that venereal disease control became sufficiently safe for the Society to take a public position on it. The Royal Commission on Venereal Diseases which reported in 1915 had several members of the Society's Council among its members. The Secretary to the Royal Commission was Sir James Crichton-Browne, first President of the Society. The Commissioners reported that 9 per cent of admissions to the London County Council asylums were for general paralysis of the insane, a late stage of syphilis. Poor Law infirmaries also contained similar cases of neurological syphilis and of chronic disease of bone and skin, many of whom might live for ten, twenty or even thirty years in a helpless state. There were also congenital syphilitics, often idiots or imbeciles. It was the Commission's argument that this social and economic burden could be greatly diminished by the state provision of free clinics where treatment with salvarsan and other medications could be offered.[103] Following the Report came the foundation of the National Council for Combating Venereal Disease, with Lord Sydenham, the Chairman of the Royal Commission, as President and with the driving force of Sybil Gotto as Honorary Secretary. The National Council was to act as 'remembrancer to the Government'.[104] The list of members of the National Council contains many familiar names. Its treasurer was Major Leonard Darwin, its Honorary Secretary, Sybil Gotto. Dr Mott, Dr Douglas White, Dr Saleeby and Dr Mary Scharlieb and others were members. Dr Edgar Schuster, Leonard Darwin and Georgina Chambers were representatives nominated by the Eugenics Education Society to the National Council. The University Settlements also sent nominated representatives: Oxford House, Cambridge House and Toynbee Hall, together with the Honorary Secretary of the Settlements Association, F. J. Marquis.[105]

The Eugenics Society and the National Association together

started a press campaign to push things further.[106] They advocated not only notification of the diseases but compulsory treatment, or, in the words of the Report, 'Detention, where necessary, of Poor Law patients suffering from venereal disease' under the existing provisions of the Poor Law Amendment Act of 1867.[107] No legislation, however, compelling the segregation of the venereally diseased ever actually came before Parliament. Venereal diseases were not a matter which affected only a powerless residuum.

In 1925, the National Council amalgamated with the Society for the Prevention of Venereal Disease to become the British Social Hygiene Council, with the object of concentrating on educational propaganda. Since the free treatment and the clinics advocated by the original National Council had now been established, venereal diseases had passed from being unmentionable to taking their place as a part of public health alongside the problems of tuberculosis and infant mortality, and were now equally freely discussed in the press. The time had come to concentrate on education for prevention. Links were now formed between the British Social Hygiene Council, and the Social Hygiene Councils of the United States and Canada.

The personnel of the new Social Hygiene Council still overlapped to a considerable extent with those of the Eugenics Society. The psychologist Cyril Burt, J. Arthur Thomson, Professor of Natural History at Aberdeen, Julian Huxley, Professor of Zoology at King's College, London, as well as Sybil Gotto, now Mrs Neville Rolfe, as Honorary Secretary, were all active in both societies.[108] After about 1920, however, Sybil Neville Rolfe withdrew from the Eugenics Society. The organisation of the venereal disease campaign, the social hygiene congresses, and the amalgamation of the National Council for the Prevention of Venereal Disease with the Society for the Prevention of Venereal Disease, as well as the social hygiene movement on the international stage, took up the time that she had been giving to the Eugenics Society.

Recent work by Greta Jones has placed the Eugenics Society among the groups belonging to the social hygiene movement, in a slightly different, less direct, sense. She suggests that social hygiene should be seen as an alternative or counterpart to the growing Welfare State of the early twentieth century. The social hygienists looked to biology for improvement in human life, while the proponents of the Welfare State looked to economic redistribution. Both groups worked for increased state responsibility for the life of its citizens. Social hygiene advocated, and brought about, a programme of health legislation. Advice to its clients was backed by the authority of the state and frequently of the courts. Greta Jones points to a number of semi-official societies that had the power to enforce through the courts the decisions of their agents. She lists the National Association for Promoting the Welfare of the Feeble-Minded, the People's League of Health, and the National Council for Mental Hygiene.[109]

Whether or not this group of societies should be placed as a right-wing alternative to the socialist goal of a Welfare State, they may certainly be placed in the context of a long history of middle-class social activism, visiting its opinions upon the less organised working class.

Up to this point, we have seen the Eugenics Society as one among many groups who shared programmes, members and methods among themselves. They had a common history which can be traced back to the legislative reformers of the nineteenth century, and which includes the major reform movements of this earlier time in education and sanitation, temperance and charity.

The problem of the differential fertility of classes, however, was one that the eugenists of the twentieth century made particularly their own. It was through this problem that their enduring influence on the history of human genetics took effect. It was the same preoccupation with the uncontrolled fertility of the poor, and especially the paupers, that linked the Eugenics Society and its colleague groups, the Charity Organisation Society, the Society for the Care and Control of the Feeble Minded, and the medical groups involved in the promotion of legislation to control venereal disease and inebriety, and, of course, the birth control movement.[110]

The history of the eugenists' preoccupation with the biology of social class goes back to a time before Sir Francis Galton's more explicit statements on the subject defined the new field of eugenics. As Farrall has said, the ideology of the twentieth-century eugenics movement should not be seen as the single-handed creation of a genius. He traces Galton's hereditarianism to ideas stated more or less explicitly between 1860 and 1890 following Charles Darwin's *Origin of Species* of 1859 by a number of writers.[111] However, although it had not always been discussed in hereditarian terms, the biology of social class was an old preoccupation. The idea of a differential fertility of classes is a tradition that goes back to the earliest writers on demography. D.E.C. Eversley suggests that it originated in the contrast between town and country life. The luxury, decadence and infertility, as well as the high mortality, among city populations was a common theme from Virgil to the seventeenth century statistician John Graunt.[112] The theme of the infertile aristocracy and the fertile poor was common, too. 'The demographic decline of ruling castes', says Eversley, 'is part of the general tradition of Western social thinking.'[113]

From 1800 onwards, the problem of the fertility of the poor was generally argued on the lines set by T.R. Malthus in 1798.[114] Malthus suggested that population growth was controlled by pressure on the food supplies which provided a limit beyond which populations could not increase. At the limit, the 'misery check' ensured that the population would be cut back by malnutrition, disease and 'misery' until it had declined to a level that could be supplied adequately by the available food. In order to prevent periodic famines and epidemics, Malthus advised prudent men to control their fertility voluntarily, for example, by marrying as late as possible. The poor, who formed the majority of any population, were likely to be the first to suffer the 'misery check'. Early marriages and large families were the chief cause of their poverty. Since they brought the population as a whole nearer to the limit, their fecundity was a threat to the rich as well as to themselves.[115]

Early nineteenth-century rulers following Malthus felt that the lower classes could not be trusted to control their own fertility by the 'prudential check'. In German-speaking Europe, several states tried to prevent poor subjects from marrying by legislation, a remarkable reversal of the eighteenth-century cameralist's policy of promoting population increase.[116] Malthus's predictions were discussed in France, too, but there seems to have been no legislative attempt there.[117] In fact, many early nineteenth-century French economists, following J.B. Say, thought that Malthus had been too negative, and that food production could always be supplemented by industrial production. However, the economists agreed that charity was dangerous: it would minimise whatever prudential check the poor were prepared to put upon their fecundity. It should never be offered to the able-bodied. As Malthus had said, economic prosperity promoted fertility, even the factitious prosperity of the recipient of charity.[118]

No direct attempt to postpone marriages by legislation was ever made in Britain. But Malthus's formulation was indirectly influential in many other ways. The *Essay on Population* of 1798 introduced a view of the biology of poverty that persisted into the twentieth century, and which prepared the way for the hereditarianism that followed Darwin's publication.

Malthus's *Essay* appeared at a particularly crucial time for class relationships in Britain. As H.L. Beales has said, it was a godsend to frightened conservatives who feared the spread of the revolutionary temper from France, but it was angrily rejected by all writers of the left, from William Cobbett to Karl Marx himself.[119] Friedrich Engels called it 'the most flagrant warlike aggression of the middle classes against the workers'.[120] Malthus provided the arguments against the traditional right to subsistence through public funds, established by the Old Poor Law of 1601. The Poor Law came to be seen as making the distress of the poor worse, not better, by subsidising their increase. Attempts to broaden its support by supplementary wages, as William Pitt suggested in 1796, or by setting a national minimum wage, as Samuel Whitehead proposed then, or by reforming the Old Poor Law, as Whitbread tried to do in 1807, were put out of court by Malthus's arguments.[121]

H.L. Beales argued that the spirit behind the Poor Law Amendment Act of 1834 was that of Malthus, even though its creators were Edwin Chadwick, the future sanitarian, and Nassau Senior, the economist, neither of whom were strictly Malthusians. Chadwick thought that the unchecked fertility of the poor was balanced by their unchecked mortality, and that the Malthus's law of population did not apply in England at that time. Senior thought that Malthus's argument that population was bound to outrun food supply did not hold in actual cases. But both thought that any kind of subsidy offered to the poor would allow their numbers to increase, as the theory had it.

The harsher provisions of the New Poor Law were intended to abolish outdoor relief, and to force those who needed help to enter a workhouse to get it.[122] The workhouse was to be an intentionally unpleasant place, so as to comply with the principle of less eligibility: no one would choose to go there in preference to anything but utter destitution. It would not allow its inmates to mistake charity for prosperity. The public housing it provided, unlike that proposed by Whitbread in 1807, would not encourage the poor to marry. Malthus himself had raised this objection to the provision of housing for the poor.[123]

The differential mortality among classes was the central problem dealt with by the physicians and statisticians of the nineteenth-century sanitary movement. The 'average age of death', which Chadwick preferred to the crude death rate because it showed up the differential mortality better (or, according to his critics, exaggerated it) was his favourite statistic. He used it to demonstrate that the 'comparative chances of life in different sections of the community' meant that the gentry lived longer than those in trade, and a fortiori, longer than the labouring classes. Statistics also showed the overall chances of life to be better in a rural than an urban area.[124] Reports such as Chadwick's of 1842, and the two Reports of the Royal Commission on the State of Large Towns of 1844 and 1845, publicised the relationship between class and mortality rates.[125] But as Cullen points out, the sanitarians did not put the whole of this difference down to sanitary conditions, to the exclusion of individual responsibility. There was a continuous discussion about the relative parts played by the moral responsibility of the poor as individuals, and the degrading circumstances in which they lived.[126]

These two threads, the Malthusian and the sanitarian, with their emphasis on the fertility and the mortality of the poor, formed the warp and the weft of the developing science of demography in Britain. The post-Darwinian emphasis on heredity as the biological feature that distinguished the poor from the rich and successful was a later embroidery upon this basic material. In this, the background of eugenics in Britain differs from that in America, where race rather than class was more important.[127] It differs from that in Germany, too, where, apart from the racist strain, the focus of so-called main-line eugenics was on the importance of weeding out the psychotic taint from the population. The emphasis on the dangerousness of the *Lumpenproletariat*, the urban poor or social problem group as a class, seems to have been peculiarly British.

It was Francis Galton's more explicit statement of the inheritance of mental qualities that the eugenists saw as the foundation stone of their movement. Karl Pearson's rhetorical fanfare for Galton expresses that loyalty:

> The little men say there was evolution before Darwin; the little men say somebody discovered logarithms before Napier; the belittlers believe that the law of the inverse square was propounded before Newton, and that somebody conceived of eugenics before Galton ... the name and the idea of a science of eugenics have become worldwide only since Galton made his appeal and showed its possibilities.[128]

The idea that the mental qualities that made up an outstanding man often ran in families, and that they must be inherited, struck Galton soon after coming across Darwin's *Origin of Species* in 1859. The paper he published in 1865 marked the beginning of Galton's vocation, as Ruth Schwartz Cowan pointed out.[129] In it, Galton described a statistical investigation of the biographies of distinguished men. He had found that the frequency of distinguished men who are related to one another is much greater than the frequency of their occurrence in the general population, and he concluded that the relevant mental traits must be inherited.[130]

These ideas were not completely new, but Galton had two personal contributions to add to them. One was his statistical approach to family histories, and the other his traveller's experience of populations 'in the field'. In 1869 he suggested that the comparative worth of a race might be judged by the frequency with which it produced men of high natural ability, defined as intellectual capacity, eagerness for work and power of doing work.[131] These were the values which he saw as contributing to the spread of western civilisation. Races that could not supply men with these abilities were destined everywhere to be swept away, no matter how well they had been adapted to their own lifestyle.

Galton also suggested that the operation of the Malthusian checks on population would be against the interests of the race concerned. Malthus stood for a prudent delay in marriage and self-control in procreation, but, says Galton, only the prudent and self-controlled would follow this pattern. The less disciplined elements would then outbreed them, and the very persons who had the needed high natural abilities would leave the fewest progeny.

This was a theme that particularly interested Galton, and he continued to develop it in successive books and articles. He summarised the passage from *Hereditary Genius* again in his *Inquiries*, and the idea that the direction of evolution of a race depended on which of its classes was the most fertile was the subject of a paper in 1891. Galton implied that classes corresponded to biological subtypes that would breed true. The most prolific would therefore set the bodily, intellectual and moral qualities of the population as a whole:

> The question to be solved relates to hereditary permanence of the several classes. What proportion of each class is descended from parents who belong to each of the other classes? Do those persons who have honourably succeeded in life, and who are presumably on the whole, the most valuable portion of our human stock, contribute their fair share of posterity to the next generation? ...
>
> Taken altogether, on any responsible principle, are the natural gifts of the most productive class, bodily, intellectually and moral, above or below the line of national mediocrity? If above that line, then the existing conditions are favourable to the improvement of the race. If they are below that line, they must work towards its degradation.[132]

This paper is the common ancestor of a whole lineage of eugenist thinking, beginning with that of Karl Pearson, Galton's devoted admirer. 'Looking round impassionately [*sic*] from the calm atmosphere of Anthropology', said Pearson in 1903, he believed that the less able and the less energetic were the most fertile.[133]

The feeling that the population was degenerating physically was at that moment being widely and seriously discussed. A memorandum from the Director General of the Army Medical Service had claimed that a high proportion of the young men who offered themselves as recruits were unfit for military service.[134] An Interdepartmental Committee was set up to look into this, and to try to discover whether there was in fact any evidence of national deterioration. They recognised that the army was recruited from the lowest levels of society, and there was ample evidence that these people were physically inferior to those of higher degree (see Figure 1.1). But the Report argued that the few figures available did *not* show deterioration. It cited

Karl Pearson's Huxley Lecture, and the comment upon it by the Edinburgh anatomist, Professor D.J. Cunningham, who scoffed both at Pearson's suggestion that there was a decline in intelligence, and also that intelligence was confined to one particular class:

> I do not think that there is a single solid fact to support such a view. I am astonished that one for whom I entertain so high an admiration as Professor Pearson should have put forward such a statement, and more especially claim for it, as he does, that it emerges from the 'calm atmosphere' which is supposed to surround the anthropologist.[135]

The general tenor of this report is in the tradition of the nineteenth-century environmentalist health reports, such as Edwin Chadwick's of 1842.[136] Its section on 'Hereditary Taint' is brief and negative and follows Cunningham's rather than Pearson's line. Almost all its witnesses, unlike those of the Royal Commissions on the Poor Law and the Feeble Minded of only four years later, concentrate on the effects of bad and insufficient food, over-crowding and dirt, and do not suggest that it is either lack of thrift or heredity which is at fault, although the group which offers itself to the army recruiting officers is, as the Committee accepts, the residuum of the population.[137] The suggestions of the Committee include action by the Local Government Board on over-crowding, the improved inspection of factories, mines and workshops, and provision of free meals for underfed children. The Malthusian point of view of the Charity Organisation Society is not evident in the main body of the Report.

However, C.S. Loch, its Secretary, submitted a separate statement to the Committee, in which he attacks Charles Booth's division of the poor into classes. Booth says that his lowest class, that of 'labourers, street-sellers, criminals and semi-criminals', is now hereditary 'to a very large extent', but he also says that the number of children in it is very small, and that it is recruited from adult men of all classes. Loch points out that Booth is confusing two different concepts of class; a statistical sense in which a class is no more than an income group, and a true social sense in which it is '[a] classification of people and their conditions in relation to social habits and organisation ... in which the charateristics of the persons classified represent real factors in the formation of society'.[138]

Although Booth describes his lowest class in terms which could apply to a 'real' social class – it is uncivilised in manner, and lives without the ordinary obligations of social habit – it is not possible, says Loch, to say from his data whether it is actually hereditary. It is this which is the important point in the question of degeneracy: are these people who simply lack means, but who could use them if they had them, or are they by nature incapable of it? Booth, says Loch, does not distinguish between the poverty of physical weakness, of weakness of mind, of inability to use means, of depravity – all these are lumped together. His classes are not accurate enough to be statistical, nor carefully enough distinguished to be real social groups. Booth, Loch thinks, does not try to distinguish the deserving from the undeserving poor.

It may not be entirely true to say that Professor Cunningham's 'astonishment' at Professor Pearson's 'unsupported' belief in the excessive fertility of the lower classes insulted Pearson into setting out to collect the figures to prove him wrong: the Report itself, after all, had suggested that the point should be investigated.[139] But within two years of its appearances, David Heron, the Galton Research Fellow at the Biometric Laboratory, University College, had produced, under Pearson's direction, the first paper in a series headed 'Studies in National Degeneration' on the relation of fertility to social status.[140]

Heron's figures came from the census for the years 1851 and 1901, from between twenty and thirty London districts. His test of superior social status in each district was the number of professional men per thousand occupied men, and the number of female domestic servants, which he took as measures of wealth and education. The number of general labourers and pawnbrokers showed the presence of the lowest class of worker and of a degree of improvidence; and for thriftlessness and poverty, he took the number living more than two to a room. These figures were related by the biometrician's usual technique of the calculation of correlation coefficients, with the number of legitimate births per 100 wives. Heron tried to define his classes socially, so that they were, as Loch would have had it, 'real'. He attempted to weigh the different social parameters to create an index of social worth. The correlations he found were very high between a low birth rate and indicators of high status, and conversely, between a high birth rate and indicators of low status. The comparison of figures for 1851 and 1901 showed the correlation between social undesirability and birth rate had almost doubled in fifty years. Heron's conclusions were the most pessimistic possible for a eugenist:

a: 25 per cent of the married population ... produces 50 per cent of the next generation;

b: physical and mental characters, tendencies to health and disease, intellectual and manual capacities, are undoubtedly inherited;

c: a higher net fertility is shewn ... to be very markedly correlated with most undesirable social factors.[141]

It is a kind of syllogism which proves that the population was degenerating, as Pearson had said. And unlike the other serial publications of Pearson's laboratory, many of which were still available in 1980 at almost the original prices, this one apparently created some interest: it sold out. Heron became a member of the Eugenics Education Society as soon as it was formed.[142] In 1909 he was elected to its Council.[143] Pearson would not join, although he was actually invited to become its President. He told the Committee that 'his work lay more in accurate statistical research, and unless the Society intended working on those lines, he would rather not be connected to it in any responsible position'.[144] A possible reason for his refusal may be guessed at from the Society's minutes: Francis Galton, whom Pearson revered, had also declined to become Honorary President.[145] But a few months later Galton changed his mind, and accepted. The Society was delighted; his approval at once raised its status.[146] Galton even drafted a statement of policy for the Society.[147] But Pearson never relented, and continued to despise the woolly-minded activists of the Society. Later work by Pearson and his group tried to avoid the accusation of class prejudice by making income an indicator of social value within a single social stratum, the working class, and showing that it was still parents of low social value who were the most fertile: the 'class' divisions of good and bad health, ability and stupidity, which were indicated by income, were not meant to be social classes in Loch's sense.[148] But it is clear that their meaning is effectively to divide the 'labour aristocracy' from the residuum, just as the Charity Organisation Society had done in the eighties, and even to put the blame on charity and the Poor Law as that Society had done:

'Sundry sentimental sociologists' have asserted that biological laws do not apply to human life, but they have made
no attempt to meet the evidence: (i) that in man physical
and mental characteristics are alike hereditary, (ii) that
under the dominating economic and social tendencies of
today the physically and mentally fitter members of each
social class leave fewer progeny, and (iii) that the physically
inferior and less fit members are directly encouraged by a
vast system of charitable and Poor Law institutions to
provide a large supply of cheap but inefficient labour ...
without the institutions wages are wholly inadequate to
maintain the large families of the low-waged working class,
while the high-waged working classes, representing by far
the most valuable element in the community – the stocks
that would propagate physique and skill – are refraining in
increasing numbers from the family warranted by their
wages. Any nation under such conditions must deteriorate.[149]

The 'sentimental sociologist' was Sir Shirley Murphy, who was
Medical Officer of Health for the County of London. He had
given evidence to the Committee on Physical Deterioration on
the effects of overcrowding on infant mortality.[150]

The Report of the Committee on Physical Deterioration
appeared in 1904, Heron's paper in 1906, and the Reports on
the Feeble Minded and the Poor Laws in 1908 and 1909. The
close relationship between them is pointed up in Sidney Webb's
1909 lecture to the Eugenics Education Society on the Minority
Report, already referred to above (note 51). Webb's line of
argument to the Society against the Poor Law is that it is anti-
eugenic, that its provision of help especially for feeble-minded
maternity encourages the proliferation of the unfit. He argues
that the answer to this is not *laissez-faire* and an abandonment of
society to natural selection. Where there is no state interference,
it will not be the fittest but the survivingest stock that is bred
from:

The question, who is to survive is determined by the
conditions of the struggle. ... Where the rules of the ring
favour a low type, the low type will survive and vice-versa.
... If, for example, it were possible for an epidemic of
malarial fever to spread all over the United States of
America, it is highly probable that the whites would be

eliminated and the blacks would survive. ... That is to say, the unfit are surviving.[151]

In the Minority Report, the Poor Law is not only promoting pauperism and feeble-mindedness, but is also a factor in the differential birth rate. For this Fabian socialist just as for the eugenists, the prolific poor are degrading the race; they themselves are a degraded race, as his comparison of them with American blacks is meant to show. The conflation of class with biological subtype, and biological with social superiority which forms the basis of the eugenics movement in Britain at this time can be found even among the Fabians.

Nothing could demonstrate more plainly the truth of Hobsbawm's description of the Fabian Society as 'middle class socialists'. The number of practising workers among them, he says, never exceeded 10 per cent of the membership.[152] The Fabians represented, in Webb's phrase, a *nouvelle couche sociale*, the salaried middle class, whose intellectual superiority fitted them to be the experts who led the working class.[153] The elitist implications of this accorded very well with the class-centred eugenics of the time.

Fertility in Europe had begun to decline during the last third of the nineteenth century. By 1900, according to the demographer Ansley Coale, about half the western European states had already experienced a 10 per cent drop in marital fertility.[154] But long before there was any evidence of a decline in fertility within marriage, western Europe had had an *overall* fertility very much lower that that of the non-western world. John Hajnal found that west of a line drawn between Trieste and Leningrad, beginning perhaps as early as the sixteenth century, only about 50 per cent of potentially fertile women were actually married. This European marriage pattern, or abstinence from marriage, is equated by Coale with Malthus's moral check.[155]

The falling birth rate had been anxiously discussed in Europe before the First World War, but during the twenties and thirties, the problem of low fertility and the projected fall in population became acute for governments in many European countries. The Fascist governments in particular feared a falling population for racial reasons and took steps to promote fertility. The Fascist regime in Italy included allowances for children in its tax system from 1927 onwards, as well as giving bonus payments proportional to the number of children to industrial workers from 1934, helping those whose incomes fell below the taxable level. In Germany, the National Socialist government set up fertility inducements as soon as it came to power in 1933. Loans were provided for couples who could show that they could not have set up house otherwise. The loans were to be remitted at a rate of 25 per cent for each succeeding child. Again, this measure would especially encourage the less well-off to be more prolific. In France too, the system chosen benefited the lower class. Firms began in the twenties to pay allowances to workers with dependent children. The custom spread until in 1932 it was made compulsory.[156] In each of these countries, the problem was seen as that of generally low fertility. The class differential was not discussed and measures taken benefited the poor more than the rich.

In Britain, the demographic trend was similar to that of Europe as a whole. A slight rise in fertility between 1841 and 1871 was followed by a steep fall of about 20 per cent between 1871 and 1901. Over the next thirty years, the fall was even steeper. According to David Glass, fertility fell by at least 40 per cent, although the net reproduction rate fell much less: female mortality in the reproductive period also declined by about 30 per cent between 1841 and 1931, which lessened the overall effect of the fall in fertility.[157] The percentage of unmarried women in the 20 to 45 age group remained roughly the same, at about 40 per cent between 1851 and 1931. Glass calculated in 1938 that the number of children needed per married woman for replacement was 2.84; the actual number was then 2.19.[158] In 1936, *The Times* in a leading article called this a 'deeply founded social predicament ... wholly new in human experience'. Malthus's claim had been disproved, said the leader writer: higher standards of living did not bring higher birth rates.[159]

The decline had been public knowledge at least since the Report of the National Birth Rate Commission of 1916. This was not a Parliamentary or a Royal Commission. It was a private and voluntary group, a subcommittee of the National Council of Public Morals, a society which defined itself as being concerned with the 'Promotion of Race Regeneration – Spiritual, Moral and Physical'.[160] A statement of its origin, constitution and scope prepared for *The Times* said that there would be four heads of inquiry. First, the Commission would look at statistics on fertility, including the relation of fertility to income and occupation. Second, it would examine possible causes of decline, including both physiological causes such as the effect of town life, and so-called prudential causes. Third, it would look at the effects of the decline upon home and family, and fourth, 'economic and national aspects' would be examined. The latter were said to be, paradoxically enough, the effects of a rapid increase of population in a land already fully cultivated, and of a permanent surplus of workers upon the condition of the working class, in overcrowding and unemployment.[161] The Malthusian point of view on population control had survived even the alarm over a falling birth rate. It would seem that it was the low fertility of the 'prudential' classes, rather than that of the population as a whole that was alarming to the members of the Commission.

Given the composition of the Commission, this alarm over the fertility of the prudential classes is not so surprising. The Commissioners included a number of the usual people to be involved in this type of social activism, members of the Eugenics Education Society and its sister organisations. Sir James Crichton-Browne, who had been the first President of the Eugenics Education Society, and Vice-President of the Society for the Study of Inebriety, was on the Commission and so was the Dean of St Paul's, the Very Reverend W.R. Inge, one of the the pauper class's most outspoken critics. Dean Inge later became the Commission's Chairman. The Commissioners also included Dr Ettie Sayer, active member of both the Moral Education League and the Eugenics Education Society, who had earned headlines in 1908 at the Moral Education Conference with her modest proposal as to what should be done with 'real moral degenerates' (above, note 71). Other active eugenists included the biologist C.W. Saleeby and Dr Major Greenwood, statistician to the Lister Institute, both of whom were teaching in the Eugenics Education Society's courses. Greenwood and Saleeby also gave evidence before the Commission.

The section of the Birth Rate Commission's Report dealing with statistical evidence mainly works through the figures linking fertility with occupation and income, using material collected by the Galton Laboratory. The figures showed that the national decline in birth rate represented an average of the steep falls of prosperous areas such as the upper middle-class suburb of Hampstead in north-west London, and the very slightest

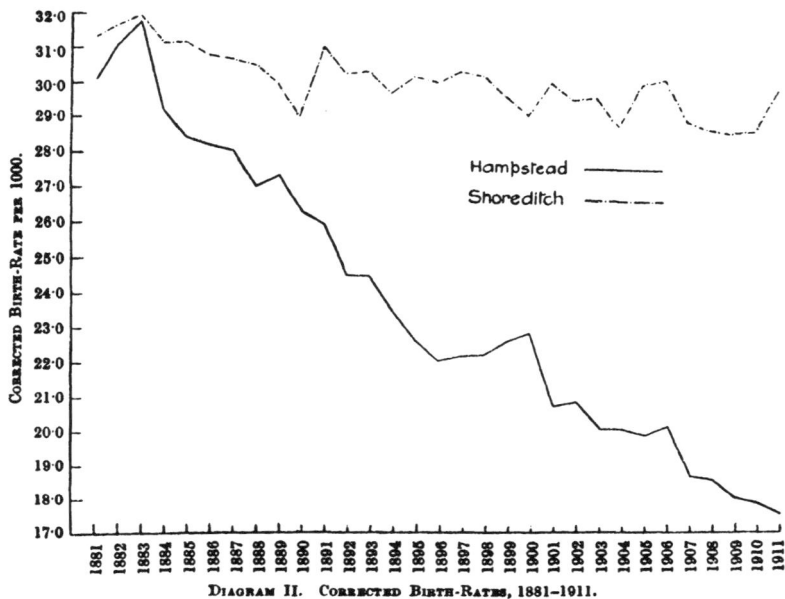

DIAGRAM II. CORRECTED BIRTH-RATES, 1881–1911.

Figure 1.2 The declining birth rate in Britain: curves by Ethel Elderton of the Galton Laboratory, showing the differential decline in upper-class Hampstead and working-class Shoreditch, both suburbs of London
Source: National Birth Rate Commission, *The Declining Birth Rate* (1916), n. 160, 4–5

of downward drifts in Shoreditch, an East End slum (see Figure 1.2). The bibliography on fertility problems that appears at the end of the Report includes a special recommendation to readers on the importance of Karl Pearson's papers, and of the series issued by the Francis Galton Laboratory of National Eugenics.[162]

Leonard Darwin, President of the Society, wrote in 1916 that the works of Malthus 'unquestionably form the starting-point for all speculation on population, and are still valid in substance'.[163] The Malthusian thread of the differential fertility problem runs through most of the Society's work of the twenties and thirties.

Possible means of counteracting the supposed dysgenic tendency were continually discussed and promoted by the Society. Attempts to reverse the differential by encouraging the economically successful to have larger families, called 'positive eugenics', included a scheme for tax rebates on children.[164] Leonard

Darwin's pamphlet of 1916, entitled 'Quality not quantity', agreed that the

> economic promotion of fertility must take the form of lessening the burden of taxation on parents and throwing it onto the childless, a method which is likely to have eugenic consequences because it will only materially affect the well-to-do classes in possession of considerable incomes.[165]

State and charitable aid to the poor as a class would 'often be harmful as regards racial qualities'. Social reforms would 'do little or nothing to render the submerged tenth less prolific'.

The Society proposed an amendment along these lines to the Finance Bill of 1917. It got as far as discussion in the House, but although the Prime Minister 'expressed sympathy', no action was taken.[166] In 1919, a memorandum was prepared for presentation to the Royal Commission on Income Tax, in which Darwin made the usual case that the poorest economic strata contained a higher proportion of biologically inferior types, and that they were multiplying the most rapidly, which he took to point straight to national deterioration. The falling birth rate among the skilled and professional classes constituted a national danger.[167] In 1927, Darwin was making the same argument for increased allowances for children of the tax-paying class, so as to check the fall in the birth rate of 'this valuable class': it was inconceivable, he said, that this valuable class could be made to multiply too quickly. The differential birth rate was 'a source of grave national danger'.[168] The society's policy statements throughout the twenties and thirties always contained sections on Taxation and Family Allowances. The Family Allowances they favoured were graded to give larger allowances to the better off: flat-rate payments were regarded as 'wholly dysgenic'.[169] But, as the statistician R.A. Fisher pointed out to the Eugenics Society in 1932, the only Family Allowance system at that time in Britain came as part of unemployment and poor relief; it must therefore be supremely dysgenic.[170] Michael Freeden has noticed the similarity in the social programmes advocated by both eugenists and progressives during this interwar period.[171] The eugenists in fact thought of themselves as highly progressive. Both Left and Right argued for family allowances of some kind, but for the eugenists, family allowances were a part of positive eugenics, and were intended to promote the fertility of the class they favoured.

Anti-Malthusians, who were afraid that the nation's best stock was controlling itself out of existence, and Neo-Malthusians, who feared the super-fertility of the 'submerged tenth', might unite in the name of a positive and negative eugenics. The economist J.M. Keynes was a member of the Eugenics Society and a Neo-Malthusian, who saw unemployment as a sign of over-population. Sir William Beveridge, one of the founders of the Welfare State in Britain, argued against Keynes that the danger was under-population, but even he felt that it was more important to encourage the fertility of *good* rather than *ordinary* people. Beveridge did not join the Society, but he was prepared to speak in public on behalf of the Society's position.[172] Views like these were widely held by the members of a class who thought of themselves as 'good' rather than 'ordinary', even when their political position was to the left of centre.[173] Class sympathies often went deeper than politics: differential fertility made the upper-class intellectuals feel uneasy, even if their politics were not strictly those of their class. Frank Allaun, later to become a Labour MP, gave the problem an anti-capitalist twist in a letter to the *Eugenics Review* in 1933:

> It is hard to imagine anything more suicidal than the differential birth rate, yet it is a natural result of the private property system, where the intelligentsia cannot devote the required time and money to rearing children.[174]

The discussion of intelligence and its relation to class was a product of the introduction of universal compulsory education, which had begun to make itself felt by the end of the century. The attempt to apply the old pattern of education to a new range of children produced a new range of problems, as well as adding a new indicator of social class to the differential fertility debate. Two psychologists, both members of the Society, contributed to this early debate on intelligence and class: they were Charles Spearman and Cyril Burt.

Spearman's inspiration was Galton's suggestion that differences in general intelligence would parallel differences in sensory acuity. He set out to test a group of children from a village school for three kinds of sensory discrimination which he then correlated with the teacher's estimate of their cleverness at school.[175] His first paper on general intelligence appeared in 1904. The technique was to perform quantitative tests of different human faculties, such as verbal or mathematical ability, and then calculate correlation coefficients for each pair of tests. The coefficients themselves were then paired and a tetrad difference calculated according to the formula:

$$r_{xy} \, r_{yz} - r_{ab} \, r_{bc},$$

where x, y and z and a, b and c were six separate tests, and r their correlation coefficients. Spearman calculated all tetrad differences and plotted a frequency distribution for them. The distribution was approximately normal, with a mean near zero. He claimed that this showed that there was a single factor underlying all intellectual abilities, a factor he called g or general intelligence.[176] Spearman was very critical of the simpler non-mathematical IQ testing that had been introduced by Alfred Binet in the first decade of the twentieth century. The collection of a miscellaneous list of tests to give a linear scale was theoretically weak, though he agreed that it did work in practice. It was a cruder way of measuring g. The late Bernard Norton very perceptively pointed out that Spearman's 'faculties' were faculties in the university or public school sense: classics, mathematics and history, for example, of which classics was the most representative of g itself. A talent for Greek was a reliable indicator of a boy's capability in any upper-class career.[177] Spearman's method of factor analysis has since become the ancestor of a group of statistical methods aimed at reducing matrices of correlation coefficients to their most important components.[178]

Writing for the *Eugenics Review* in 1914, Spearman applied his method to the Galtonian problem of the inheritance of general intelligence as he defined it.[179] By 1927, he expected that the mental energy he associated with g would soon be found to have a material or physiological equivalent. Stephen Jay Gould remarked that this is the ultimate reification of a mathematical term.[180]

The Mental Deficiency Act was passed in 1913 (above, note 61). It made mentally deficient children the responsibility of the education authorities, who were to transfer them out of the elementary schools into special schools. Cyril Burt, who had been working in Liverpool on the application of Spearman's tests to schoolchildren there, was appointed by the London County Council to identify children to be transferred, sorting out the defectives from the merely backward.[181] At first, he was supposed to test only the children thought to be subnormal. Two years later, by 1915, he had set up a general programme for investigating the distribution of backwardness in children and designing and standardising practical intelligence tests.[182]

In one of his first papers, written for the *Eugenics Review* in 1912, Burt had already said that the evidence was conclusive that intelligence was inherited.[183] This was the position that he was to defend to the end of his long life. It led him first into adjustments of real data, and finally to the point of faking data, results and even, perhaps, collaborators.[184]

As part of the Eugenics Society's scientific weaponry, intelligence testing fitted very neatly into the discussions on population and fertility. It had in fact become an additional parameter of social class, as well as a significant factor in the tailoring of education to class in Britain.[185]

The *Eugenics Review* in 1936 gave a special number to the discussion of population and fertility. In it, Raymond Cattell, the Society's Leonard Darwin Research Fellow, applied the new measure, the intelligence quotient, to the old problem. Cattell was well enough aware of the implications of his discussion to disclaim them:

> The present results are not based on any assumption of a social stratification of intelligence or of a differential birth rate between social classes. They cut across classes and study directly the relation of intelligence and fertility.[186]

But he suggests, and quotes figures to support it, that both unemployment and petty delinquency are the result of the excessive supply of workers with low intelligence. The residuum of 1936 is found to be lacking not in thrift nor in character, but in intelligence. And as Malthus had predicted, and the eugenists continued to endorse, the group with the lowest IQ had the expected high fertility. The British Population Society was formed in 1929. It was a small group of twenty, mainly distinguished academics: economists, statisticians, sociologists and biologists.[187] Fourteen of the twenty were members of the Eugenics Society: their high academic status emphasises the high standing of the Eugenics Society among intellectuals. The Chairman was Sir Bernard Mallet, KCB, Registrar-General from 1909 to 1920, President of the Royal Statistical Society and President of the Eugenics Society; other members of the

Eugenics Society included the statistician R.A. Fisher, the biologist Julian Huxley, the economist J.M. Keynes, the anthropologist G.L.F. Pitt-Rivers, and the sociologist A.M. Carr-Saunders, a Vice-Chairman of the Society. Those not members of the Eugenics Society included Sir William Beveridge, the Director of the London School of Economics, and Bronislaw Malinowski, the anthropologist. It is a list of brilliant names; one can be in no doubt of the status of the Eugenics Society: it could count among its own members, or coopt when necessary, some of the most distinguished men and women of its age.

The British Population Society had its offices within the Eugenics Society's rooms. It was affiliated with the International Union for the Scientific Investigation of Population Problems, whose headquarters were at the Institute for Biological Research at Johns Hopkins University in Baltimore, but whose Chairman was the animal geneticist Frank A.E. Crew of Edinburgh, a member of the British group and of the Eugenics Society. In 1930 Crew outlined the problems to be investigated by 'Commission II' of the International Union: it was to work on differential fertility, fecundity and sterility.[188]

In 1934 the Eugenics Society itself set up a Positive Eugenics Committee to draw up 'a statement of a factual character' on the steps taken in other countries to promote fertility; the Committee was interested particularly in the political measures taken by the Fascist governments in Germany and in Italy.[189] In these countries, the fertility problem was seen in racist rather that class terms, or, as the Society expressed it, these countries were interested in quantity rather than quality; but fears about the falling birth rates had by this time become general all over Europe. In 1936 the Society formed an eighteen-member Population Investigation Committee. Its Chairman was Alexander Carr-Saunders, who was also a member of the British Population Society, and its Research Secretary was David Glass.[190] The Committee arranged for Glass to visit France, Belgium and Germany to look at population policies, and to go to the International Population Conference in Berlin in 1935 on the Society's behalf. His survey was published in 1936 as *The Struggle for Population*, and submitted to the Society's Council as the Report of the Positive Eugenics Committee, though in fact it says nothing at all about positive eugenics. It was also circulated free to members of both Houses of Parliament.[191] Carr-Saunders hoped that it would help towards the construction of a population policy for Britain. Awareness of the differentially falling birth rate had led already, he wrote, in the past year, to changes in income tax and increases in children's allowances.[192] In Continental Europe, Glass found that the population problem was seen in very different terms. He quotes a speech by the Italian dictator Benito Mussolini:

> To count for something in the world Italy must have a population of at least 60 millions. . . . It is a fact that the fate of nations is bound up with their demographic power. . . . Let us be frank with ourselves: what are 40 million Italians compared with 90 million Germans and 200 million Slavs? Let us look at our western neighbours: what are 40 million Italians compared with the 40 millions of France and the 90 millions of her colonies, or with the 46 millions of England and the 450 million inhabitants of her colonial possessions? . . . With a declining population a country does not create an empire but becomes a colony.[193]

German marriage and birth rates had increased during 1933 and 1934 following legislation designed to promote marriage and fertility, the *Gesetz über Förderung der Eheschliessungen*. Glass felt that the loans given out under this law could be shown to have played only a very limited part in this, though when combined with increased severity in the enforcement of anti-abortion laws, he thought that they might have had some effect in reducing abortions.[194] Glass's report on the Berlin Population Congress shows that although he was interested in the demographic problems of the Fascist states, he was disgusted by the political rac sm demonstrated at the Congress, and did not like to see his organisation having anything to do with it.[195]

In spite of its interest in the population policies of the European states, the Society does not seem ever to have moved towards a racial-state principle: it continued to advocate both negative and positive eugenics, rather than to look for a way to increase the British birth rate as a whole. Its class emphasis was never lost.

It supported by grants in the year 1936–37, for example, several birth-control organisations, which would have been illegal in either Italy or Germany.[196] The Society for the Provision of Birth Control Clinics was one of them; its secretary,

Evelyn Fuller, was also a member of the Society. Its objects were stated as follows:

> in the interests of social welfare, and for the relief of poverty, to establish and support clinics in which instruction will be given to men and women in poor circumstances by registered medical practitioners (preferably women).[197]

The Society had already set up forty-eight clinics, all over Britain, and the Eugenics Society's grant was to help establish five new ones. Although the eugenists knew that, from their point of view, the practice of birth control in the last seventy years had acted dysgenically rather than eugenically, they seem to have hoped to change this, and to even up the differential fertility rate by persuading the poor to adopt it too.[198]

The Population Investigation Committee stayed at the Eugenics Society's headquarters at 69 Eccleston Square, with David Glass as its Research Secretary, until 1948, when it moved to the London School of Economics. Glass then became Professor and Chairman in succession to Carr-Saunders. Although the Society as a whole continued to be faithful to its class, in Glass's own work, the class-centredness disappears. The lack of it was noted with surprise and disapproval by the reviewer of Glass's book for the *Eugenics Review*. The reviewer presumed, he said, that since the subject of eugenic principles was not mentioned anywhere in the book, it must be being kept for future discussion in some other work.[199]

The work of the Population Committee can be traced intellectually back to Heron's original paper of 1906 on differential fertility, which continued to be cited as late as the thirties. Glass's re-examination of differential fertility in 1938 continues Heron's work, but Glass explicitly rejects social definitions of class in favour of purely economic ones, with none of the pejorative remarks about improvidence and lack of culture which Heron had made in 1906. After correcting Heron's figures in various ways – demography had become a little less easy in the meantime – Glass concluded that the differential had probably increased between 1851 and 1911 as Heron had said, but that it might have decreased since then.

In this chapter I have tried to show that the Eugenics Society formed a part of a broad social complex, which itself was part of the long tradition of meliorism stretching back into the nineteenth century, at least as far back as the Poor Law Amendment Act of 1834. The interests of the meliorists both of the nineteenth and twentieth centuries focused on the lives of the poorest stratum of the community. Under the aegis of the Social Science Association, the causes of their poverty and the remedies for it were discussed by a class which was itself immune from all such problems. The educationists tried to socialise them with specially designed schools, some of them fairly coercive; the Malthusians and their successors saw their excessive fertility as the underlying cause of the misery of their lives. The sanitarians tried to control their mortality by cleaning up their streets and houses. The Charity Organisation Society tried to build up their moral life into something more consonant with the ideals of the Charity donors themselves: they offered a subsidy to those willing to take part in the organised and disciplined lifestyle favoured by the Society. All groups felt that crime would be diminished by the application of its particular remedy.

Although nineteenth-century social activism concentrated on environmental problems, it would be a mistake to assume that its advocates were any more sympathetic to the class in which they were interested that the eugenists were to be in later years. As Trygve Tholfsen emphasised, nineteenth-century reformers found the lower classes just as repulsive as their twentieth-century successors were to do.[200] The link between a left-wing sensibility and an environmentalist point of view was not to be made until the late twenties, in Britain as in the rest of Europe.

The twentieth-century Eugenics Education Society itself shared both ideals and members with a network of other societies, all devoted to improving the lives of the poor, and at the same time explaining the nature of their defect and pressing for remedial legislation. Each of the Societies had some specific pathology to suggest: alcoholism, venereal disease or ineducability, all causes of pauperism that had been discussed for many years by the social activists of the middle class. The Eugenics Education Society undercut them all by proposing that pauperism was biological, and that a hereditary defect underlay all the rest. This opinion was echoed by those who thought that alcoholism, too, was constitutional, and that both alcoholism and syphilis could affect the germ plasm and produce degenerative change. To the eugenist, class lost its fluid sociological connection with property, income, status or power, and acquired the meaning of a permanent biological subtype. The lowest class or residuum was a degenerate subspecies whose *differentia* were low social worth, low intelligence and high fertility, as well as those seemingly social diseases, alcoholism, venereal disease and in-educability. It was on the linked problems of feeble-mindedness and differential fertility that the Society focused its efforts.

It was a conception of poverty that could only have arisen in a society so deeply divided by class that the upper classes, even those members of the upper classes who, like Helen Dendy, spent their time doing casework in the slums, could have very little personal experience of the life of the lower. But it was also a conception that arose at a time when these class relationships were changing. It is a measure of the extent and the speed of this change that we, only a few decades later, can find it so strangely easy to distance ourselves from their class-centredness. It is hard now for us to appreciate the serious innocence of intention of that generation of progressives, trying to explain the nature of their own superiority, and to persuade the state into taking responsibility for those lives that they found so rebarbative.

It was within this context of social activism that the Eugenics Education Society's problematic was formed, and its members worked and agitated. Human genetics was primarily a matter for legislative pressure groups.

2

THE AGE OF PEDIGREES
The methodology of eugenics, 1900–20

Eugenics was a movement that attracted people who felt themselves to be serious and responsible, concerned about the civic duties of science and its application to human problems. Their teaching was to spread a new understanding of society in terms of biological law. During the first forty years of the twentieth century, almost every geneticist in Britain, the United States and Germany who was interested in human studies at all was involved in the eugenics movement: human genetics was synonymous with eugenics. It is legitimate, then, to look at the methodology of eugenics as a paradigm for genetics as a whole during this period. In the terms of my analysis, the Eugenics Society is both a tool for the historical investigation of human genetics in Britain and a sample which takes in almost the whole of the field to be investigated.

The methodology of eugenics as a science involved both theoretical teaching and practical research. As I shall show, the theory taught in Britain was an even balance of Mendelism and biometry, and the practice was that of the pedigree study. Pedigrees were felt, as Karl Pearson put it, to give the raw facts of heredity, free of all more or less contentious interpretations.[1] They could demonstrate that something was clearly hereditary without implying that it was either a Mendelian unit-character or part of the quantitative spectrum of blended inheritance in the biometric style. Conversely they could be used to demonstrate both of these theories, and even the influence of environment on an inherited constitution. Quite often there was no analysis of the pedigree in terms of any theory of transmission at all: it was the simple fact that like produced like that interested the eugenists. In the period from 1900 to 1930, the period when the

Eugenics Society dominated the field, the methodology of human genetics in Britain was in practice the uncommitted pedigree study. In the United States too, the collection of pedigrees was the main method of study. American eugenists standardised and refined the symbolism used, and the British group adopted their conventions. But to the Americans, the pedigree implied a Mendelian interpretation of heredity. Its usefulness lay not only in the straightforward claim that it showed something to be inherited, but also in its ability to distinguish at a glance the dominant and recessive modes of transmission. Skipping a generation at once suggested, or even proved, that a condition was inherited as a Mendelian recessive.

German eugenists too began work at the turn of the century with a methodology based on the collection of pedigrees. Many years before either the Americans or the British, the German eugenists began to develop the mathematical models of Mendelism that were to supersede scientifically the simple *ad oculos* demonstrations of the English literature. But though the pedigree had come to the end of its reign in Germany as a scientific tool, it gained a new significance as the official proof of Aryan descent under the race laws of the Nazi racial state.

It is now often said that Mendelism and biometry represented two distinct and incompatible ways of explaining inheritance and evolution and that they were practised in two different camps by different groups of people who saw themselves as enemies. W.B. Provine has suggested that these camps were kept apart by the personal enmity of their leaders, Karl Pearson of the biometricians and William Bateson of the Mendelians.[2] But, as we shall see, this enmity did not involve everyone in the field. A look at the Society's teaching in the courses it arranged as part of its education programme shows that the Eugenics Education Society was quite prepared to sponsor either method. Its lecturers included some of the most outstanding members of both groups.

The biometric group was the creation of Karl Pearson, the protégé and admirer of Francis Galton, whose statistical methods he took up and developed. The Galton Laboratory at University College began in 1905 as the Eugenics Record Office, personally funded and personally directed by Francis Galton, and with a single worker, Edgar Schuster, who was Research Fellow in Eugenics. It was taken over in 1907 by Karl Pearson, and renamed the Francis Galton Laboratory for the Study of National

Eugenics. Pearson was already director of the Biometrical Laboratory at University College and from 1907 the two were run as one unit. In 1911 a Chair of Eugenics was established for Pearson, funded by a bequest from Galton. The funds became available in 1911, but activity did not get started until after the end of the First World War. Pearson was to hold the chair until he died; his successor in 1933 was the statistician R.A. Fisher.[3]

Pearson used his department mainly for the collection and statistical analysis of data on inheritance. The statistical tool which was most typical of the biometric style was the calculation of correlation coefficients, for example, between the measured heights of relatives of different degrees. It was fundamental to biometry that population data such as height formed a continuous normal distribution and that evolution took place by natural selection which gradually shifted the population mean.[4]

William Bateson, leader of the Mendelian camp, was Professor of Genetics at Cambridge; it was Bateson who discovered and promoted Mendel's laws in Britain. He emphasised particularly the law of dominance and recessiveness of discontinuous unit-characters, and introduced his own modification of it in the so-called presence-and-absence theory, a theory which interpreted dominance as the presence of a unit-character and recessiveness as its absence.[5] In Bateson's hands, Mendelism, in spite of its original quantitative or statistical nature, became almost entirely visual: a matter of the inspection of pedigrees. Evolution was by selection for the favoured unit-character and was therefore sharply discontinuous.

It is Provine's thesis that Mendelism and biometry were assumed to be mutually antagonistic explanations of the same material until they were united by R.A. Fisher in his famous paper of 1918.[6] But within the Eugenics Society, there is little evidence of antagonism between Mendelians and biometricians. The President of the Society, Montague Crackanthorpe, KC, in his Presidential Address for 1910 arranged his discussion of eugenics as a science around the theme that both Mendelism and biometry were needed:

> The Mendelian thesis that inherited characters may either be 'patent' or 'latent' militates somewhat against Prof. Pearson's results, which being based on the statistical line of inquiry are derived from the observation of patent

characters only. But I beg you not to infer from this that Mendelism has therefore superseded Biometry. It would be a thousand pities if the Mendelians were to say to the Biometricians, 'We have no need of you,' or if the Biometricians were to say to the Mendelians, 'We have no need of you,' for Eugenics requires the services of both, as a little reflection will show.[7]

The lectures arranged by the Society for its first public series included a very even distribution of clearly Mendelian and clearly biometric lectures. During the first year, G.P. Mudge, the Society's regular lecturer, spoke on 'Mendelism and human society', and the young geneticist A.D. Darbishire gave a talk on 'The inheritance of sex', on behalf of the Mendelians. For the biometricians, two of Pearson's colleaguesn from the Galton Laboratory lectured to the Society: Ethel Elderton spoke on 'The marriage of first cousins', and David Heron on 'The work of the Eugenics Laboratory'.[8]

This fair-minded distribution with equal time for both parties was kept up in the training course on the 'Groundwork of eugenics' that was organised at Imperial College, London, in January 1913. The syllabus was set by a special committee consisting of Adam Sedgwick, Professor of Zoology at Imperial College, Dr Major Greenwood, head of the Department of Statistics at the Lister Institute, Edgar Schuster, who had been the first Galton Research Fellow, and the gynaecologist and obstetrician, Douglas White, who had an interest in the birth-control movement.[9] The course began with a term of introduction covering general biology, given by the protozoologist Clifford Dobell.[10] Dobell must have been an entrancing teacher: his textbook *Intestinal Protozoa of Man* is beautifully written.[11] The following term, Reginald C. Punnett, who had the Chair of Genetics in Cambridge, taught Mendelism. For the final term, biometry was taught by Udny Yule, a statistician from Pearson's unit at University College. The course was entitled 'Lectures on the Biological and Statistical Basis of Heredity' – that is, on Mendelism and biometry.[12]

The representatives of both parties were well trained and fairly distinguished. Professor Punnett was student, colleague and successor to William Bateson at Cambridge and a Mendelian *pur sang*. His thinking was very close to that of his teacher, even to adopting Bateson's presence and absence theory, and he was convinced that an understanding of Mendelian laws was essential for the eugenist:

It is coming to be more clearly recognized that the eugenic ideal is sharply circumscribed by the facts of heredity and variation and the laws which goven the transmission of qualities in living things. What these facts, what these laws are, I have endeavoured to indicate ... for I feel convinced that if the eugenist is to achieve anything solid, it is upon them he must build.[13]

Udny Yule, who gave the lectures on biometry, was one of the statisticians from the Biometrical Laboratory.[14] He was a particularly good choice for the Society, since he had been interested for many years in the statistical analysis of pauperism by biometrical techniques and had used them to show up the statistical naïvety of Charles Booth, famous for his collection of material about the London poor.

The statistical investigation of pauperism, like most of the Society's interests, had a certain tradition behind it, and it was to remain for many years one of the Society's main concerns. Charles Booth's collection of statistics on the life of the lower classes was in some ways a quantative continuation of Henry Mayhew's *London Labour and the London Poor* of 1861. Concern abot the problem of the 'casual poor' had been revived by the worsening economic conditions of the 1880s. 'The bitter cry of outcast London', a pamphlet of 1883, was a product of that concern. Its horrifying details of 'moral corruption, heartbreaking misery and absolute godlessness' concentrated on the overcrowded housing of the poor as an important factor in their degradation.[15]

In 1887, Booth presented the Royal Statistical Society with figures on the inhabitants of the East End of London, well known in Booth's words as 'the most destitute population in England'. He divided the population into eight classes, the first three of which included the 'criminal or semi-criminal' class, the casual labourers, and the irregularly employed, together about 20 per cent of the inhabitants of the area. Booth remarked that the numbers in the very lowest class were affected by the economic condition of the classes above them, and by 'the discretion of the charitable world'. Although its children were mainly to be found in pauper or industrial schools, or in Dr Barnardo's Homes, separated from their parents, it was also, he thought, 'hereditary to a very large extent'. But Booth's statistics of poverty showed that the frightening residuum was smaller than the middle-class activists of the time had expected: class 1, the 'vicious element', was no more than 1.5 per cent of the whole population.[16]

Booth took his figures to show that the level of poverty and the number of paupers depended to a large extent on the proportion of people over 65 years of age in the population. As an indicator for the level of poverty, he used the extent of over-crowding – that is, the proportion of people living more than two to a room. Booth's statistical method was very simple. He grouped his Poor Law unions across the country into rural, half rural, mostly urban and urban, and set up tables for each type showing the cost of relief, and the number of old people per 10,000 population. In each case he found that maximum relief coincided with maximum number of old people, and minimum with minimum. His London figures showed a very rough relationship between pauperism and crowding.[17]

Booth's rather compassionate conclusions were attacked instantly by C.S. Loch, of the Charity Organisation Society. Loch claimed that the percentage of pauperism would go down is stricter administration of the Poor Law made it more difficult to get relief without going into the workhouse.[18] It was the Society's principle that it was easy access to charity that created pauperism, even though Booth's figures did not appear to show it.

It may have been Loch's assertion about Booth's figures that drew the attention of George Udny Yule to the problem of pauperism, a problem upon which he could use the new technique of correlation recently invented by Francis Galton and improved upon by Karl Pearson[19] In 1894–95, Udny Yule had been one of Pearson's first students, and he had immediately become an enthusiastic exponent of the new statistical method.[20] He was easily able to show from Booth's own figures that C.S. Loch has been right: there was strongly positive correla-tion between the amount of outdoor relief given and the amount of pauperism. The correlation had become closer over the last twenty years. The enthusiastic young biometrician crit-icised the elderly Booth's statistical amateurishness: the only generalising process adopted, said Yule, seems to be 'looking down the list'.[21]

Charles Booth's lack of sophistication in statistics was the occasion for Yule's presentation to the Royal Statistical Society of a lesson, which he himself had just learned, on the power of the new technique. No apology was necessary, he wrote, 'for bringing before the society a method that whatever its difficulties exceeds in completeness and generality any other that covers the same ground'. The working example that he used came from Booth's figures: his diagrammatic statistical array shows 'rows' of the percentage of males over 65 years of age in receipt of relief, versus the 'columns' of the number relieved outside the workhouse for each one inside. He uses the figures to explain standard deviations, regressions and coefficients of correlation, Pearsonian style.[22] 'Looking down the list' had had its day.

Yule was particularly excited by this socially useful application of his statistical technique.[23] He also used the pauperism figures as an example in the courses on statistics that he gave at University College between 1902 and 1909. They appear in his textbook *Introduction to Statistical Theory*, based on those courses, where he works out examples on the causation of pauperism as one of the practical applications of this method.[24]

With this background in an area that was of such prime importance to the Eugenics Education Society, Udny Yule was the perfect choice for their statistics course. His lectures covered the usual statistical methods of biometrics: frequency, sampling and, of course, the correlation coefficient, the biometrician's master key. His college lectures and his textbook had used the causes of pauperism as his example but for the eugenists he added some new examples from Mendelism to illustrate his methods. His discussion of fluctuation in sampling was applied to cases from Mendelian breeding experiements, and his correlation coefficient to cases of inheritance in a Mendelian breeding population. His last lecture discussed the analysis of inheritance from both the Mendelian and the biometric standpoint.[25]

To return to the problem of the relation of Mendelism and biometry: there is nothing here to suggest that within the Society, there was a personal hostility keeping biometrics and Mendelism apart. It was the Society's policy to join them together whenever possible. The only concession to Pearson's dislike of the Society itself that one can detect here, is that

Udny Yule, the loyal Pearson student, never became a member of it.[26]

From 1914 onwards, the organisation of the Society's eugenics courses was taken over by Ernest W. MacBride, Professor of Zoology at Imperial College, who incorporated the Society's eugenics and genetics training programme into the College's normal biology course. MacBride's style in genetics and evolution was out of the ordinary in two ways. First, he was more interested in race than in class, and second, he was a Lamarckian environmentalist. As a young man, MacBride had spent a year in Germany, where his mother had been educated. His postgraduate work had been on embryology, under Adam Sedgwick at Cambridge, and from there he had gone on to spend the year 1891–2 with the Austrian Anton Dohrn at the Naples Marine Biology Station, working on invertebrates. Between 1897 and 1909 he was Professor of Zoology at McGill University in Montreal, but when Sedgwick moved to Imperial College, London, MacBride joined him there. In 1913, he succeeded Sedgwick as Professor of Zoology at Imperial College.[27]

Since MacBride's work up till this time had been in zoology rather than in human biology, belief in the potency of biological law came easily to him:

> The lessons which the eugenist seeks to enforce are written out in flame across every page of zoology: the wiping out of the less perfectly developed and less adaptive tribes is going on daily under our very eyes. If this sort of mental pabulum were supplied to those who are likely to become our public men and leaders instead of the exclusively classical education on which the last generation has been reared, the eugenist would not preach to deaf ears.[28]

MacBride's German background, too, remained a determining influence throughout his life. His *Introduction to the Study of Heredity* of 1924 harps with Germanic emphasis on the subject of race, a subject which seldom came into the eugenists' discussions in Britain; he never mentions class.[29] His position was that races had acquired their characters as adaptations to different environments, and that these acquired characteristics were then inherited. This was an important part of the belief system of German race science and folkish anthropology, and of many

65

German eugenists. According to the political philosophers of Aryanism, the Nordic race was a product not only of its genes for tallness and fairness, but also of its prehistory as a settled argicultural folk. The race had learned its self-discipline and far-sightedness while putting by its seed corn or patiently waiting for harvest in a cold climate.[30]

As laboratory evidence for this guiding effect of environment, MacBride cited the experiements of the Viennese biologist Paul Kammerer, which demonstrated an environmental influence on transplanted ova, and the inheritance of learned behaviour. It was MacBride who interpreted for Kammerer on his visit to the Cambridge Natural History Society in 1923. Kammerer expounded his experiments on the midwife toad to a hostile and sceptical audience, while MacBride, committed to Kammerer's point of view, stood fast by his side.[31] Lamarckianism and the formation of the Nordic race sat well together:

> the assumption of new habits, that is, the adaption of the organism to new situations, has been the guiding force that has brought about evolution, ... when animals take on new habits, their descendants tend to assume these habits more readily and on slighter stimulation than their parents. ... The change of habit preceded change of structure and was the cause of the latter change.[32]

But in spite of the power of habit as a determining force, MacBride thought it futile to imagine that education or environmental change could in a few years cancel the work of thousands of generations:

> Each of these races has its unborn psychic qualities. The Nordic race ... learnt in their struggle with the bleak climate of their old home the virtues of indomitable courage, bold adventure and justice between man and man. Is not the word 'fair' a tribute to their virtue?[33]

MacBride's position was that of a true Lamarckian: it was the 'biological memory' of that old struggle that was fixed in the Nordic germ-plasm. He goes on to say that under the 'pernicious doctrine of the equality of man', the doors of immigration were opened wide and North America became filled with a vast crowd of Mediterranean peoples, who with characteristic imprudence were outbreeding their Nordic

66

neighbours.[34] Very un-British sentiments indeed, and not heard very often in London, where it was the poor who were dangerously fecund, not the Mediterranean races.[35]

Peter Bowler has commented that MacBride's Lamarckian stance comes as a surprise from a eugenist, since environmentalism is generally supposed to be a left-wing point of view.[36] But there are many other examples of it, particularly in Germany, when leading eugenists, such as Max von Gruber, Professor of Hygiene in Munich, were supporters of Kammerer and his work. The left-wing reaction against eugenics, and its adoption of environmentalism as its own particular weapon, were not to take place until around 1930, either in Germany or in Britain. The Eugenics Society's literature simply put aside the environment as being dealt with elsewhere, by some other society, perhaps:

> The Society ... desires to awaken public opinion to the vital importance of heredity as a factor of both racial degeneracy and racial improvement.
>
> Eugenists do not deny the great importance of *environment* as a factor in progress, but this is the only society in this country which emphasizes the importance of heredity.[37]

Both MacBride, however, and the psychiatrist A.F. Tredgold, his colleague on the Society's Research Committee, gave the environment primary importance in their emphasis on the deleterious effect of town life.

MacBride was unusual among the British eugenists with his emphatic and explicit Lamarckianism and his Germanic views, but he remained a loyal and active member of the Society until 1931. The proximate cause of his resignation is not quite clear, but he had taken a stand against the Society's sterilisation campaign, which the Council found embarrassing.[38] In his published work, MacBride maintained the even-handed tradition of the Society's teaching programme, by giving equal time to Mendelism and biometry. His Mendelism is Bateson's; he explains Bateson's experiments and his presence-and-absence theory, and he suggests a probable physical basis for it.[39] His biometry is very simplified, he says, because it is a difficult subject for an elementary course, but he explains the ideas of probable error, standard variation, coefficients of regression and correlation, and regression to mediocrity using

Galton's measurements of stature as an example.[40] Like its courses, the Society's more popular Monthly Meetings also covered both Mendelism and biometry. The lectures were designed not to teach any particular theory of inheritance, but to promote the broad hereditarianism that was the groundwork of eugenics, and to apply it to the Society's usual social problems. The balance was maintained even in its political work: the Society's Poor Law Report Committee, at a council meeting in 1909, recommended that a subcommittee be set up to inquire into the eugenic bearing of Poor Law reform, and suggested that its members should include an advocate of the Majority and of the Minority Reports, and a Mendelian and a biometrician.[41]

The evidence of the syllabi of these courses and the work of the people who taught them, shows that the Society's public position on the proper theoretical approach for human genetics was one of careful even-handedness between Mendelism and biometry. Mendelism and biometry were not incompatible, they were complementary: both were important for eugenics. R.A. Fisher's famous synthesis of 1918, which I shall discuss in the next section, is in line with this official policy (see Chapter 3, n. 50)

In private, however, some of the members were not nearly so even-handed. The combat of Mendelians and biometricians that forms Provine's theme did make an appearance, though not a very lasting one. Pearson at this time rejected Mendelism as having no application to most of human inheritance, for example, to skin colour in race crosses, or to coat colour in animals.[42] He and his group also attacked the American eugenist Charles Davenport for his crude use of Mendelian theory to explain the inheritance of feeble-mindedness.[43] The substance of their criticism was that Davenport's use of Mendelism was not only crude, but inappropriate for a character such as intelligence that could not be defined sharply enough to be seen as a unit-character. The Pearsonian or biometric point of view was that mental defect was a continuously graded character, and that defectiveness formed part of the lower tail of the normal curve for three types of test: intelligence, memory and maturity (see Figure 2.1).[44] Classification of defectives was a social matter, depending on the availability of so-called help schools – Pearson uses the German term for them – and the transfer of the children out of the ordinary classes into these special schools.[45]

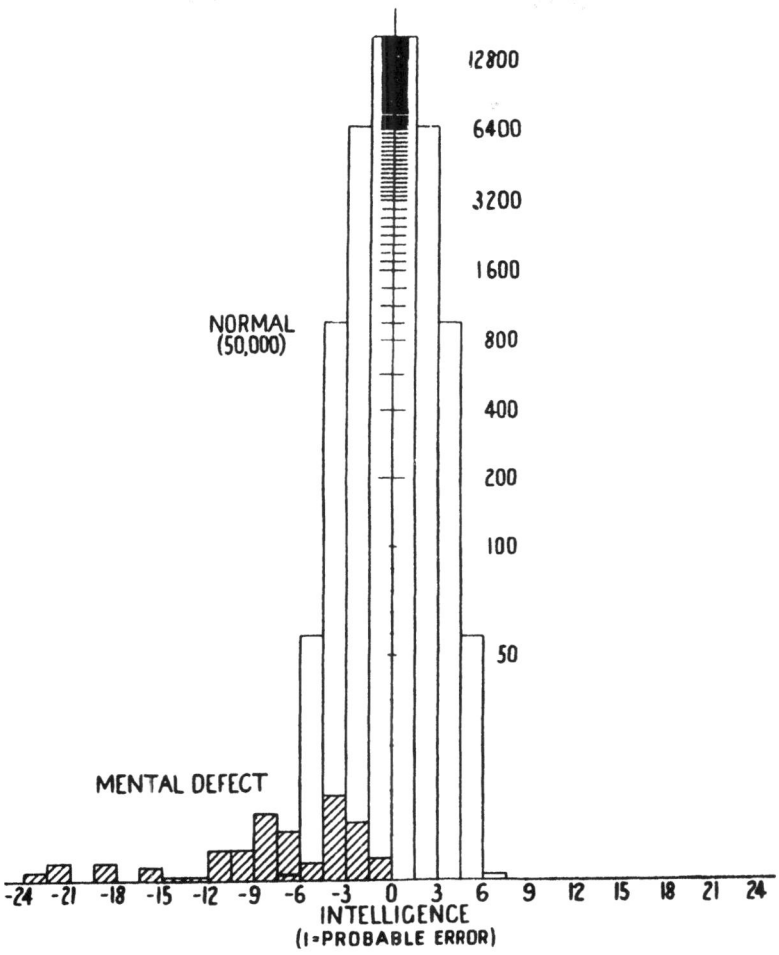

Figure 2.1 Pearson's view of intelligence as a graduated parameter following a normal distribution. Mental defect occupies the tail of the curve

Source: Pearson, *Mendelism and the Problem of Mental Defect* (1914), 33, n. 96

It seemed to the biometricians absurd to see this process as a discontinuous recessive unit-character, or absence of normality. It is odd that, as Charles Rosenberg noticed, Davenport was originally working in biostatistics, but after coming across

Mendelism, he abandoned quantitative or statistical thinking completely.[46]

Davenport's trust in Mendelism was fairly representative of the American view. He himself was in a powerful position to propage that view, since he was director of the Eugenics Record Office, established in 1910, and the Station for the Experimental Study of Evolution, established in 1904, both at Cold Spring Harbor. There were other organisations concerned with eugenics in the United States, notably the American Breeders Association, with its Eugenics and Immigration Committees, but Davenport's were the only institutions that had their own buildings and laboratories.[47]

In Britain, Pearson's anti-Mendelian sallies were returned with gusto, but not by the Society's members in their official capacity. There was in the Society's library a single number of the *Mendel Journal*, which ran in all for only three years from 1909 to 1912, the organ of a group called the Mendel Society. Of the four signed articles in it, three were by members, or future members, of the Eugenics Education Society. There were also several unsigned articles, possibly by the editor, whose name does not appear anywhere, and there was one with the signature 'Ardent Mendelian'. This writer called his paper 'Present postion of Mendelians and biometricians', and wrote in the form of a military dispatch:

> Opposed to the Biometrical Army is the Mendelian. More recent in origin, less martial in organization, but very vigorous, the Mendelian army had already turned the flanks and pierced the centre of the other one opposed to it. For signs of surrender on one wing, and of retreat, very skillfully covered, on the other, are visible in the biometric ranks. The broken centre, encouraged by the boldness and coolness of its eminent Field Marshal — who like the kings of old personally fights on the battle-field — is making a rally on the high grounds to the rear — they are named the hills of 'Masked Segregation.' On the biometrical map they are marked as impregnable, when once occupied and entrenched, and are named 'Continuous or Fluctuating Variants,' or in their more recent maps, as 'Intermediates.'
>
> The great battle of the future is that which will be fought along this rugged range of the 'Intermediates.' The task of

the Mendelian army is to take it. And, already in the plains below its brigades are beginning to deploy.[48]

The hills of Masked Segregation were actually captured in 1918 by a double agent, Ronald A. Fisher. The Mendelians, in the person of Punnett, did not understand that the heights were now theirs. Punnett turned down Fisher's paper when it was submitted to him for publication.[49]

That, then, was the Eugenics Society's theoretical methodology for human genetics, as it was expressed in the Society's teaching and the work of its teachers. In public, the Society tried to keep a fair balance and to teach both Mendelism and biometry in equal proportion. In private, it seems that there were a number of enthusiasts who leaned unofficially towards Mendelism.

Just as the Society had a collective theoretical position, it had also a collective practice in research on human genetics, and in this practice neither Mendelism nor biometry played very much part. The fact of heredity itself could be demonstrated independently of theory by the collection of family histories and their reduction to pedigree diagrams. Here British and American practice came together, although the theoretical underpinnings differed. For the American eugenists, with their insistence on seeing everything in Mendelian terms, the pedigree was a means of demonstrating Mendelian inheritance.

In Britain, pedigrees were used by both Mendelians and biometricians. They presupposed no particular theory of heredity, yet made the visible fact of heredity easy and convincing to demonstrate. Pedigree studies implied only the basic hereditarianism that underlay all eugenics, and were used by eugenists of all theoretical camps. It is the conjunction of pedigrees and ideology which is so typical of the eugenists of this period and it is demonstrated exquisitely in the work of the Society's Research Committee. The research programme originated in an examination, by the Society's Committee on Poor Law Reform, of the eugenic implications of the Majority and Minority Reports of the Royal Commission on the Poor Law. According to the Annual Report of 1910–11:

It soon appeared that before anything could be ascertained concerning the existence of a biological cause of pauperism, research must be made into a number of pauper family histories.[50]

The relieving officers of three workhouses had cooperated with about twenty members of the Society in tracing the family histories of paupers, and the Annual Report particularly thanked Ernest J. Lidbetter, one of the relieving officers, for his help. A special Poor Law number of the *Eugenics Review* was got out, containing the 'Report of the Committee on Poor Law Reform'. The Report makes the Society's position clear. The Majority Report had claimed that pauperism was caused by lack of character and produced by indiscriminate charity, a position that was supported both by the Charity Organisation Society and by Udny Yule's statistical analyses. The Minority Report, like Charles Booth, had claimed that the root cause was economic. According to the eugenists, neither charity nor economics was the fundamental cause. Both were secondary to an inborn biological deficiency:

> That element in pauperism which represents and transmits original defect ... almost wholly neglected in the recommendations of the Commission, is the one we wish to be taken into consideration. [The defective] affords the chief burden on the public purse. He is not the man who responds to a call upon manly independence or stands ready to take a place made available through the labour exchange.
>
> He is born without manly independence ... he does not respond because there is nothing in him to respond. His mainspring came into the world broken. His reproductive instinct however remains intact.[51]

E.J. Lidbetter found this a memorable phrase: 'As Dr Slaughter has said so well, "He was born without manly independence ... he came into the world with his mainspring broken," and no sort of virtuous appeal can reach or move him.'[52]

He was to cite it again twenty-two years later, when he finally published his book on pedigree studies.[53] It was the able-bodied pauper that the Committee was interested in, a man for whom the status of industrial employment was too high an aspiration. His degenerate tendencies

> do not manifest in transmission a single set of characteristics but take on a great multiplicity of forms. A single family

stock produces paupers, feeble-minded, alcoholics and certain types of criminals. If an investigation could be carried out on a sufficiently large scale, we believe that the greater proportion of undesirables would be found connected by a network of relationship. A few thousand family stocks probably provide this burden.[54]

The eugenic solution for this problem is the same as that for the feeble-minded, from whom these unemployables are, in the Committee's phrase, barely differentiated. The solution is that the Poor Law Guardians must have legal power of detention. The old Poor Law principle of less eligibility should be reversed; the paupers should not be made to elect to get out of the workhouse whenever they could. They should be kept there in detention, like the feeble-minded, and their prolific breeding brought to an end.[55]

It is the point of view typical of British eugenics, the class-centredness that was laid out in the first chapter of this book. The so-called residuum, that sub-human class whom the Charity Organisation Society had defined as unhelpable and consigned to the Poor Law, was believed by the eugenists to live isolated both socially and biologically, out of contact with the normal industrial working class. The able-bodied unemployed only *seemed* to be physically helathy; they wre really too inefficient to compete as industrial workers. Both the Charity Organisation Society and the Eugenics Society defined the group by reference to Booth's lower three grades – the criminal class, the casual labourers and the irregularly employed (see note 16 above).

Ernest Lidbetter had been with the Poor Law Authority in London from 1898, living in its institutions and doing the job of investigating the case histories of applicants for poor relief.[56] He seems to have come into contact with the Society when it started investigating pauper case histories and he joined it almost at once, in 1909–10. From 1911 onwards, he was a frequent speaker at public meetings, lecturing mainly on eugenics and social problems. During the year 1912–13 he spoke ten times, at both the Society's own meetings, and at 'Propagandist Meetings', to conferences, universities, debating societies and political groups.[57] His lecture on 'Eugenics and the Poor Law' was repeated four times in one year.[58] In 1913 he is listed as having gone to the Society's course on 'The groundwork of eugenics'

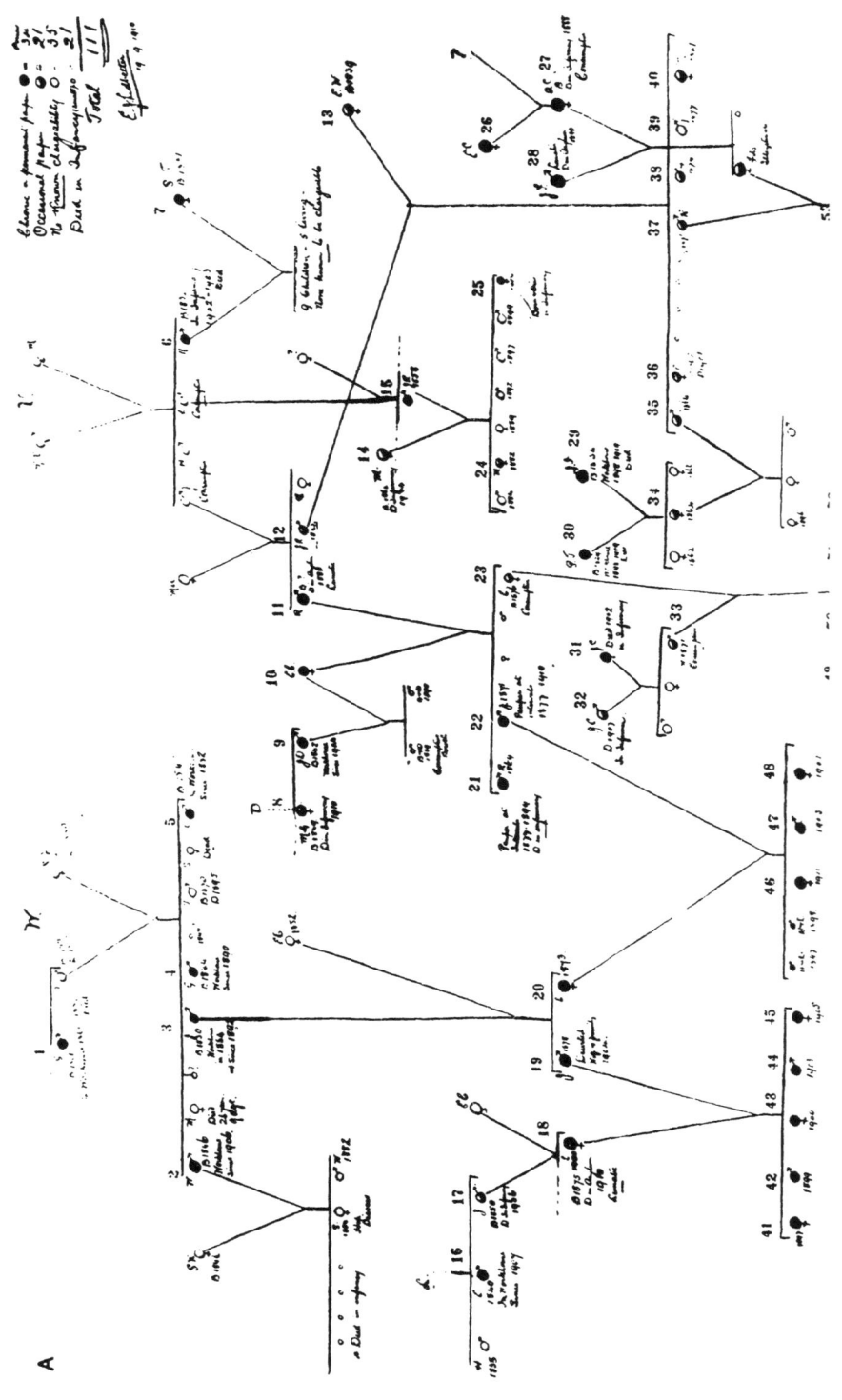

A

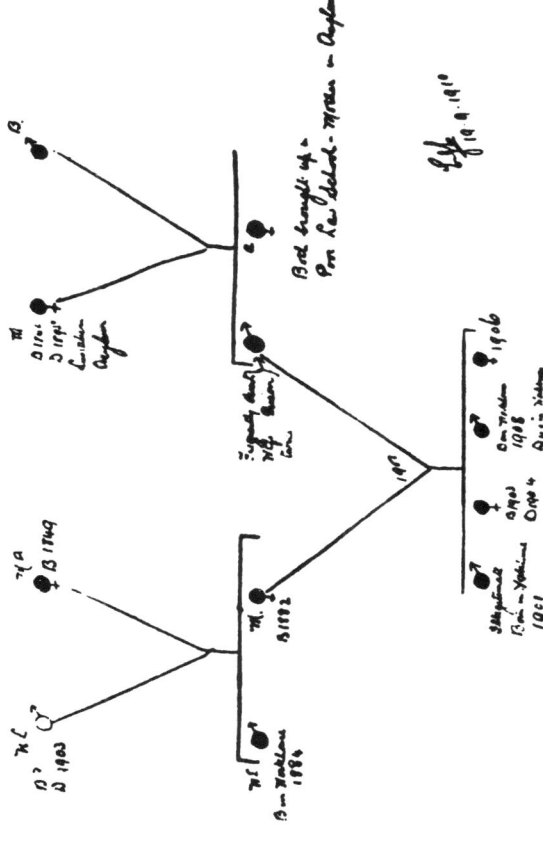

Figure 2.2a and b Standardisation of the pedigree diagram: Lidbetter's pauper pedigrees in their original unstandardised form, showing a complex network of genetic relationships between the pauper families, extending over several generations

Source: E.J. Lidbetter, 'Some examples of Poor Law eugenics', *Eugen. Rev.* 2 (1910–11): 202–28

B

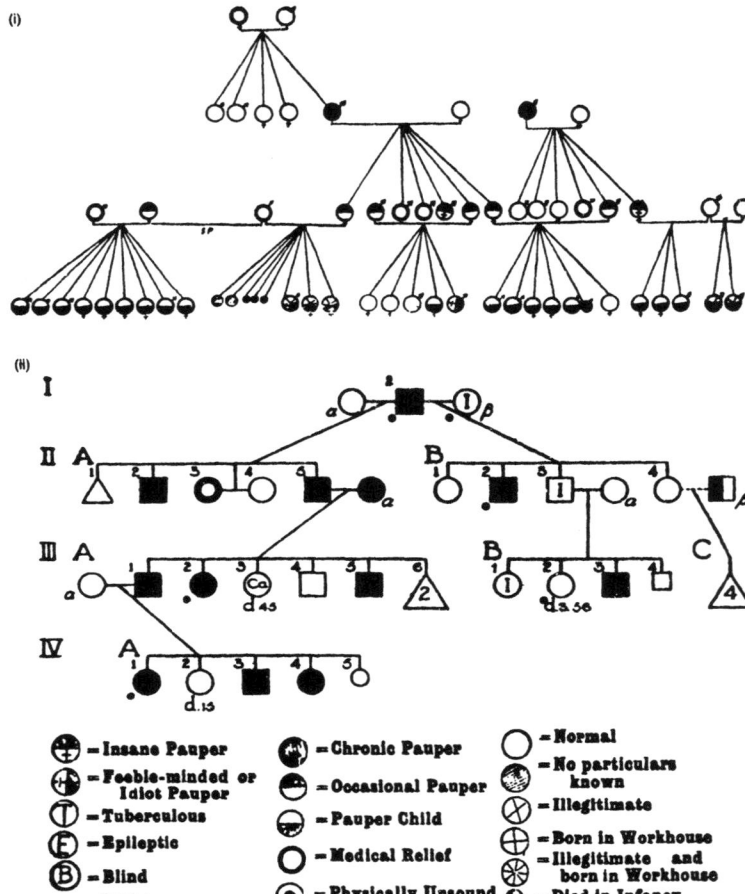

Figure 2.2c The standardised pedigree. i) Lidbetter's diagram is designed to show the familial concentration of failing individuals, and the interrelationships of the pauper families. It does not imply any particular theory of inheritance, or even that natural inheritance alone is responsible for human failure. ii) The committee's standardised pedigree, based on the usage in the US and Germany. The symbols for male and female are replaced by a square and circle; the siblings are all attached to a single line, with a special symbol for twins (II A 3 and 4). Other symbols are to be defined on the page as in Lidbetter's diagram

Sources: i) E.J. Lidbetter, 'Nature and nurture – a study in conditions', *Eugen. Rev.* 4 (1912–13): 54–73. ii) A.M. Carr-Saunders, Major Greenwood, E.J. Lidbetter and A.F. Tredgold, 'The standardisation of pedigrees: a recommendation', *Eugen. Rev.* 4 (1912–13): 383–90

given by Dobell, Punnett and Yule. Lidbetter was one of those who got a certificate for passing all three parts: in general biology, Mendelism and biometry.[59] He was the Society's own product, both in his Poor Law background in his genetics. The Research Committee founded in 1912 to work on the pauper pedigrees adopted him at once. He began work on the preliminary large-scale investigation suggested by the Committee on Poor Law Reform.[60]

The pedigree method seemed a new and promising way of attacking the old problem of pauperism and its causes. Techniques were changing: Booth's rough analysis by 'looking down the list', had been superseded by Yule's correlation coefficients. In the view of the Research Committee, both Booth's and Yule's methods were to give way to the newest, latest technique, that of pedigree study.

The Committee was the proposal of Major Leonard Darwin, one of the sons of Charles Darwin, who succeeded Montague Crackanthorpe as President in 1911.[61] Darwin suggested that pedigree work and pedigree symbols be standardised and that the matter be referred to a Research Committee.[62] The standardised form for the pedigrees that was eventually adopted was based on the one used by Davenport's Eugenics Record Office at Cold Stream Harbor.[63] The standard form of pedigree was published in the *Eugenics Review*, over the signatures of four members of the committee (Figure 2.2, a, b and c).[64] Lidbetter was soon reported to be working on a set of pauper pedigrees as part of a collection of slides and charts for lectures (Figure 2.3, a, b and c).[65] He was to give a series of four lectures to the Haslemere Branch of the Society, one of which later appeared in the *Eugenics Review* illustrated with the new standardised pedigrees.[66] They seemed specially suitable for 'the illustration of popular lectures and articles'; an ideal means of educating the public with an irrefutable demonstration of the inheritance of pauperism.[67]

The Society's Research Committee had six founding members. Its chairman was Edgar Schuster, who had been the first Galton Research Fellow in National Eugenics, appointed by Francis Galton himself to 'carry out investigations into the history of classes and families', so as to 'build up a sentiment of caste among those who are naturally gifted'.[68] Galton had planned to prepare a biographical index of both gifted and

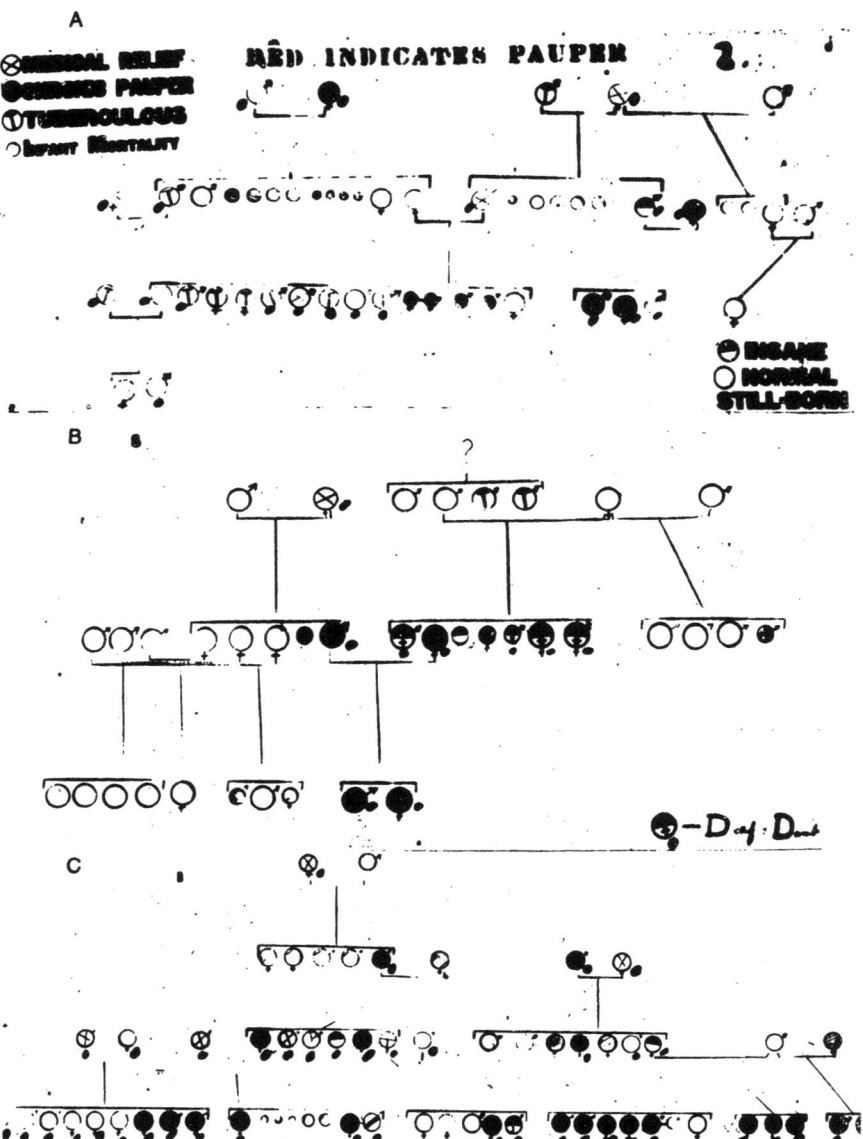

Figure 2.3a, b and c Lidbetter's pauper pedigrees from lantern slides of
pedigrees prepared for International Eugenics Congress, 1912
Source: Eugenics Society Papers, Wellcome Institute, Contemporary Archive
Collection, G38

defective families, which was to include 'the families of persons in asylums, hospitals and prisons'. The book that he completed, with Schuster's help, covered only gifted families, and perhaps Schuster felt that the Society's pauper pedigree study was going to carry out the rest of Galton's plan.[69] Schuster had stayed on at University College under Pearson for some time and produced two more very Galtonian memoirs, but by the time he became Chairman of the Research Committee he was no longer based in London but in Oxford.[70] The Secretary of the Research Committee was Alexander M. Carr-Saunders, who was soon to become Charles Booth Professor of Social Science at the University of Liverpool, and later to hold the Chair of Sociology at the London School of Economics. His 1935 lecture, 'Eugenics in the light of population trends', was to be the stimulus which resulted in the setting up of the Population Investigation Committee. He was also President of the Society from 1949 to 1953.[71]

The members of the Research Committee, besides Lidbetter, were Dr Major Greenwood, the statistician from the Lister Institute, Sybil Gotto, the social activist who was the effective founder of the Society, who served as Honorary Secretary from 1907 to 1920 and gave many public lectures on its behalf, and the psychiatrist A.F. Tredgold. Tredgold was the author of a famous and extremely influential textbook on mental deficiency. He was consulting physician to the National Association for the Feeble-minded and expert witness to the Royal Commission on the Feeble-minded. His view of inheritance rather resembled E.W. MacBride's in that he accepted that environment could produce hereditary defect: Weismann's theory of the inviolacy of the germ-plasm applied only to mutilations, not to general disease and debility:

> I think ... that it cannot be questioned that the germinal plasm shares in those alterations of the body protoplasm which result from disease and environment. ... Consequently, each individual is a potent influence for good or ill in the development of the race. The environment of today becomes the heredity of tomorrow. ... I believe that there are certain diseases which bring about a deterioration of the germ-plasm. The chief of these are alcohol and consumption, although it is probable that other poisons, sexual

excesses and many factors may be lowering the general vitality produce a similar effect. In consequence there results a pathological change in that part of the offspring which is at once the most vulnerable and of the most recent development, the cerebral cortex.[72]

The neuropathic heritage thus produced is passed on, and progresses from generation to generation if drunkenness, disease and sexual excess persist, until amentia and the other stigmata of degeneration appear. Tredgold feels that amentia is both a moral and a class matter, and, like the members of the Charity Organisation Society, he feels that it is being encouraged by the community that supports the children of the diseased, the criminal and the pauper.

> So long as our law-makers and would-be philanthropists are blind to the folly of transferring the burdens and penalties inevitably following carelessness, improvidence, indifference, drunkenness and unlimited selfishness from the shoulders of those upon whom they should rightly fall, to the careful, the provident members of the state, then so long will these classes (and these qualities) continue to be perpetuated.[73]

He demonstrates his thesis with a series of pedigrees in which the causes, – alcoholism, tuberculosis and general ill health, – are shown with the effects, – amentia, insanity and epilepsy (Figure 2.4). Statistics, he says, are compiled from case books or official returns, and lack the accuracy and completeness of these family histories which were obtained by detailed personal enquiry and persistent questioning of the patient's relatives.[74] The subject of family records was one on which Tredgold lectured for the Society in 1912. In that same year, E.J. Lidbetter too is recorded as explaining his charts at a display at a 'Social and Missionary Need Exhibition'.[75]

The pedigree method that Lidbetter and his committee were using was the eugenist's most typical and effective instrument. It had been introduced to them by Francis Galton in his *Hereditary Genius* of 1869, though neither Galton himself nor his young research assistant, Edgar Schuster, used it in its visual form of the pedigree diagram.[76] After the turn of the century, pedigrees became the classic instrument of eugenics argument and demonstration.

CHART I.

SHOWING GOOD HEREDITY CONTAMINATED BY SLIGHT ALCOHOLIC HEREDITY AND TOWN LIFE.

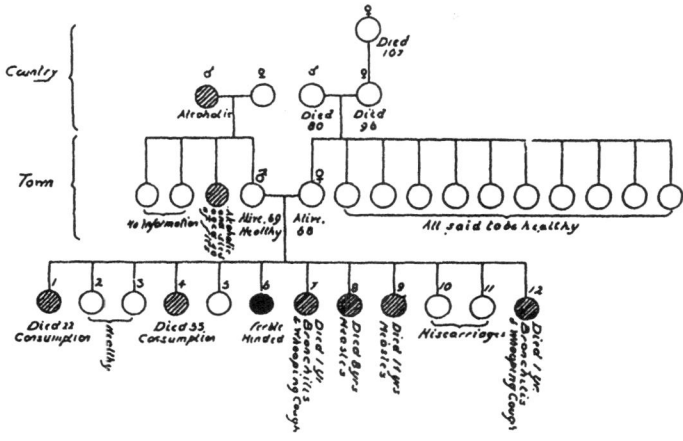

CHART II.

SHOWING GOOD HEREDITY CONTAMINATED BY MORBID HEREDITY.

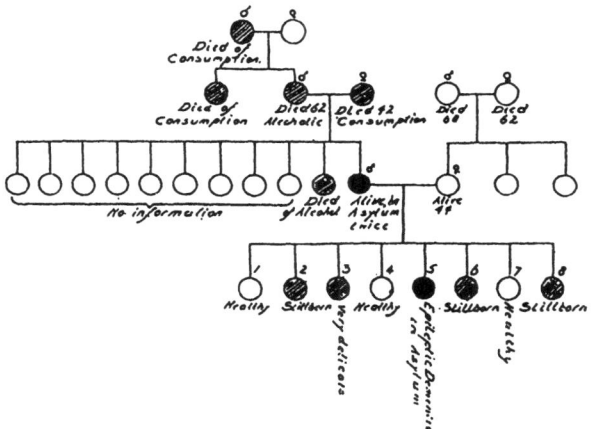

Figure 2.4 Two charts by Tredgold showing alcoholism, tuberculosis and town life as *causes*, and amentia, insanity and epilepsy as *effects*
Source: A.F. Tredgold, *Mental Deficiency (Amentia)* (1908), London: Ballière

In America, the eugenists used the pedigree almost exclusively with the assumption of Mendelian inheritance. Charles B. Davenport, Secretary of the Eugenics Section of the American Breeder's Association, and Director of the Eugenics Record Office at Cold Spring Harbor, New York, a position which made him 'chief eugenist', organised a collection of pedigrees at the Record Office, and wrote about them in many publications.[77] His *Heredity in Relation to Eugenics* of 1911 first explains Mendelian inheritance in a non-quantitative way, and then goes on to apply it to the inheritance of human character traits, such as memory, temperament, handwriting, general bodily energy, criminality, as well as pathology. Davenport argues that these can all be put down to Mendelising unit-characters, even though the complexity of human behaviour makes the analysis difficult. There are already many cases in which the method of inheritance is quite clear, and Davenport predicts that there will soon be many more. Many of his pedigrees come from H.H. Goddard of the Training School for Defectives at Vineland, NJ. Low mentality is a recessive condition, which according to the Batesonian presence-and-absence theory which Davenport supports, is due to the *absence* of some factor: if it is lacking in both parents it will be lacking in all of their offspring (Figure 5a and b).[78] Davenport, of course, was not the only 'vulgar Mendelian' in America. Other eugenists used the same methodology of pedigree displays and look-and-say Mendelism. H.H. Goddard, the Principal of the Vineland Training School in New Jersey, used his students' pedigrees to prove that feeble-mindedness was a Mendelian recessive.[79] Harry H. Laughlin, Davenport's appointee as Superintendent of the Eugenics Record Office, campaigned for sterilisation on similar grounds.[80]

Although the style of the Eugenics Education Society's pedigrees was modelled on that of the Eugenics Record Office's formalised notation, their analysis was not. None of the members of the Society's Research Committee was an ardent Mendelian; the pedigree study as they used it was a demonstration of hereditability *per se*, and not of a theory of transmission.

There are innumerable examples of pedigree studies from this period which were used in this uncommitted way. The most striking is Pearson's massive collection, *The Treasury of Human Inheritance*, a series which he organised and edited at the Galton

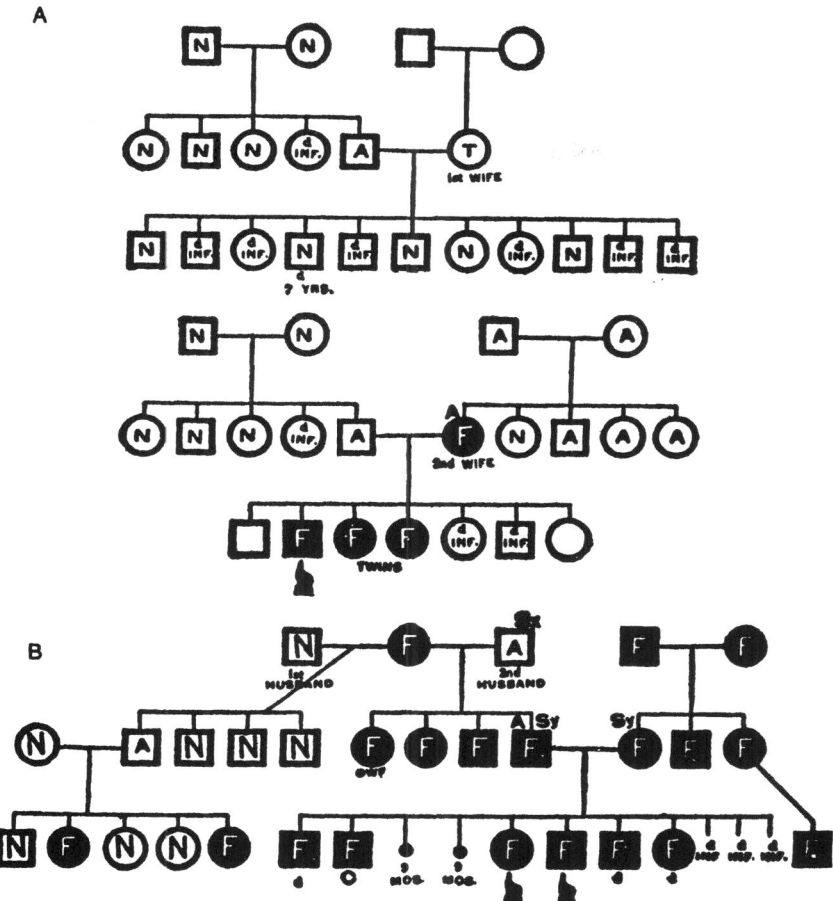

Figure 2.5a and b Pedigrees demonstrating the inheritance of feeble-mindedness as a Mendelian recessive. In A the central mating is of an alcoholic man with a normal woman who died of tuberculosis. Of their eleven children, five are known to be normal; the others died early. This man then married a feeble-minded woman and of seven children three are certainly feeble-minded and two were, as young children, killed at play in a fashion indicating a lack of ability to avoid ordinary dangers. In B a feeble-minded woman (of the first generation) has married a normal man and has four normal children (except that one is an alcoholic); then she marries an alcoholic sex offender (who is probably also feeble-minded) and has four feeble-minded children. Here the mental strength of the first husband brought the required strength into the combination, so as to give good children

Source: C.B. Davenport, *Heredity in Relation to Eugenics* (1911), New York: Holt

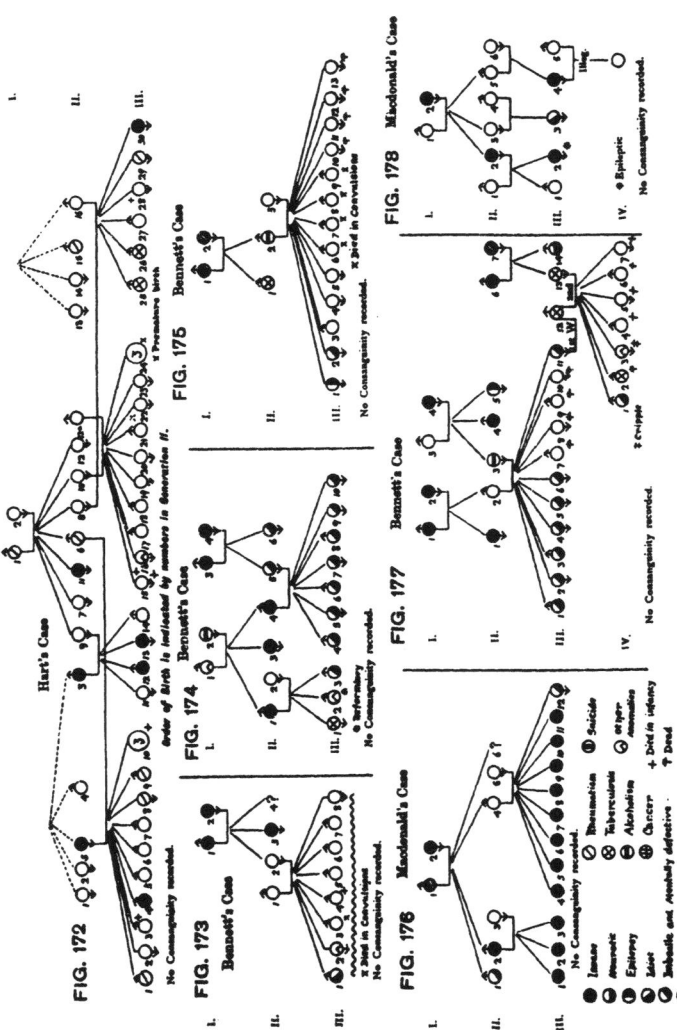

Figure 2.6 Pedigrees collected from the medical literature by Pearson and his group, the biometricians, 'entirely free from controversial matter'. They show families with a variety of mental conditions, including insanity neuroses, epilepsy, mental defect, paralysis, alcoholism and suicide; there are also a few cases of cancer and tuberculosis

Source: K. Pearson, J. Bell *et al.*, *A Treasury of Human Inheritance: Pedigrees of Physical, Psychical and Pathological Characters in Man*, Part III (Angioneurotic oedema, Hermaphroditism, Deaf-mutism, Insanity, Commercial Ability), no. 9 in series, Eugenics Laboratory Memoirs (1909), London: Dulau

Laboratory, in which case histories with family data on all known inherited human conditions were collected.[81] The verbal histories of the *Treasury* came partly from the published medical literature, some of it going far back into the nineteenth century, and partly from the Eugenics Laboratory records. The standardised pedigrees were worked out by the authors of the *Treasury* (Figure 2.6). They were supposed to contain no reference to theoretical opinions: according to Pearson, the series was to be 'entirely free from controversial matter'.[82] For Pearson, the use of a pedigree format obviously did not suggest that the defect shown was inherited as a Mendelian unit-character, as he personally did not believe in Mendelism.

The Report of the Committee on Poor Law Reform of 1910 contains many examples of eugenist pedigrees. In the section on 'The eugenic principle and the treatment of the feeble-minded', for example, there are two pedigrees of feeble-minded families.[83] It is their prolific breeding, the large families richly studded with miscellaneous kinds of defect, and not the pattern of inheritance, which the pedigrees are supposed to show. In the next section on the pauper family histories, an enormous six-generation fold-out pedigree is illustrated (see Figure 2.7). The point of its inclusion is to show the intermarriage of the pauper stocks, as well as to demonstrate beyond all doubt that pauperism is inherited.[84] The writer comments:

> Several broad features are at once discernible. ... First among these is the fact that one pauper family has a tendency to marry into other pauper families. In this way half a dozen or more pauper families may be related to each other. Secondly, the evidence is clear that successive generations of the same family contain a due proportion of paupers. This points to the conclusion that pauperism is due to inherent defects which are hereditarily transmitted. Thirdly, the experience of the Committee is quite clear that the paupers whom they have seen and examined individually are characterized by some obvious vice or defect such as drunkenness, theft, persistent laziness, a tubercular diathesis, mental deficiency, deliberate moral obliquity or general weakness of character, manifested by want of initiative or energy or stamina and an inclination to attribute this misfortune to their own too great goodness and generally to bad luck.

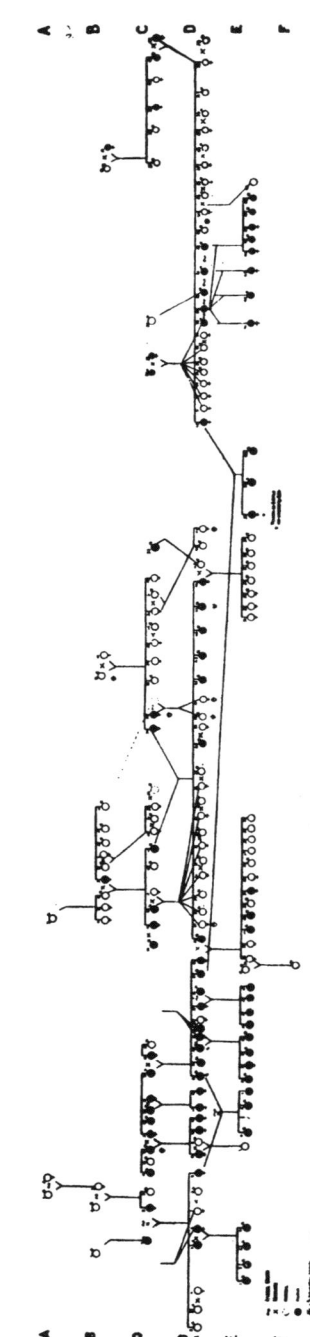

Figure 2.7 Part of a six-generation pedigree, showing the prolific breeding and the intermarriages of 'pauper stocks'. It was this kind of pedigree that Leonard Darwin called 'rivers, flowing steadily on wide fronts, carrying on their surface patches of refuse'. They represent a kind of non-quantitative population genetics

Source: Report of the Committee Appointed to Consider the Eugenic Aspect of Poor Law Reform, Section 1, *Eugen. Rev.* 2 (1910–11): 167–77, n. 51

... There is no doubt that there exists a hereditary class of persons who will not make any attempt to work or to continue in work so long as charitable funds, even of small amounts, are forthcoming.[85]

Later in the *Report* there appears the comment:

When we find it possible to trace four generations of paupers there can be little doubt as to the hereditary transmission of these defects. More perhaps than anything else such a fact speaks forcibly as to the real nature of pauperism.[86]

The pedigree is a network of relationships, demonstrating inheritance of defect in terms of the biological connections within a social class. The hereditary transmission of the defects which are the characteristics of this class is made obvious at a glance, a demonstration *ad oculos* of the *fact* of heredity. Theoretical interpretations such as the Mendelian or the biometric are subordinate, second-order problems. The pedigrees are not arranged like diagrams of Mendelian inheritance, with two parents and two filial generations. They are more like huge kinship networks, spreading often across several fold-out pages, with several couples even in the first generations. Leonard Darwin wrote that they were like 'rivers, flowing steadily on wide fronts, carrying on their surface patches of refuse'. (See Figure 2.7.) The wide front samples two or three generations of the class. It does not show single families traced to a unique defective ancestor, the 'vulgar Mendelism' of the American eugenists, but a kind of non-quantitative population genetics, the interrelatedness of the entire pauper class as well as the transmission of its civic defects.[87] The Eugenics Education Society was relying on the pedigree to educate its audience about the characteristics of the pauper class, the hereditary source of pauperism and feeble-mindedness, as well as a whole range of physical defects. The laws of heredity were not part of that lesson. They were reserved for the Society's academic courses.

In theory, then, the eugenists taught both Mendelism and biometry; in practice they used the method of pedigree study. Their class-centredness called for the investigation of a whole class, not simply a few individual families showing single defects; the interrelatedness of the paupers was as important to them as

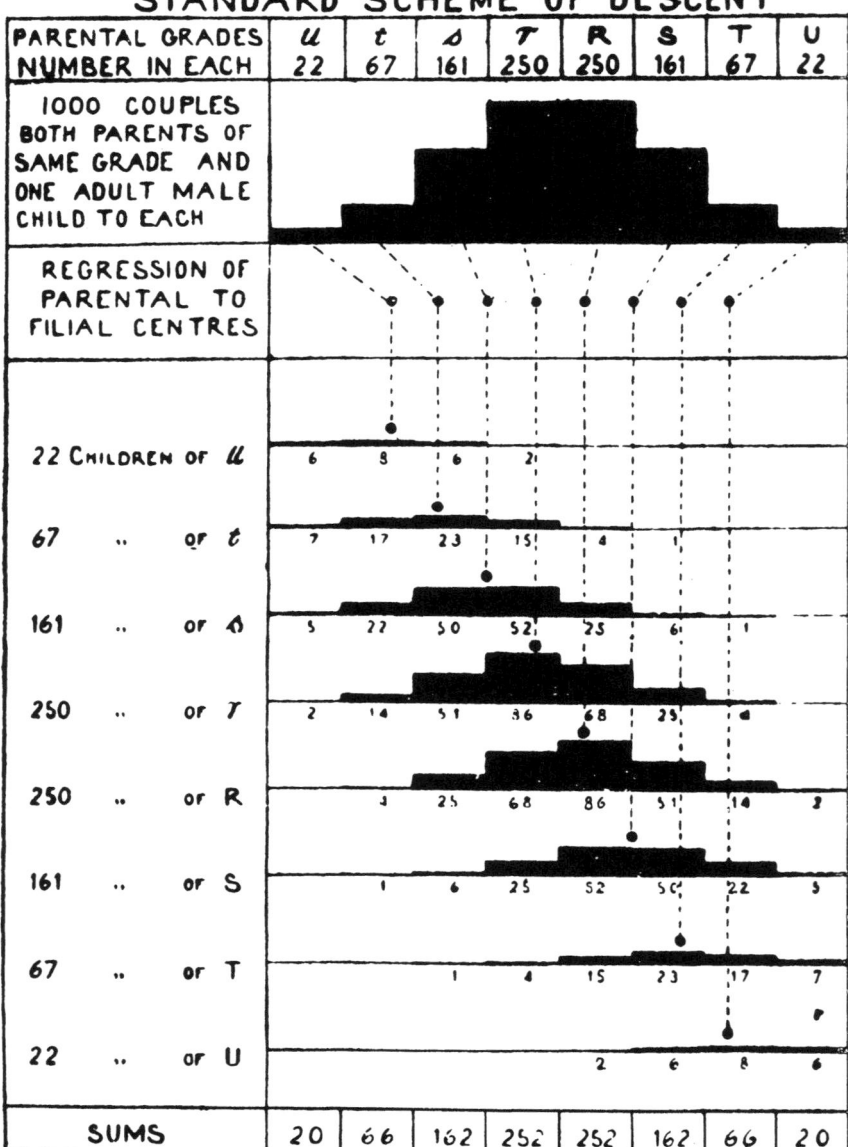

Figure 2.8 Galton's 'standard scheme of descent', showing how regression to the mean population value takes place.
From a lantern slide

Source: Eugenics Society Papers, G.38

the defect itself. The pedigrees demonstrated the interlocking of biological descent with the social failure of a group.

The exhibition which accompanied the First International Congress of Eugenics of 1912 was rich in examples of all kinds of pedigrees. The biometricians were not personally represented: Pearson boycotted on principle anything organised by the Society, especially something involving exposition of science to the public, but, as usual, the Society included both Mendelism and a little biometrics. A series of charts showed the theory of Mendelian inheritance as illustrated by peas.[88] Another series showed Mendelism with dominance, no dominance, and the theory of gametic purity as illustrated by blue Andalusian fowls, a type of fowl whose classic blue plumage only appears in heterozygotes, and which pleasingly shows the recovery, unstained, of the genes for pure white and black, in the F3 generation. By the side of these hung Galton's 'Standard Scheme of Descent', an example of the original meaning of the statistician's regression to the mean (Figure 2.8), and, as an example of the inheritance of ability, a pedigree of the Darwin, Galton, and Wedgwood families (see Frontispiece). There was also a chart 'comparing Mr Booth's classification of all London with the normal classes', presumably meant as an explanatory comment on the collection of Lidbetter's pauper pedigrees drawn from Booth's three lowest grades.[89] Lidbetter's pedigrees themselves were there in large numbers, 'showing their pauperism is associated with mental and physical defect, and justifying the inference that a high proportion of pauperism is to be attributed to the transmission of defect'. With the last one, showing 'insanity, epilepsy and infant mortality', Lidbetter cautiously commented, 'a Mendelian suggestion'.[90] This was his only reference to Mendelism. It was the intermarriage of the defective families, not the mode of inheritance, that Lidbetter wanted to show.[91] The pauper pedigree project, and some of the pedigrees, also formed the subject of a talk given to the Medical Section of the Congress by Frederick Mott, pathologist to the London County Asylums, who was to be one of Lidbetter's most loyal supporters for many years to come (Figure 2.9).[92] (See Chapter 3, n. 84.)

The American Breeder's Association put on a similar exhibition.[93] Their list of items includes charts of the statistics of defectives, and of the principles of heredity, followed by a group

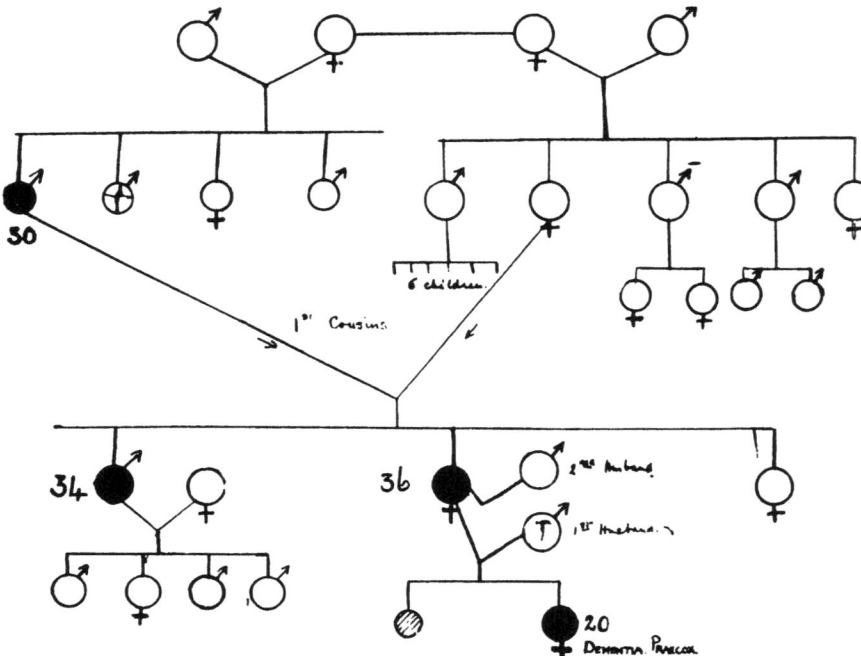

Figure 2.9 A Lidbetter pedigree used by Frederick Mott
Source: Lantern slide, Eugenics Society Papers, G.38

of sixteen pedigrees collected by field workers in America. Their section had been put together by C.B. Davenport; so presumably the pedigrees represented mental defect to be a Mendelian recessive as Davenport had said in his *Heredity in Relation to Eugenics*, which had come out in 1911, and was to be so ferociously denounced by Heron and Pearson in 1913.

The largest section of the exhibition, in terms of the catalogue at least, was the German. The consultative committee arranging the German contribution to the Congress itself was a distinguished one; it included the names of most of the country's leading eugenists: Eugen Fischer, Max von Gruber, Ludwig Plate, Ernst Rüdin, and Wilhelm Schallmayer and Alfred Ploetz, with the statistician Wilhelm Weinberg as secretary. His Excellency General von Bardeleben, President of the Verein Herold, the official genealogist to the German nobility, was a honorary member, who together with Alfred Ploetz, made

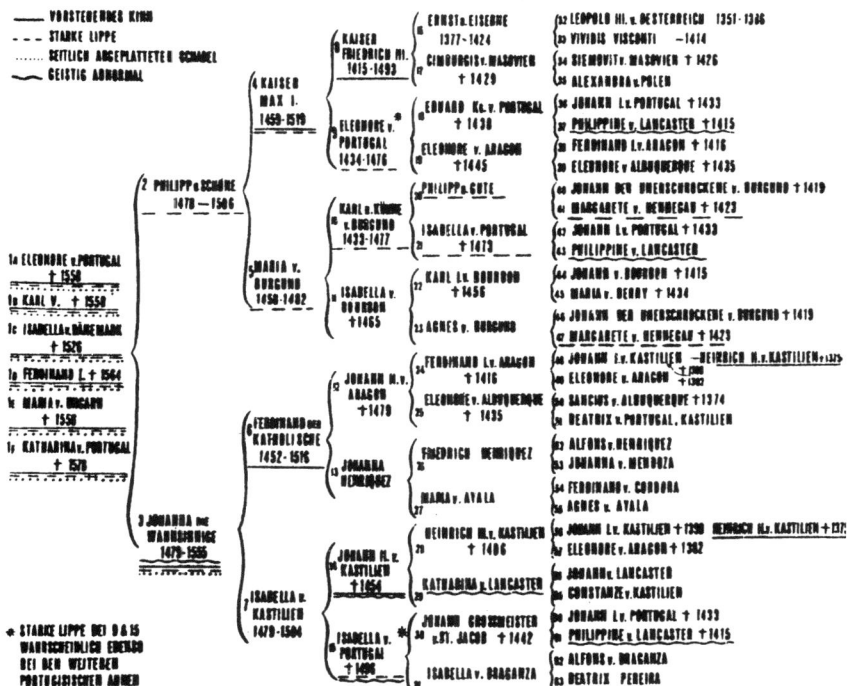

Figure 2.10 An *Ahnentafel* showing the inheritance of the peculiar lip, the overshot jaw and flattened skull of the noble Habsburg family. It also shows the phenomenon of *Ahnenverlust*, or loss of ancestors. Instead of thirty-two ancestors in the sixth generation, the young Habsburgs had only twenty-four

Source: Dresden Hygiene Exhibition (1910) and published in von Gruber and Rüdin (eds), *Fortpflanzung, Vererbung, Rassenhygiene* (1911), n. 94

the journey to London in person along with the exhibit in July 1912.

Much of the material for the show was conveniently ready, after having been used at the *Internationale Hygiene-austellung* in Dresden the previous year, organised by Max von Gruber.[94]

Perhaps this accounts for Ploetz's insistence on the importance of environment for eugenics:

> Many theoretical workers hold that the most important mission of race-hygiene is to fight against therapeutics and hygiene of the individual, for about these they have the most serious misgivings. They consider that by maintaining inferior variations up to the age of reproduction, the average quality of the race must suffer. ... This point of view, short-sighted as it may be, must be examined into. It appears to be forgotten that on the one hand hygiene is powerless in cases of a high degree of degeneration and that on the other hand hygiene by prevention of illness, does away with a number of causes of inferiority. Finally it appears to be entirely overlooked that with the best inherent qualities and unfavourable surroundings, the individual development may be poor and stunted. Of what use are high potentialities if they remain latent?[95]

This piece of catalogue text was to accompany two charts by Ploetz showing 'race-hygiene amongst other sciences, and what the various branches consist in', placing race-hygiene as it was to be taught in the German university courses in the context of social and personal hygiene. The first of these courses were to start in Berlin and Munich within the next two years.

Even more insistently environmentalist was Gruber's own exhibit, a demonstration of the experiments of Paul Kammerer with the fire salamander and the midwife toad, showing the hereditary changes that Kammerer claimed to have established in them by teaching them new habits in the classical Lamarckian manner. Like the British eugenist MacBride, Gruber found Kammerer's work both important and convincing.[96]

The German exhibit also contained pedigrees, some of them in the typically German form of the studbook style *Ahnentafel* (Figure 2.10), and its variant, the *Sippschaftstafel* (Figure 2.11), which showed the heaping up of the *erbliche Belastung*, the genetic loading that crushed beneath its weight the unfortunate final recipient of the degeneration of several families, like a circus strong-man supporting too many acrobats on his shoulders. The aristocratic families showed the phenomenon of *Ahnenverlust*, or loss of ancestry, a feature which today's breeders of pedigreed cats, such as the author of this book, always check out

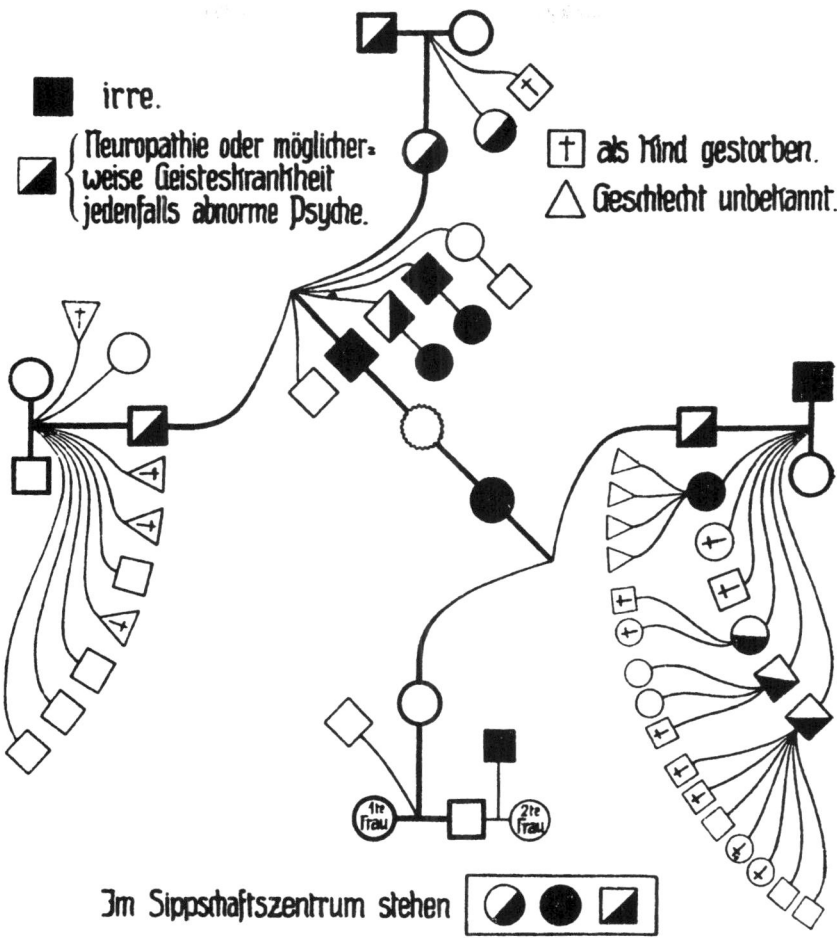

Figure 2.11 An *Ahnentafel* of the type known as *Sippschaftstafel*, showing the *propositus* as the focal point of the family's genetic load
Source: Dresden Hygiene Exhibition (1910) and published in von Gruber and Rüdin (eds), *Fortpflanzung, Vererbung, Rassenhygiene* (1911), n. 94

very carefully when arranging a mating for a queen. The young Habsburgs inherited their peculiar face from both sides of their family; one couple occurred three times in their sixth generation. The family of Kaiser Wilhelm II was a particularly extreme example of this: at twelve generations back, he had only one-eighth of the possible number of ancestors, a shocking demonstration of aristocratic inbreeding. There was also a huge pedigree of the 'Zero family', sprung from 'good German peasant stock', but now comprising the 'largest family of degenerates the world has ever known', according to the man from the *Pall Mall Gazette*, reporting on this 'interesting little side-show' to the main meeting.[97]

One further group of charts in the German exhibit must be mentioned for its future significance. It is the contribution of Wilhelm Weinberg, Secretary to the German Consultative Committee.[98] His charts are not pedigrees, although they are a demonstration of heredity. They are quantitative, although not Mendelian or biometric. Using histograms, Weinberg demonstrates the inheritance of 'constitution', showing that with increasing age of death of parents, child mortality declines, especially in the case of children from tuberculous families. He also attacks Pearson's claim of the 'Handicapping of the Firstborn', using data from 3,129 tuberculous families and 1,830 non-tuberculous families, collected from his own practice in Stuttgart between 1873 and 1889.[99] Weinberg's table, comparing the maternal and paternal sides of each family, shows that in both cases mortality of the last-born is higher than that of the first-born. His method probably owes something to his colleague on the German Consultative Committee, the Rostock clinician Friedrich Martius. Martius was the leader of a clinical movement that argued for an inherited constitution, rather than environmental exposure, as a determining factor in tuberculosis.[100] Weinberg felt that he was 'correcting for environment' by using the maternal and paternal branches of the family as internal controls for each other. He presumed they lived in approximately the same social environment but were not genetically related. Weinberg's empirical data-collecting, his comparison of observed deaths with expected, and most particularly, his use of very large samples, were not to be seen again until the 1920s in human genetics. These features were to reappear in Germany, in the work of the blood group geneticists, and the psychiatric eugenists around Ernst Rüdin in Munich.

The exhibition that went with the First International Eugenics Congress is a neat microcosm of the human genetics practised by the eugenists before the First World War. It is dominated by pedigrees of all kinds. Davenport's, Lidbetter's, and the *Ahnentafel* of the Germans. To each of these groups of workers, the pedigree represented the most convincing demonstration of the basic hereditarian claim that like produces like. But beyond that, each had its own interpretation of how that came about.

Lidbetter was content simply to show that it did come about. The complexity of his large intermarrying families suggests that he expected in the end to index every member of the pauper class, and to be able to show that every one of them was linked to all the others in a single loose family structure. Davenport's claim was that social failure was inherited in a Mendelian pattern, as the recessive absence of a normal gene, an explanation that fitted well with its with its occasionally skipping a generation in his families. The German *Ahnentafel* was soon to be of tragic significance in the Nazi racial state as a passport to the privileges not of nobility, its original purpose, but of Aryan ancestry. It seems to show the whole burden of an individual's forebears crushing a single, final victim beneath its weight; it is no accident that in German a family showing the transmission of a deleterious gene is called *belastet* or 'loaded'. The *Ahnentafel* suggests a more profoundly deterministic attitude to heredity than the broader form of pedigree used by the British and American eugenists, whether or not they were ardent Mendelians, in which it could be seen that at least some of the siblings of a 'tainted' family would probably be lucky. There are no siblings in an *Ahnentafel* to lighten the burden on the *Propositus*.

3

IDEOLOGY AND METHOD
R.A. Fisher and research in eugenics

The years before the first world war were a time of robust confidence for the eugenists. Lidbetter's pauper pedigree project linked ideology and method in perfect union. The changes that began to take place in the twenties were not the results of attacks from outside the movement, but of an internal evolution. As the ideology began to soften, the pedigree method was no longer able to give answers to the new questions that began to be asked.

Ronald Aylmer Fisher's association with the eugenics movement began in 1911 and went on until the late 1930s. The case study of his doings in the Society during the first period of my chronology, the period of the dominance of the Society and its methods in human genetics, reflects the transition from the certainties of the Society's first decade to the uncertainties of the twenties, when changes were happening within the Society itself, and its members were groping for a means of adapting the old methodology to answer the new questions.

R.A. Fisher, who died in 1962, was one of the most important and productive thinkers in statistics of this century. Any current textbook is full of his methods; they are used in every field in which data are collected and analysed, from agriculture to economics.

Fisher went up to Cambridge in 1909 to read mathematics as an undergraduate; it was one year after the foundation of the Eugenics Education Society, and two years before the death of its founder, Francis Galton. His official biographers in the Royal Society memoirs, and after them W.B. Provine, simply say that at Cambridge he came across Karl Pearson's 'Mathematical contributions to the theory of evolution', and so became interested in the mathematics of evolution and in genetics.[1] But his interest in evolution and genetics was a good deal more active than that would suggest. In 1911, the year before the first International Congress of Eugenics in London, and Fisher's last year as an undergraduate, he helped to start the Cambridge University Eugenics Society. For two years, from May 1911 to May 1913, it was one of the most active of the Eugenics Education Society's outposts.[2]

The Cambridge branch society was one of many; there were branches at Oxford, Liverpool, Manchester, Birmingham, Southampton, Glasgow and Belfast, as well as in Australia and New Zealand. The Annual Reports give details of them: the lists of members, the topics of their meetings, which were often addressed by speakers from the parent body in London.[3] The Cambridge Society's minute book, preserved in the Eugenics Society's library, shows it to have been fairly typical in its choice of speakers and topics, though it seems to have been rather shorter-lived than some of the others, as student societies often are. But no minute books are to be found among the Society's papers for these other groups. This one is interesting both as an example of a branch society and as a demonstration of how deeply involved the young Fisher was in the eugenics movement at this time. The first public meeting of the Cambridge Society took place on 22 May 1911, when the Reverend Professor Inge, Dean-designate of St Paul's, gave an address entitled 'Some social and religious aspects of eugenics'.[4] Professor Inge's speech, reported in the *Cambridge Daily News*, brought up most of the basic eugenists' problems: the feeble-minded, the degeneration of the race, the differential birth rate and positive eugenics, the responsibility of those 'possessed of a particularly fine organism' to do their part towards improving the quality of the next generation.[5] He was thanked after the speech by Mr R.A. Fisher of Caius College, the student chairman of the Society's Council.[6] Professor Inge was a reliable choice as an inaugural speaker. The committee which invited him already knew his views, as he had published a paper in the first number of the new *Eugenics Review* in which he had made plain his opinions. His paper is a model of that upper-class horror of the urban poor which was so typical of the eugenists:

> I cannot say I am hopeful about the near future. I am afraid that the urban proletariat may cripple our civilization

97

as it destroyed that of ancient Rome. These degenerates, who have no qualities that confer survival value, will probably live as long as they can by 'robbing hen roosts', as Mr Lloyd-George truthfully describes modern taxation, and will then disappear. Meanwhile we must do what we can, which is not very much.[7]

It sounds fairly extreme, but the founding members of the Cambridge Society must have felt it to be a proper statement of their position, and they invited him to be their inaugural speaker.

The first meeting of the undergraduate section of the Society was held in Fisher's rooms at Caius College, with C.S. Stock, the Secretary, giving a paper.[8] At the next meeting, R.A. Fisher gave a paper on 'Heredity'; he explained it first as Mendelism, then as biometry, then said that the eugenist needed both and that they did not exclude each other.[9] It is a foreshadowing of his 'Correlation between relatives on the supposition of Mendelian inheritance' of 1918, but it is also the Eugenics Society's party line.[10] As we have noticed in Chapter 2, Montague Crackanthorpe's Presidential Address of 1910, the arrangement of the Society's public lectures, the pattern of the Society's teaching from 1912 onwards, and the Society's discussion of the Majority and Minority Reports, all show that the Society's public policy was to teach both Mendelism and biometry, and to harness both in the service of 'heredity', and that was what Fisher wished to do. C.S. Stock put it thus: 'Statistics (e.g., Biometry) will tell us what result to expect in the aggregate. Genetics will tell us what result to expect in the individual.' But, he goes on to say,

the outcome of the research on Mendelian lines is likely in the near future to provide us with the knowledge of how to rid society of a great incubus of disease, crime, deformity and many other 'ills the flesh is heir to'.[11]

It was Mendelism, not biometry, that Stock, the Cambridge undergraduate, expected to provide answers in the near future. In Cambridge, things were not as evenly balanced as in London. In Cambridge, where William Bateson was the first Balfour Professor of Genetics and R.C. Punnett the second (Fisher was the third), the eugenists' teaching tended towards Mendelism.

The second public meeting of the Society was a lantern lecture by Professor Punnett, called 'Genetics and eugenics', and for Punnett the genetics was, of course, Mendelian.[12] The undergraduate committee of the Society found Punnett's exposition of Mendelism so important that, at a meeting in Fisher's rooms the following term, Fisher as chairman proposed that they should make it a rule that each academic year one paper be devoted to an elementary exposition of the principles of heredity, meaning, of course, Mendelism.[13]

That same term, another of the Society's lectures was given by L. Doncaster, on 'Sex-limited inheritance', a subject which Doncaster may be said to have 'discovered' in Mendelian terms.[14] Before Doncaster's lecture, the committee arranged for a preliminary lecture on Mendelism to be given to the members by Mr Kidd, one of the undergraduates.[15] Stock sent round the announcement with the paternal remark on it that 'it is hoped that all those not familiar with the simplest ideas of Mendelism will attend'.

Professor Punnett's public lecture was not simply a teaching exposition of Mendelian genetics. It was reported and summarised, with considerable sympathy, in the *Cambridge Daily News* with the headlines:

> *Lecture by Professor Punnett*
> *Facts about heredity*
>
> Legislation required

The article started with an introduction to Mendelism in Punnett's Batesonian manner. In the reporter's words:

> Heritable characters, continued the lecturer, are represented by something definite in the gamebes [*sic*] and with respect to any such character two and only two conditions of the gamebe are possible: whether the gamebe contains the character on which the development of the character depends, or it does not.

It ends with a call for social action based on this new understanding of the laws of heredity:

> We may object to the way in which God made some people; we may decide the world would be better without them.

But it must be done calmly and without prejudice, in the clear light of reason, and not under the cloak of righteousness or of doing a thing that is pleasing to any but ourselves. ... It is in the interests of the majority but if the majority are to recognize their interests, they must have some knowledge of the workings of heredity.[16]

Punnett has adopted Bateson's Mendelism and Bateson's 'presence and absence' theory, and believes that Mendelism can now be accepted as fact and natural law. The majority can do away with those whom the world would be better without, and they can do so 'calmly and without prejudice', that is, without guilt, in the 'clear light of reason', if they know the natural laws of heredity.

Throughout the nineteenth century, the natural laws of economics were appealed to in similar fashion: if the lower classes had not been so ignorant, they would have understood that their condition was determined by simple natural laws, the laws of supply and demand. Writers of popular tracts wrote to explain to the lower class that they could do nothing but submit to laws like this. Harriet Martineau, the well-known Unitarian, wrote her stories dramatising the plot of John Stuart Mill's economics textbook to persuade working men by poignant examples that combinations could only injure the working man and could never improve his position.[17] E.P. Thompson has called this appeal to natural law to hide the exploitation of man by man 'the greatest evasion of all' in the 'complex of involuntary evasions and inhibitions which made up Victorian middle class sensibility'.[18] It is the same appeal to natural law that this news report shows Punnett making to his Cambridge audience, but there is a difference. Punnett is not trying to educate the lower classes; he is explaining to his own class where their interests lie. They need not pretend to be doing something that is pleasing to anyone but themselves; the 'cloak of righteousness' of earlier natural law givers can now be let fall. The upper class should attack its class enemy with the enemy's own weapon, that of fertility.

This awareness of the conjunction of the aims of eugenics and the feelings of class interest comes out again in the third public lecture to the Cambridge Society, this one given by Major Leonard Darwin. He says:

the poorest classes, though containing many persons of the highest excellence in every respect, do nevertheless contain a larger proportion of the naturally unfit than do the richer classes. ... [It is] consistent with known facts to hold that to the presence of the naturally unfit, with their want of self-control the great fertility of the poorest classes ought in large measure to be attributed. ... We eugenists in fact assert that the problem we are dealing with is largely a biological one, and that it certainly has no relation to class prejudices.[19]

The *Cambridge Daily News* again reported the lecture.[20] The headline repeated Major Darwin's assertion:

Not class prejudice

These three public lectures – Inge's, Punnett's and Darwin's – give a good picture of the ideology of the Cambridge Society. Their common ground is in the class-centredness which they all show, with greater or lesser awareness of it in themselves. Dean Inge is the least self-conscious; he can damn the proletariat without turning a hair. Punnett and Darwin, a little more gentle, have to argue themselves out of their awareness of their own inhumanity.

Their line was evidently popular at Cambridge. The reports in the *Daily News* are never critical in tone; they are seriously informative, long and very detailed. Attendance at the public meetings was very high; Stock gives the figures:

May 22nd [Inge] The room was full, 200 persons, many of them women ...
December 5th [Punnett] ... room full, 250 ...
February 8th [Darwin] Rooms quite full, about 300.[21]

The Cambridge Society had been the result of an under-graduate impulse: Stock gives an account of its beginnings in his secretarial report.[22] The 'Provisional Committee of Under-graduates', which was presumably himself and his best friend, Fisher, with one or two others, had started by approaching Inge, Punnett and W.C.D. Whetham, FRS, dons who were members of the London Society. From this beginning, it drew in, among other senior members of the university, three more Darwin sons

– Horace, Francis and Sir George (all Fellows of the Royal Society); the Reverend the President of Queen's College; the Reverend the Master of Magdalen; the Master of Christ's, Professor Sir Joseph Larmor, FRS, MP, a physicist and Secretary of the Royal Society; the palaeobotanist Professor A.C. Seward, FRS, who later became Master of Downing College and was Chairman of the Society; Sir Clifford Allbut, KCB, FRS, the Regius Professor of Physics; F.G. Hopkins, FRS, later the first Professor of Biochemistry at Cambridge; the anthropologist and ethnologist A.C. Haddon, FRS, and the psychologist and ethnologist W.H.R. Rivers, FRS.[23] In addition there were some more junior members of the university, such as the economist J.M. Keynes, who acted as the Society's treasurer. For its second year, the Lord Bishop of Ely, and Lord Rayleigh, Chancellor of the university, agreed to act as patrons.[24]

Distinguished Cambridge scientists, churchmen and dignitaries, the local press reviews, and the packed meetings all show that eugenics was extremely well supported in the years before the Great War. There was no quarrel between the biological scientists and the churchmen here; both were content to accept that man's immortal soul was inherited as a quasi-Mendelian character, which might, it seemed, be either present or absent, according to class. It is not possible to dismiss this historically as prejudice and snobbery, although these words were soon being used to attack it.[25] It is an indication of the very restricted nature of the English intellectual leadership; here is no *freischwebende Intelligenz*, to use a famous phrase.[26] The English intelligentsia clearly and consciously represents the class from which it is drawn.

R.A. Fisher was a dedicated supporter of the Society. He was one of its founders, its chairman and a frequent speaker at its meetings, and when Fisher went down from Cambridge, the Society seems to have withered away. But the tone of frightened loathing of the lower class which is so plain in the writing of most of the eugenists is not so blatant in Fisher's work. Fisher is a more romantic and enthusiastic elitist, the feeling of a young man who had been agreed by all to be a genius since he was a child. His is a predominantly positive eugenics, the encouragement of mankind to breed for a cultured upper class, rather than the suppression of the undesirables at the bottom.

In the Michaelmas term of 1912, Fisher had just graduated in mathematics and had decided to stay another year at Cambridge, with a studentship in physics at Caius. The paper he read at the Society's second annual meeting was called 'Some hopes of a eugenist'. His hope was not that the pauper classes or the feeble-minded might finally be extinguished, but that mankind should evolve further, beyond the level of his present elite:

> When men were first assured that there were reasons for believing that their ancestors of a certain period would be classified as apes, they appear to have been for the most part either shocked or amused. It has taken a long while for the extreme optimism of the view to manifest itself. Yet the optimism is very necessary and obvious. 'What man is to the ape', says Zarathustra, 'a joke and a sore shame: so shall man be to beyond-man, a joke and a sore shame'. We can set no limit to human potentialities; all that is best in man can be bettered.[27]

But there is an obstacle to this steady evolutionary improvement. It is that small families have a social advantage which lets them rise in the social scale, so that the highest class, the class which should have the highest intelligence, beauty and taste, will also have the smallest number of descendants. Infertility, as well as talent, produces success. In the highest class, hereditary talent breeds with hereditary infertility, and the upper class continually die out at the top. Fisher quotes Dean Inge, who says, 'We need a new tradition of nobility', a tradition which will come from the eugenists. Fisher continues,

> Eugenists will on the whole marry better than other people: higher ability, greater beauty. They will on the whole have more children than other people. Their biological type characterized by their solicitude for human betterment, their scientific insight, above all their intense appreciation of human excellence, has a strong tendency to improve and survive. ... [They will] absorb more and more of the best qualities of our race, will become fitted to spread abroad ... the doctrine of a new natural ability of worth and birth.[28]

For Fisher, 'a new natural nobility of worth and birth' means that it is not we the members of the upper class who are fittest to survive, or even we the members of the Aryan race, but we the

103

members of the Eugenics Society, who will give us Nietzsche's race of *Übermenschen*, beyond-man.

Fisher had been interested in Nietzsche before he formed the Cambridge Eugenics Society. Joan Fisher Box, his daughter, speaks of him reading Nietzsche with a group of college friends in his early undergraduate days.[29] An interest in Nietzsche was not uncommon among the eugenists. Maximilian Mügge, a founding member who occasionally lectured for the Eugenics Education Society, wrote in 1909 in the first volume of the *Eugenics Review* that Galton had founded a racial religion: the ideal of the super-man would supply the religious feeling of responsibility which would give the science its popular support.[30] Havelock Ellis, another founding member of the Society, was also one of Nietzsche's most prolific exponents in English; Ellis found in him both a philosophy and a poetry of eugenics.[31] The library of the Eugenics Society in London contains the early series of Nietzsche translations, and several books on his work.[32] The commentators at this time generally saw Nietzsche as the philosopher of Darwinism and evolution, whose *Übermensch* was the forerunner of a new human race, a master-race.[33] A later generation of commentators has radically reinterpreted him.[34]

One of the Nietzschean commentators who was given a notice in the *Eugenics Review* was the young Geneva sociologist and social-Darwinist Georges Chatterton-Hill. His exposition of Nietzsche's philosophy has just the same tone of visionary aristocratic elitism as Fisher's essay; it is dated 1912 and Fisher's essay was first read in November of that year. But there is no need to force a connection; Chatterton-Hill's interpretation was not an unusual one:

> It is the mass of humanity which is justified by the existence of the over-man who *creates* new values and thus adds to the power of the race. It is just and it is necessary that *humanity should also be made to suffer for the over-man* [Chatterton-Hill's emphasis].[35]

Chatterton-Hill finds in Nietzsche too the eugenist's feeling that the race is degenerating, but he puts it into the Continental form of race, rather than class conflict: 'The aim, of the modern state, of modern sciences, of everything modern is the greatest happiness of the greatest number, the most vile ideal ever presented to man.' He then quotes Nietzsche's own words, which make the transition from the social to the racial:

In the whole of Europe, the inferior race has now triumphed, in regard alike to their colour and their brachycephalic features and perhaps even in regard to their intellectual and social instincts. ... The race of the Masters and Conquerors is decaying even in a physiological sense.[36]

The critic for the *Eugenics Review* says a little nervously that Nietzsche's thought has affinities with the general doctrine of eugenics, though the eugenists may find him a dangerous ally: 'Nietzsche is not good meat for immature minds, but there are some to whom he may be a useful tonic, or at least good red pepper.'[37]

Fisher went down from Cambridge at the age of 23 in 1913, with no planned career.[38] He spent a few of the early months working on a friend's farm in Canada, then came back to a job in the City, sharing rooms in London with his friend, C.S. Stock. They worked together for the Eugenics Education Society; together they wrote a paper for the *Eugenics Review*, lectured and reviewed books.[39] Fisher later worked on the bibliography of eugenics that the Society was making.[40]

When the war began, Fisher was rejected for the army because of his very poor eyesight. It was a profound disappointment for him. Army life had appealed to him as embodying the 'physical fortitude, the adventurous mind and the courageous spirit of the primitive hunter or the Nordic explorer'. When he was turned down by the army, he went in for farming instead, which, as Joan Box has written, satisfied both his eugenic ideals and his desire to serve during the war. The farmer succeeded or failed by nature's own criteria of fitness to survive.[41] He spent the four years of the war in schoolteaching, which he hated, but at the same time he and his young wife worked at subsistence farming on a smallholding. Eileen Grattan-Guinness was just 17 when they were married, and she shared Fisher's romantic eugenic ideals. Joan Box interprets Fisher's 1915 essay on sexual selection to show how he felt his own love to be an experience of the direct contact with nature, freed from the learned contamination of nurture. In the growth of sexual passion, all inappropriate aesthetic and moral teaching falls away, and we feel a freedom and certainty, a 'mystical appreciation of the human personality' through which we act for nature in our instinctive selection of the mate who matches our unconscious eugenic ideal. If this describes his own experience, so does his sense that this ideal will lead us beyond man:

> Here we pass, like Nietzsche, beyond Good and Evil. Morality ceases to be arbitrary and dogmatic, but takes its place as a particular formulation of the requirements of the Highest Man – of our ultimate judgements of human value.[42]

Joan Box says that Eileen, her mother,

> felt the need to give her life to some worthy cause, as she had seen her parents serve God. She could find no proof of the existence of God ... then Ron [Fisher] presented himself, an idealist with very real and worthwhile ambitions, and she found her life's work in him, in his person and in the pursuit with him of great aims for the increase of human excellence and the advance of scientific truth.[43]

In the evenings, after days of hard work on the land, hard enough to produce sufficient to keep the family without bought food, they read aloud history and philosophy of science, with the emphasis on the rise and fall of civilisations. They read Frazer's *Golden Bough*, Gibbon's *Decline and Fall*, Norse sagas in William Morris's translations, Plato and Nietzsche, Darwin and Rabelais. It is hard to see in this passionate and idealistic naturalism any connection with the fear and class-hatred shown by so many others among the eugenists. But Fisher had been educated at Cambridge and the pattern of his social thought was formed in that mould. His intellectual elitism is the eugenist's class-centredness in a less horrifying form. He assumes, just as they do, that all the virtues worth breeding for in the human race are to be found in the upper classes; there should be a downward social mobility of excellence produced by a highly fertile upper class. Wealth, culture and political power should spread naturally from above.[44] The professional classes, lawyers, doctors and skilled artisans, have formed professional societies to protect the honour and status of their members by excluding all inferior types. These societies, he suggests, could also protect their members from the dysgenic effects of the expense of educating their children to their own status, by providing scholarships for the children of their colleagues and by restricting entry to the profession not just by examination but by requiring the nomination of each candidate by several senior members.[45] Fisher is suggesting that professional associations should become hereditary castes, that upward nobility should be controlled to prevent the dilution of upper-class morality by the *arrivistes* from below.

The assumption that environment was of negligible importance even in such physical parameters as height was one which was fundamental to eugenics, but new to British social thought. We have seen in Chapter 1 that the *Report of the Committee on Physical Degeneration* assumed the very opposite, and that Pearson and his group wished to prove them wrong (p. 40 and Figure 1.1). One of the methods the biometricians used was to show that correlations between the heights of relatives were approximately the same as the correlations for eye colour. For eye colour, no environmental effects could be claimed.

As we shall see below, the Society's research projects continued to emphasise heredity at the expense of environment. Its official position was that the environment might have some effect, but even if it did, it was not the Eugenics Society's business to worry about it. The Society's problem was nature, not nurture. Some of the British eugenists, such as Ernest MacBride, A.F. Tredgold and Frederick Mott, believed that the conditions of town life were responsible for the degeneration of the germ-plasm (pp. 66, 80 and Figure 2.4). But Ronald Fisher was not one of them: Fisher felt that the environment was of vanishingly little significance, from either the Lamarckian or the social point of view. That assumption was a fundamental part of his 'synthesis of Mendelism and biometry' of 1918.

When Fisher first wrote on Mendelism and biometry, the argument that they were compatible had already been put forward by George Udny Yule, whom we have seen in Chapter 2 teaching biometry with Mendelian illustrations in the Eugenics Education Society's course (p. 64). Yule had suggested that the discontinuity of Mendelian unit-factor inheritance could be reconciled with the smooth distributions of biometric measurements by assuming that many factors were involved in the determination of quantitative characters like height.[46] But the measured heights of relatives gave correlation coefficients of

0.54 for fraternal and 0.46 for parental correlation, and it was argued by Pearson that these correlations were too high to be accounted for by Mendelian laws. Pearson calculated that if dominance were assumed, so that only half of the genetic factors available showed up in the measured heights, the calculated parental coefficient would be only 0.33 instead of 0.54.[47] Yule, writing in 1907, then calculated a coefficient using a different model, in which there was no dominance, and the heterozygote was intermediate in height between the homozygotes. He found a fraternal coefficient of 0.50, but, he says, it is impossible to distinguish between the effects of dominance and those of environment; he assumes that both will reduce the coefficient.[48] It is to be noted that for environment to have this effect on the correlation coefficient, it has to be assumed to be randomly distributed throughout the population. Yule's unspoken implication is that the environment of parents is no more like that of their *own* children than it is like that of anyone else's.

It was this problem, the reconciliation of the observed correlation between the measured heights of relatives with the predictions of Mendelian theory, that Fisher wanted to solve. He wanted to do so because, as we have seen in Chapter 2, it was the official position of the Eugenics Society that both types of analysis were valid; and he wanted to do it in the way approved by both the biometricians and the Society; that is, by accounting for all the variance by hereditary factors, to the exclusion of environmental effects. In 'The correlation between relatives on the supposition of Mendelian inheritance' of 1918, he achieved these aims.

Like Yule in 1907, Fisher in 1918 assumes that the effects of environment are randomly distributed; he makes this clear in a lecture he given at the London School of Economics in 1924, in which he explains the arguments he had used in 1918:

> Any factor, or experience, which affects stature independently in parent and child, as for example the age of onset of infectious diseases might be supposed to do, will tend to lower the correlations between relatives; so that if we had two populations similar in respect to inheritance, one living under a very uniform environment and the other under very diverse environmental conditions, we should expect that latter to show lower correlation, if environment were

at all influential upon the characters studied. Equally, if we had two populations with the same range of environmental influence, one of great genetic uniformity and the other of great genetic diversity, we should expect the latter to show the higher correlation coefficients. In this sense, it may be said that the correlation coefficient provides a measure of the relative importance of hereditary and environmental influences upon the character studied.[49]

Fisher goes on to say that there may be other factors involved as well, which affect the value of the correlation coefficient, but nowhere does he point out that for the environment to have this effect, it must be assumed to be randomly distributed. If it is not, and there is any correlation between the environment of parents and the environment they in turn produce for their own children, and if this differs between families, then this correlation will *increase* rather than decrease the correlations between relatives.

The fraternal correlation coefficient of 0.54 meant to the biometricians that 54 per cent of the variance in the population could be put down to differences in ancestry and 46 per cent to differences between people of the same ancestry. As Fisher pointed out, although this 46 per cent of the variance was not accounted for, the biometricians still claimed that inheritance was all-important.[50] It was Fisher's intention to demonstrate what the biometricians had only been able to assert. The additional 46 per cent, which did not show in the correlation of measured heights, could also be accounted for on the Mendelian system by taking into account the segregation of Mendelian factors, dominance, and the resemblance between parents, a feature which introduces another positive component into the correlation. Using three values, the parental correlation, the fraternal correlation and the marital correlation, Fisher estimated the extent of the effect of dominance, and the effect of the environment, in the case of measurements of stature, forearm length and span. His calculations showed the environmental effect to be no more than 2 to 5 per cent in each case.

Fisher defined environment as 'arbitrary external causes independent of heredity'.[51] By using this definition, as his commentators Moran and Smith noted, Fisher tacitly supposes that the effects of environment can be represented by an addition to the measurement which is independent of the genotype value, so there is no interaction between genotype and environment. This environmental deviation is supposed to be normally distributed with zero mean and constant variance and is not correlated among relatives so that

observed height x = genetic component y + environmental component

$$\text{coefficient } c = \frac{\text{variance without environment}}{\text{variance with environment}}$$

$$= \frac{\text{var (y)}}{\text{var (x)}}$$

Fisher is able to show in each case that this coefficient c is more or less 1 for the three measurements, stature, cubit and span, and that there is nothing left to be accounted for by environment.[52] It is this part of his conclusion that Fisher, as he explained in some lectures that he gave at the London School of Economics in 1924, felt to be an advance on previous work. The biometricians had generally ignored 46 per cent of the variance; Pearson had thought that the correlations between relatives in man could not be reconciled with the predictions of Mendelism; and Yule, in trying to reconcile them, had not been able to separate the influence of Mendelian dominance from that of environment in their effect on the correlation coefficient.

William Provine, in his *Origins of Theoretical Population Genetics*, has brought out very well the importance of Fisher's solution to Pearson's problem.[53] But for Fisher and his colleagues in the Society, the problem of heritability versus environmentally determined variance was almost as important as that of Mendelism versus biometry since they had never recognised a contradiction between these last two. Fisher had dealt with these problems and solved them in a way that was in the direct line of Eugenics Society policy. His low estimate of the effect of environment as well as his use of both Mendelism and biometry must be placed within the context of his eugenist background.

In 1921, Fisher took up his first real job, as statistician to the Rothamsted Agricultural Research Station, an experience which was to work a profound change in his way of thinking about the old problem of the seed and the soil. The seed and the soil were now no longer to be a metaphor for human nature and nurture, but real seed and real soil, whose relationship could be measured in terms of grain yields per acre.

The Rothamsted Experimental Station was founded in 1843 by John Bennett Lawes (afterwards Sir John) to investigate the effect of fertilisers, especially artificial fertilisers, on crop yields. In 1834, when Lawes took charge of his family farm at Rothamsted Manor, he had just come down from Oxford. He had been reading chemistry under the then Professor of Chemistry, C.G. Daubeny, who was interested in the chemical and geological history of the earth.[54]

Lawes began by using the traditional fertilisers, farmyard manure, guano or bird manure, and bone meal. He could not understand why the bone-meal dressing, a good source of phosphate, was ineffective on his clayey soil although it worked on peats and limestones. Applying his knowledge of chemistry, he found that grinding the bone meal with vitriol (sulphuric acid) converted inert dicalcium phosphate to the active monocalcium form and made it work very well.[55] In 1842, Lawes patented his superphosphate and its manufacture from bones and from rock phosphates, which had been recently found in Spain.

The main interest of the Rothamsted Station was the demonstration of the value of superphosphate and nitrogen fertilisers. The work of Lawes, and his colleague, the chemist J. Henry Gilbert (afterwards Sir Henry), played a large part in promoting the use of these artificial manures, an important change in agricultural theory and practice.[56] Lawes were also concerned to disprove the theory of Justus von Liebig, that the only added fertiliser ever needed was a mixture of minerals to substitute for those taken up by plants. According to Liebig, the proper mix for each plant type could be found by ashing the plants and analysing the ash. Liebig patented an artificial manure of plant ash, which Lawes and Gilbert took pains to show was inadequate.[57] At first the work on the response to fertilisers was paid for by Lawes himself from the profits of his fertiliser factory. He was later to set up a trust fund, the Lawes Agricultural Trust, through which the money was funnelled. Lawes died in 1900, and Gilbert in 1901. They were succeeded by Sir Daniel Hall, who added new departments of botany, bacteriology and soil science, and a connection with the University of London,

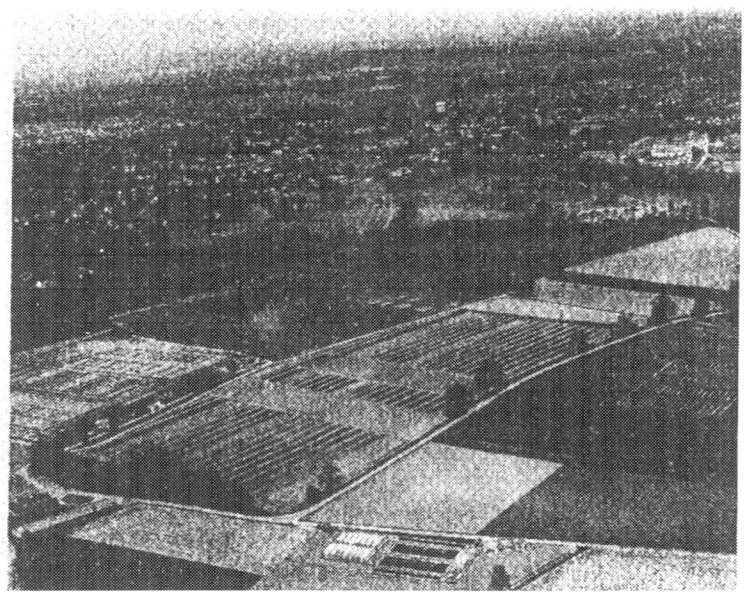

Plate I Rothamsted Experimental Station, showing the large systematically arranged strips of Broadbalk field in the centre, flanked by modern randomised experiments. Some of the simplicity of the old Broadbalk has now been lost visually since each plot was divided into ten sections
Source: Letter to the author from J. McEwen, Head of the Field Experiments Section, Rothamsted. Photograph, 22 August 1986

modernising an institution whose nineteenth-century project was essentially completed. Hall was succeeded in 1912 by Sir John Russell, who was director until 1943, covering the period when R.A. Fisher was associated with Rothamsted.

Lawes's classical experiments on the effects of artificial fertilisers on the yield of wheat were carried out on the field named Broadbalk. From 1852 on, it had been divided into long strips 17 feet wide, of half an acre each. The same wheat variety was sown all over the field, but each strip was dressed differently so as to show the effects on yield of treatments with plant ash or the minerals contained in it, and with nitrogenous fertilisers (Plate I). Two controls were used, a negative strip left unfertilised, from 1839 onwards, and a positive, dressed with farmyard manure, representing a very early use of this technique in any science.

112

Table 3.1   The Broadbalk wheat experiment, 1852–1920: soil dressings and resulting wheat yields – the material analysed by R.A. Fisher at Rothamsted Agricultural Research Station

Lots and treatments	Yields in bushels/acre	
Controls:		
No. 2 Farmyard manure	1852–1920	35
No. 3 Nil since 1839	1844–52	16
No. 4 " "	1853–1903	
	falling to	
	1904	4
Test of Liebig's theory:		
No. 5 Plant ash (minerals) alone		14
No. 6 Plant ash + 100 lb ammonium		23
No. 7 Plant ash + 200 lb sulphate		31
No. 8 Plant ash + 300 lb per strip		36
		(lodges)
Effect of different dressings:		
No. 10 Ammonium sulphate only		20
No. 11 " " + superphosphate		22
No. 12 " " + sodium		28
No. 13 " " + potassium		30
No. 14 " " + magnesium		28
Effect of times of application:		
No. 15 Ammonium sulphate		
applied in autumn only		20
autumn 100 lb + spring 300 lb		23
Residuals:		
No. 18 Ammonium sulphate alternating with minerals:		
mineral years:		14
ammonium sulphate years:		29
(i.e., mineral persists, ammonium sulphate does not)		

Source: From R.A. Fisher, 'Studies in crop variation, I' (1921), n. 65; Rothamsted, *Experimental Farms* (1962), n. 56

The yields from the unfertilised strips had remained at about 16 bushels per acre for the first thirteen years, but then over the next seventy years fell steadily to 4 bushels by 1904. In contrast, the strips given farmyard manure kept up an average yield of 35 bushels between 1852 and 1920. These yields were used as base lines to assess the effects of the new chemical fertilisers alone and combined, given at different times of year, and in alternate years (see Table 3.1, Figure 3.1 and Plate II).

The programme at Rothamsted was concentrated on the soil, and the influence of soil chemistry on plant growth. Hall had

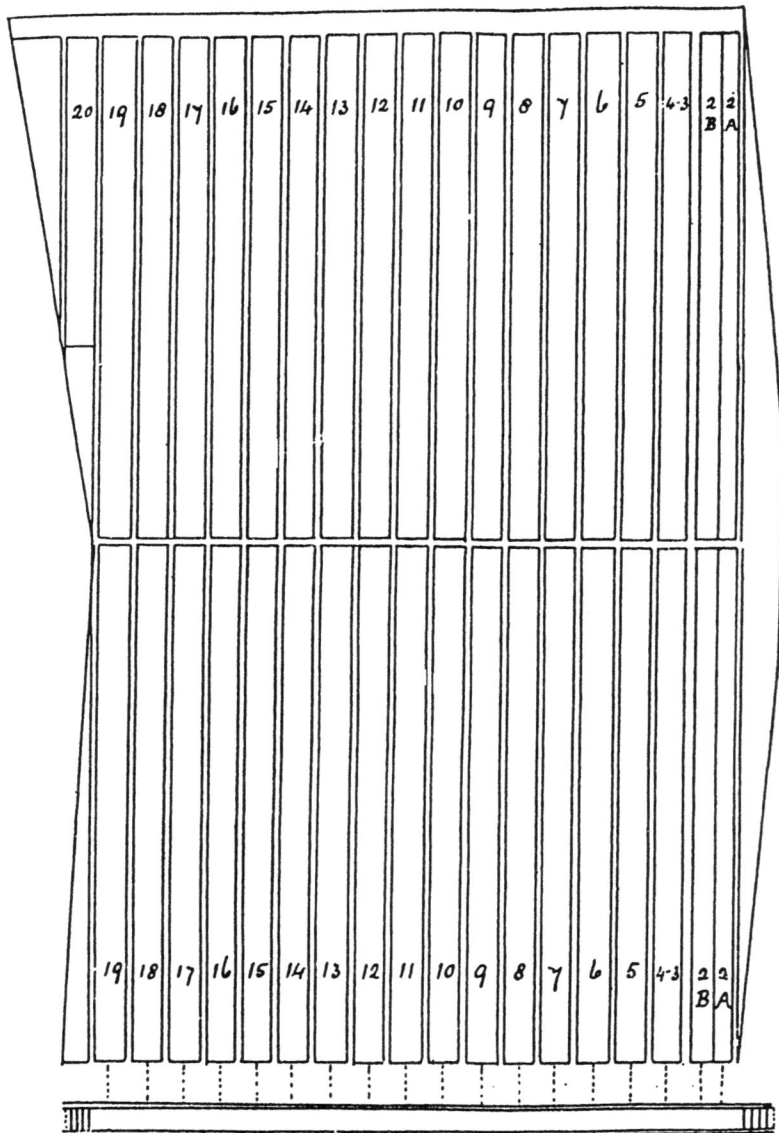

Brick Trench for collecting the Pipe Drainage from each Plot.

Figure 3.1 The Broadbalk experiment: a plan of plots in 1905
Source: Lawes Agricultural Trust, *Rothamsted Experiments* (1905), xii

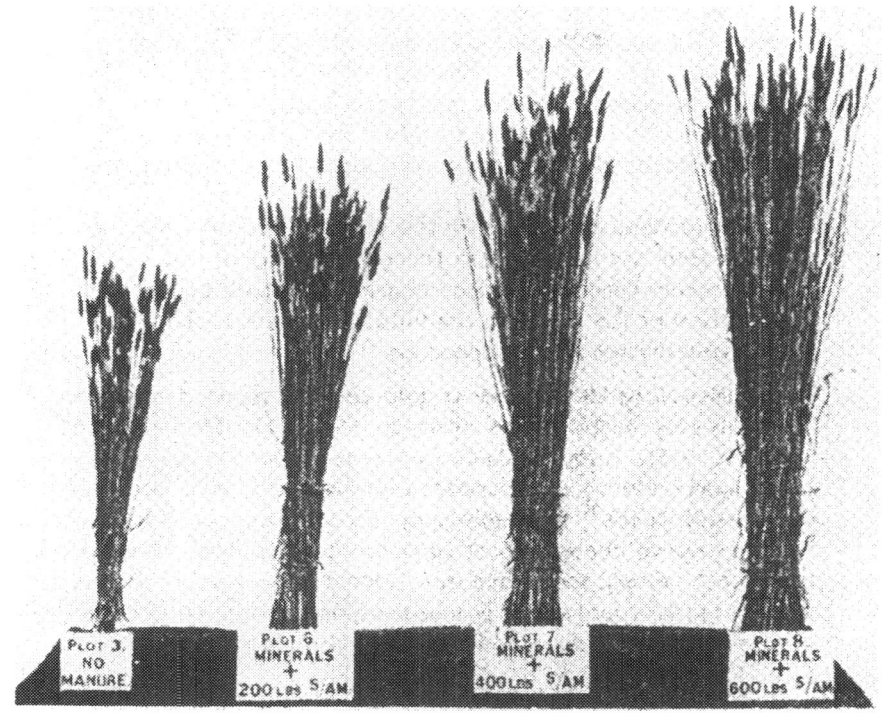

Plate II The Broadbalk experiment: Lawes and Gilbert's demonstration of the effects of a nitrogenous dressing on plant growth. The photograph shows sheaves of wheat from plots 3, 6, 7 and 8 (see Table 3.1). Plot 3 has had no manure of any kind since 1839; plots 6, 7 and 8 have had increasing quantities of ammonium sulphate. The harvest was that of 1920

Source: E.J. Russell, *Plant Nutrition and Crop Production* (1926), Berkeley: University of California Press

followed Lawes and Gilbert's direction in working on the soil and its fertility.[58] Sir John Russell after him had taken the same line. With Russell, work on the soil had come to assume an elevated romantic patriotism. In his autobiography, *The Land Called Me*, he expresses his feeling for and understanding of the local landscapes of the English home counties of Kent, Surrey and Sussex that he had worked on during his thirty years as Director at Rothamsted.[59] In his *Soil Conditions and Plant Growth* of 1921 Russell defines the work at Rothamsted:

115

1. Observations are made in natural conditions as accurately as feasible and repeated sufficiently frequently to allow of treatment by modern statistical methods. These enable the investigator to study the variations, and hence to make deductions as to the numbers and properties of the factors involved. The factors can then be studied in the laboratory. ...

2. Experiments are made on the soil and from the results, deductions are drawn as to the probable nature of some new factor. Direct experiments are then made to test the operation of the factor in the field, and precise laboratory experiments are also undertaken.[60]

When Russell invited Fisher to join the Rothamsted group in 1919, his responsibility was to be the use of 'modern statistical methods' on the huge mass of nineteenth-century material from Lawes and Gilbert's experiments on what the station now calls the classical fields.[61] The experimental problem was obviously the question of the effects of environment on yield. However, the wheat variety sown had not been kept constant; a great number of different varieties had been used, some for relatively long periods at a time, some for only a year or two (see Table 3.2).

Table 3.2 Wheat varieties planted in Broadbalk, 1852–1921

Date	Variety	Period
1852	Old Red Cluster	1 yr.
1853–81	Red Rostock	29 yrs.
1882–99	Red Club	18 yrs.
1900–04	Squareheads Master	5 yrs.
1910	Browick Red	1 yr.
1911–12	Little Joe	2 yrs.
1913–16	Squareheads Master	3 yrs.
1917–21	Red Standard	Future

Source: R.A. Fisher, 'Studies in crop variation, I' (1921), n. 63, 53

Fisher, in spite of his current hard-line position on human nature, did not try to emphasise the nature of the wheat as opposed to its nurture.[62] He dismissed this as a red herring in a few lines of his report:

When the varieties are changed infrequently, any effect due to genetic difference of constitution would be included in the slow changes. During the latter period it would appear partly as annual variation. That these genetic differences are not at any rate a principle cause of the slow changes observed, may be seen from the great changes in mean yields which occurred during the use of Red Rostock.[63]

Fisher distinguished three types of variation in the wheat yield: annual variation, steady deterioration in the soil, and a third group of 'slow changes other than deterioration'. Curves of the yields all showed two peaks, one about 1860 and one in the late 1890s, with a trough of minimum yield following each

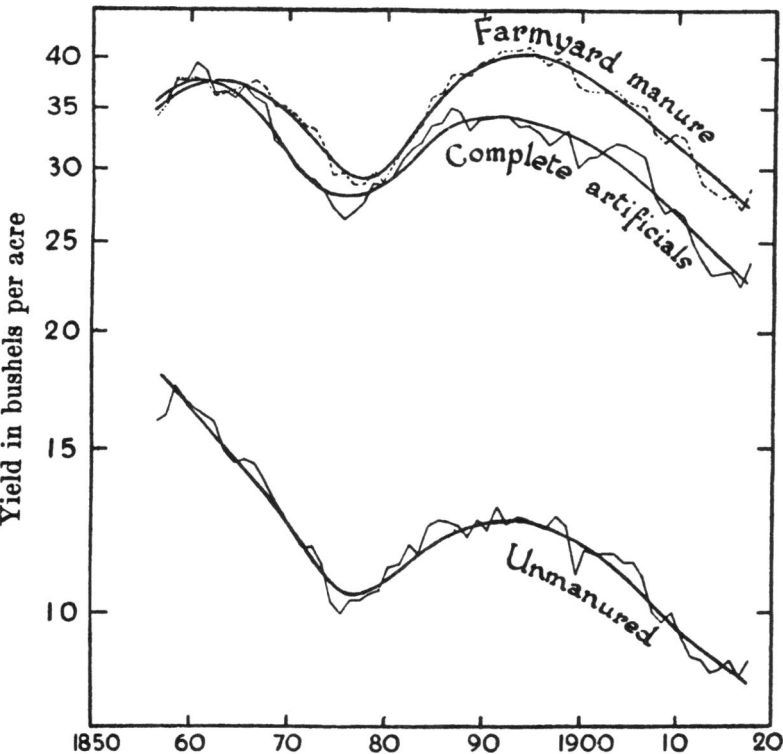

Figure 3.2 Yields of wheat from Broadbalk Field, Rothamsted, ten-year means, 1852–1922
Source: E.J. Russell, *Plant Nutrition and Crop Production* (1926), Berkeley: University of California

one (Figure 3.2). The period 1853–81 when the variety Red Rostock was being used, covered the rise of the first peak of 1860 and the trough of the mid-seventies, as well as the beginning of the recovery taking place through the eighties. There was no discontinuity in Fisher's curves. When the variety was changed in 1882, there was only a slow rise in yield, which had already peaked and begun to fall off before the variety was changed again.

The cause that Fisher proposed for the slow changes was the competition of weeds with the wheat. The records showed that weeds had been a continuous problem. The field was particularly vulnerable to them because it had been sown year after year with wheat, with no rotation, and with only two months for cleaning between harvest and re-sowing in autumn. The wheat was already known to be very sensitive to competition from weeds. At the harvest of 1882 a strip had not been cut, but fenced off and the corn left to face the weeds on its own. Within four years, only a few stunted wheat plants could be found amid a rich ground cover. They were hardly recognisable as cultivated wheat.[64] Ironically, some of the successful competitors were wild oats, *Avena fatua* and *A. ludoviciana*. Fisher correlated the falling yield of the seventies with the loss of boy weeders following the 1870 Education Act, and the fall after 1900 with the relaxation of effort following Sir John Lawes's death.

An agricultural scientist who had had experience of the new rice and wheat varieties beginning to be developed at experimental stations in Japan from 1900 onwards, varieties that were bred for fertiliser response, might have been paid more attention to variety and the varietal sensitivity to fertilisers.[65] It was this line of research that was to lead to the production of high-yielding modern varieties, the so-called MVs of the post-war Green Revolution in cereal growing.[66] But Fisher, in spite of his continued preference for nature rather than nurture in human genetics, did not try to sail against the prevailing wind at Rothamsted. It was the soil that counted there, not the seed.

Fisher's explanation of the slow changes was the occasion for the first appearance of a new statistical technique, the analysis of variance. The new procedure was a variation on the correlation method that the biometricians had used for many years in situations ranging from pauperism to the correlation between the heights of relatives, adapted to a situation in which the variation of the quantity (yield) was produced by the simultaneous action of several different causes, rather than a single pair as in the earlier methods. The variance produced by all the causal factors acting together was the sum of the individual variances resulting from each separately.[67]

The so-called factorial analysis of variance quickly became an important tool in agricultural experimentation, particularly where several factors which might interact with one another were tested. The type specimen of such experiments is one where the effects of added nitrogen, phosphate and potash, separately and together, are to be tested on a field given a basal treatment with farmyard manure. There are eight combinations, each representing a single treatment. They can be broken down into three main effects, those of nitrogen (N), phosphate (P) and potash (K), and the four possible interactions:

Effects of:
$$4 \text{ N} = (n-1)+(nk-k)+(np-p)+(npk-pk)$$
$$4 \text{ P} = (p-1)+(np-n)+(pk-k)+(npk-nk)$$
$$4 \text{ K} = (k-1)+(nk-n)+(pk-p)+(npk-np)$$

Interactions:
$$4 \text{ NP} = (np+npk)-(p+pk)-(n+nk)+(k+1)$$
$$4 \text{ NK} = (nk+npk)-(k+kp)-(n+np)+(p+1)$$
$$4 \text{ PK} = (pk+npk)-(p+np)-(k+nk)+(n+1)$$
$$4 \text{ NPK} = (npk+n+p+k)-(1+pk+nk+np).\text{[68]}$$

Joan Fisher Box has pointed out that Fisher himself said that he did not derive the idea from the problem of the yields of Broadbalk field, but from Mendelian genetics. She quotes him in 1951 as writing that:

> The 'factorial method of experimentation now of lively concern so far afield as the psychologists or the industrial chemists, derives its structure and its name from the simultaneous inheritance of Mendelian factors'.[69]

This suggestion lets us trace Fisher's conception of the idea of summing the variance produced by independent but interacting causes back to his paper on the correlation between relatives of 1918. There, Fisher had written that

> The contributions of imperfectly additive genetic factors divide themselves for statistical purposes into two parts: an additive part which reflects the genetic nature without

119

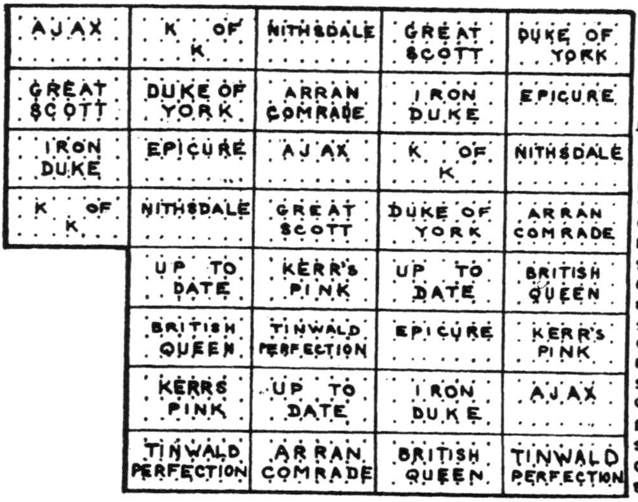

AJAX	K. OF K.	NITHSDALE	GREAT SCOTT	DUKE OF YORK	S C B
GREAT SCOTT	DUKE OF YORK	ARRAN COMRADE	IRON DUKE	EPICURE	S C B
IRON DUKE	EPICURE	AJAX	K. OF K.	NITHSDALE	S C B
K. OF K.	NITHSDALE	GREAT SCOTT	DUKE OF YORK	ARRAN COMRADE	S C B
	UP TO DATE	KERR'S PINK	UP TO DATE	BRITISH QUEEN	S C B
	BRITISH QUEEN	TINWALD PERFECTION	EPICURE	KERR'S PINK	S C B
	KERR'S PINK	UP TO DATE	IRON DUKE	AJAX	S C B
	TINWALD PERFECTION	ARRAN COMRADE	BRITISH QUEEN	TINWALD PERFECTION	S C B

Diagram 1   Plan of experiment. Farmyard manure series

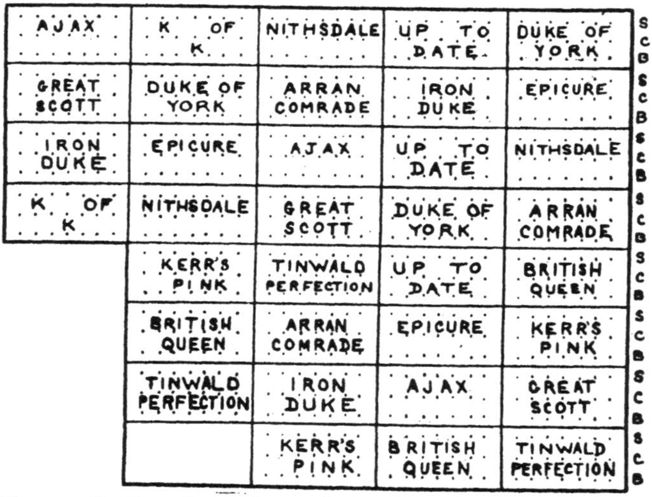

AJAX	K. OF K.	NITHSDALE	UP TO DATE	DUKE OF YORK	S C B
GREAT SCOTT	DUKE OF YORK	ARRAN COMRADE	IRON DUKE	EPICURE	S C B
IRON DUKE	EPICURE	AJAX	UP TO DATE	NITHSDALE	S C B
K. OF K.	NITHSDALE	GREAT SCOTT	DUKE OF YORK	ARRAN COMRADE	S C B
	KERR'S PINK	TINWALD PERFECTION	UP TO DATE	BRITISH QUEEN	S C B
	BRITISH QUEEN	ARRAN COMRADE	EPICURE	KERR'S PINK	S C B
	TINWALD PERFECTION	IRON DUKE	AJAX	GREAT SCOTT	S C B
		KERR'S PINK	BRITISH QUEEN	TINWALD PERFECTION	S C B

Diagram 2   Plan of experiment. Series without farmyard manure

Figure 3.3 Fisher's experiment on the response of potato varieties to different fertilisers. S = sulphate row. C = chloride row. B = basal row. The layout shows a preliminary attempt to allow for non-uniformity of the field by replicating the plots in triplicate and distributing them over the field in a roughly random manner

Source: Fisher and Mackenzie, 'Studies in crop variation, II' (1923)

120

distortion, and gives rise to the correlations which one obtains; and a residue which acts in much the same way as an arbitrary error introduced into the measurements.[70]

It was this arbitrary error that represented random disturbances due to environment in the Mendelian paper. In the Rothamsted material, the controllable environmental effects were to be the factors. The arbitrary error was introduced by the uncontrollable non-uniformity of the fields. In these experiments, instead of *assuming* that the error was random (and very small) as he had done it in the genetics paper of 1918, Fisher designed an experimental layout that was to make certain that the disturbance really was random.

His next project dealt with the possibility of varietal differences in response to manures, but in the case of the twelve varieties of potato with which he was working, he was able to show that the differences between them were no more than the normal error of field experiments.

The experiment was laid out as in Figure 3.3. The area was divided into two plots, one to be treated with farmyard manure, and one not. Each plot was divided into thirty-six smaller plots, for triplicate study of each of twelve varieties of potato, arranged rather haphazardly over the plot with the intention of minimising the effect of differences in the field conditions. In each of the thirty-six, three rows were set, to be dressed with sulphate chloride, and nothing.[71]

Fisher's analysis separated the variation within triplicates (due to experimental error alone) from the variation between triplicates treated differently. Yield was the product of two factors, the variety and the manure, but though there were substantial differences in yield, due both to variety and to manure, there was no sign of a differential response. The varieties stood in the same order with or without manure. There was none that completely failed to respond to manure, and none that became outstandingly good with manure after being outstandingly bad without it.

The interest of this paper lies in its foreshadowing of a technique, part experimental and part statistical, the method of randomisation by the Latin square. For the experimental comparison of very similar dressings, there was a need for a highly accurate method of estimation. Multiple replication was

1925

M 444	P 422	O 173	S 398
O 279	S 439	M 423	P 409
P 436	M 428	S 445	O 212
S 453	O 237	P 410	M 393

1926

M 584·0	S 557·0	O 461·5	P 498·5
S 519·5	P 485·5	M 477·0	O 389·0
P 474·5	O 378·5	S 467·5	M 491·5
O 464·0	M 511·0	P 507·0	S 492·0

Figure 3.4 The Latin square method of randomising the distribution of fertiliser treatments to correct for heterogeneity in the field environment. Each row and column contains each treatment once. S = sulphate. P = phosphate. M = farmyard manure. O = no treatment. The figures represent yields

Source: Eden and Fisher, 'Studies in crop variation, IV' (1929): 201

no use, since enlarging the experimental plot simply made it more difficult to ensure uniformity of the field.

Fisher's method was effectively to randomise the distribution of fertiliser treatments over the whole area of the experimental field.[72] Each field contained as many replications as there were treatments; each row and each column contained each treatment once. Applying the analysis of variance, an estimate of the effects due to treatment, to position and to random variation of parallels could be worked out. Position variance due to soil heterogeneity could be eliminated from the calculation, freeing the result from the muddling background noise that would have made comparison of closely related treatments impossible.[73] The analysis of variance used in this way makes possible a comparison between the mean square deviations for treatments and the mean square deviations for error; in other words, it leads to a general test of the statistical significance of experimental differences (Figure 3.4).

These techniques, the analysis of variance due to multiple interacting factors, randomisation as a means of dealing with the background noise of practical experiments, the Latin square method and the test of statistical significance were all new and original ways of dealing statistically with experimental design problems.[74] At their original appearance, all these new techniques were developed by Fisher to disentangle in the most delicate way possible the effects of experimental environmental changes from the raw results of experiments involving real plants in real, irregular fields, fields with wet patches and dry, shaded areas and exposed, pests and scattered clumps of weeds. He had taken up where Lawes's strip system with its negative and positive controls had left off.

His work was appreciated at Rothamsted, and his results led to changes in the field experiments. Between 1925 and 1929, the weeds in Broadbalk were brought under control by fallowing. The long strips were divided into five sections, and a four-year fallowing cycle, three years on and one off, with one plot left unfallowed, was started. The yields of a plot in the year after fallowing were 44 per cent up on the year before. The numbers of weed seeds in the ground fell: the poppy seed to half, and black bent to almost nothing. The wild oats still had to be pulled by hand, as they had been in Lawes and Gilbert's time. Fisher's randomised Latin squares formed the basis for the modern field experiments that began in the twenties, many of them using his factorial designs.[75]

The force of this is that Fisher at least from 1921 onwards was clearly aware of the importance of environment on plant growth. In 1918, he had been prepared to assume – and in 1924 to repeat – that it was a random variable with a negligible effect on human growth, which could all be put down to genetic factors. His 1918 paper kept within the Eugenic Society's traditional guidelines. But his work at Rothamsted now took him out of the human field, away from the area where his assumptions were guided by the loving pressure of the eugenists. With this experience, and perhaps because of it, his conventionality within the human field was loosened; he began to question the eugenists' assumptions on environment, and to find that their methods could not deal with the questions that he wanted to raise. As the questions changed, assumptions previously unquestioned began to seem arbitrary; methods began to give inadequate answers. Ideology and method, previously so well-matched, began to move apart.

The problem that demonstrated the inadequacy of the Eugenics Society's old methods was one taken up by the Society's own Research Committee, re-constituted in 1923 after a gap of ten years to continue and complete the pauper pedigree study, which had been begun in 1910 and interrupted at the outbreak of war in 1914. In those days it had perfectly embodied the eugenists' class-centred ideology, with its assumption that a class was a breeding isolate whose characters, being genetically determined, bred true. If the class did have a characteristic environment, that too was a product of its genetically determined character. The pauper pedigree study embodied the classical eugenist's methodology, the collection of pedigrees, independent as it had always been, of both biometry and Mendelism, and of the problem of nature versus nurture.

The new Research Committee consisted of R.A. Fisher, statistician for Rothamsted Agricultural Station; Ruth Darwin for the Board of Control;[76] C.M. Lloyd for the London School of Economics; Alexander Carr-Saunders, just appointed Professor at the School of Social Studies at Liverpool University; Dr F.C. Shrubsall, a member of the Royal Anthropological Institute, as well as of the Society's Council; Dr Douglas White, who also belonged to the National Committee for the Control of Venereal

Disease; Professor H.J. Fleure of the Biographical Association, also on the Society's Council; and H.N. Fallaize. It was a committee of experts, but the project itself was essentially E.J. Lidbetter's, as it had been before the war. He appears on the printed protocols only as Secretary of the Committee, but in fact the field research continued to be his. The object of the study was still to show that paupers were not simply people who happened to need economic assistance at some time or another, but a network of interrelated families within which pauperism was passed on, along with other heritable moral and physical failings. The eugenists were convinced that most pauperism could be abolished by cutting down the breeding of this group, as we saw in Chapter 2.

Lidbetter restarted his old study on 3 March 1923 by taking a new census of the paupers of his old East End parish of Bethnal Green. The paupers that day on relief in workhouse, infirmary and special schools numbered 1,174.

A new element however, had entered into the project. The Council of the Eugenics Society now felt that for any conclusion to be drawn from Lidbetter's survey, there must be a control group. Cora Hodson, the Society's General Secretary, wrote to Cyril Burt, then psychologist to the London County Council's Education Department:

> With the meagre help of one volunteer he [Lidbetter] has taken a fresh census of the chargeable population. ... The scope of what we desire covers a very wide field; namely, we should like ... to carry on a 'Control' enquiry on a less specialized part of the population. ... It is proposed that a Committee of at least four competent workers or competent supervisors should be authorized to undertake this work with Mr Lidbetter.[77]

A sketch of the proposed study shows the uncertainties surrounding the control group problem.[78] It was difficult to decide how to choose controls, whether by taking a census of a whole street, of certain house numbers in a number of different streets, by working from a single school, or from given classes of specific schools. According to Cora Hodson's letter to Burt, the questions to the two groups, paupers and controls, were not to be identical. Besides the negative qualities sought in the pauper group, some positive ones should be enquired after; such as income tax payment, support of dependents, scholarships, prizes and degrees, or attendance at evening classes.[79] Naturally, in view of the original purpose of the the study, these questions had not been asked of the pauper group. The uncertainty over the proper choice and handling of the control group was a product of the uncertainty over its function in the new experimental design.

Cyril Burt wrote back with great enthusiasm, promising to interest influential members of the London County Council in the project. He suggested that the features discovered in the paupers – chargeability, mental defect, epilepsy, lunacy, tuberculosis, criminality and infant mortality – should not be treated as forming simple heritable units in themselves, but that 'one might find what I would call temperamental deficiency running through a whole stock, and appearing variously as so-called mental deficiency (moral imbecility, nervousness (hysteria), criminality) and so forth'.[80] Burt's views coincided nicely with those of the Society. By the time of the first meeting of the Research Committee set up by the Society's Council to direct the project, Burt had been asked to serve as Chairman.[81] He was also to represent the British Psychological Society's Committee for Research in Education.[82]

The Committee's most difficult problem was the control group. They had very little funding available to them, and the collection of survey material was expensive. A donation of £20 allowed them to engage a young woman graduate, Mrs Cartwright, to start work that summer in the Bethnal Green schools.[83] Sir Frederick Mott was co-opted after being heard to speak favourably of the old study at a meeting of the British Medical Association.[84] He in turn suggested that he might organise a parallel study in Birmingham.[85] Professor Carr-Saunders thought his new department might have funds as yet unspoken for. A further co-opted member of the committee, Harold Peake, Vice-President of the Royal Anthropological Institute, opened up another source of control material. Early in 1925, he and Cora Hodson travelled to Oxford, where a meeting was held at the Anthropological Laboratory. Several members were enthusiastic and suggested using the laboratory as a clearing house for a number of sociological surveys, this one among them, which could then share one another's data.[86] Cora Hodson next made a trip to Scotland, to try to win support from the Scottish universities, and from funding sources there, the Child Life Investigation Committee and the United Kingdom Trust.[87] But the financial problems were not solved by all this hard work and effort on Cora Hodson's part. Mrs Cartwright was to have £225 per year, which was reduced when she became pregnant and worked shorter hours. Miss Greenhalgh, helping Lidbetter, required £150 per year. In addition, Mabel L. Clark was to collect data in Edinburgh. Money contributions were meagre. In 1925, the Royal Society, the Medical Research Council and Henderson Trust gave £100 each.

The Society's Council tried harder still to raise funding. Cora Hodson wrote to the well-known social activist Eleanor Rathbone in Liverpool, telling her that the need was for only £300 a year, and that it might be possible to raise the amount in 'lumps of £10 or £20'.[88] Eleanor Rathbone, an experienced fund-raiser for her own Family Endowment scheme, sent a list of local notables who might perhaps help: judges, justices of the peace, aldermen and military men.[89] In a letter to one of them, Cora Hodson tries to make the thin funding sound as respectable and promising as possible:

> We want naturally to compare two industrial areas, and the social study carried on in Liverpool makes it in my Committee's opinion an especially suitable place. ... I have spoken to a number of those concerned at the settlements and in the various social organizations and find them much interested. ... We have been supported financially by the Medical Research Council (for the Board of Control) and the London School of Economics, and this year the Royal Society is making a grant of £100 ... while the Anthropological Department of Oxford University is making itself headquarters for the rural samples in Oxfordshire. Further, the Committee of the Child Life Investigation is prepared to cooperate by allowing us to use their material collected largely under the Carnegie Trustees over the past five years for a sample from one of the Scotch industrial towns. Funds for this are being asked from the Scottish Trustees.[90]

As she wrote to Professor Elton Mayo in the Department of Psychology at Harvard 'Since the coal strike [1926] English finances are indescribable, and we greatly fear our work will be brought to a standstill for want of the small sum needed, namely £300–£500 a year.'[91]

The final effort made by the Society was an appeal to City firms. In an attempt to draw on a network of like-minded men, the members of the Society were asked to tell the Secretary if they knew anyone in the City who might have influence, and circulars were sent off to these selected people:

> At this moment when one of our most important social institutions, namely the Poor Law, is due for drastic revision, this work is becoming, we feel, of national importance as it reveals some aspects of pauperism and public health never hitherto adequately recognized. It has been generally assumed that destitution was in the main due to exceptional circumstances or to accumulation of misfortune and it is only by this careful and intimate study that we are able to show conclusively that heredity is a prime factor. It appears that a considerable proportion of the destitute represent a fraction of the community who are lacking in innate powers, mental and physical, to the extent of being incapable of self-support, and this maintenance secures similar recurrent misery in the next generation.[92]

Funding the collection of the control group, however, was not the only problem. The design of the 'experiment' itself was a problem. A few months after the Committee began meeting, in the autumn of 1923, R.A. Fisher asked some hard new questions of the old study. The minutes of this meeting say: 'Mr Fisher gave some carefully thought-out questions on the aim and scope of this research for the consideration of the Committee.'[93] At the end of the minute book a typewritten sheet headed 'Note from Mr Fisher' is stuck in. It asks,

> A. What questions is the research scheme to be designed to answer? e.g., to what extent is the causation of pauperism to be ascribed to a) heredity b) environment?
> B. What classes of facts can supply the answer to our question? E.g. what facts can give us a) a measure of the extent of pauperism in the individual? b) a measure of the extent of pauperism among relations? c) a measure of the association of pauperism with environmental factors? – *what factors?* [Fisher's emphasis]

Is it possible to discover environmental factors which shall eliminate the effects of i) example, ii) traditional moral outlook, as possible causes of the association of pauperism among relations?[94]

These questions show Fisher knocking against the barriers of both the ideological commitment to a straightforward genetical cause of pauperism and of the eugenist's simple pedigree methodology. By 1923, the date of these meetings, Fisher's experience had grown enormously; his thinking was now focused on the effects of environment in determining agricultural yields, and upon the use of factorial analysis in analysing this type of data. It was from this new experience that he drew his criticisms of the design of the experiment. In his insistence on factors we can see that he thought that at least one aspect of the problem might be quantified: the yield, as it were, of pauperism. The environmental factors might then be dealt with on the presence-and-absence system. It was as if they and not the inherited pauperism corresponded to Mendelian factors, like the presence-and-absence of nitrogen, phosphate and potash in the field experiments.

To see a social class in purely biological terms, as a closed mating group, was not, in itself, at all rebarbative for Fisher. He had done it in a short article which was published in the *Eugenics Review* of 1924 and later reprinted as a pamphlet by the Society's Committee for Legalising Eugenic Sterilisation.[95] R.C. Punnett in 1917 had published some calculations which suggested that it would be impossible to eliminate feeble-mindedness by either segregation or sterilisation. To reduce its incidence from 1:100 to 1:1,000 would take twenty-two generations, and to achieve a ratio of 1:1,000,000 would take 994 generations.[96] Fisher's argument was that this assumed that feeble-mindedness was a single Mendelian recessive, which was *probably* wrong, and also that the population mated at random, which was *certainly* wrong:

Mating is very largely controlled by social class, and the feeble-minded undoubtedly gravitate to the lowest social stratum. Further, within each class, there is a decided tendency for like to mate with like. If instead of regarding the feeble-minded as 1 in 320 taken at random in the general population, we were to regard them as constituting one-sixteenth of an intermating group constituting 5 per cent of the general population, then the effect of segregation would be to reduce the incidence by 36 per cent in one generation. This is what might be expected from an effective policy of segregation, and it is of a magnitude which no one with a care for his country's future can afford to ignore.[97]

Seeing the pauper class as a variety however, did not mean that environment would have no effect on it. The effect of soil treatments upon plant growth was profound, and Fisher was just then engaged in developing the statistical methods for measuring it.

Lidbetter, on the other hand, had no experience outside the Society's training and the Society's thinkirfg, the thinking of pre-war days when he had gone to the course at Imperial College. His response to Fisher's 'carefully thought-out questions' was both indignant and defensive. It is headed:

Memorandum on scope to research:

The syllabus drawn up by the Research Committee does not specifically state as an object the disintegration of heredity from environmental factors in the population to be studied, not out of oversight but designedly.[98]

The pauper records do not contain material for an assessment of the effects of environment, he says; their value lies in their extending over three or four generations, for which there is obviously no information on the details of environment.

It is suggested that to make a statistical statement of certain advantageous and disadvantageous qualities, as between paupers, would in itself make clear the extent to which paupers may be an isolated group, and pauperism not a sporadic characteristic of the population as a whole but a differentiating character of a small but clearly defined group.

And he repeats in a second, longer document: 'It was never contemplated that this research would make any precise contribution to the subject of heredity vs. environment.'[99]

He then quotes a talk given on the wireless by Professor MacBride, who had been one of his earlier teachers, in which

MacBride said that this question was not one that could be settled by observations on men and women.[100] In Lidbetter's opinion – and it was his project – the purpose was not to find out the cause of pauperism, but its incidence: and whether there was a real degeneracy of the race, or instead, whether 'this undesirable group is a kind of pocket in the community propagated from within and not recruited from the normal population'.

It is the same proposition that Fisher himself put forward in his paper on the segregation of the feeble-minded; indeed, since Fisher's paper came out the year after this committee started to meet, it is quite likely that Lidbetter's study was the source of Fisher's idea. A population, says Fisher, does not mate randomly: the feeble-minded may constitute one-sixteenth of an intermating group which in turn may constitute 5 per cent of the population.[101] But where Fisher speaks in terms of percentages of population, Lidbetter continues to rely on pedigrees showing the family connections of individual paupers, a technique which makes the use of statistics difficult. He admits rather unwillingly that the 'chargeability in days' for the pauper families *could* be compared to that of normal controls, but he is so sure of the result that it is not really worth doing. The problem of environment is not excluded by the pedigree method but for Lidbetter it does not really exist.

But the collection of pedigrees alone no longer seemed to the scientific world to be an adequate analysis. Early in the project's new life, Sir Frederick Mott had suggested applying to the Medical Research Council for a grant.[102] The MRC's response was to ask for an outline of the statistical treatment proposed.[103] Their request was answered by Lidbetter, who wrote:

While contemplating the use of normal statistical methods, they feel that some of the material which is being collected will be so different in its features from any other with which they have previously dealt that they expect to bring together a small group of statisticians to advise as to the best treatment. ... The committee particularly desires to draw attention to the fact that the new feature in this enquiry into [*sic*] pedigree treatment which makes it possible to compare the individuals alive today in groups whose progenitors for 3–4 generations back are ascertained. This should give the following facts: 1. For the characteristics investigated – incidence in the population as a whole compared with the incidence in different social groups. 2. The scatter of these characters: whether it can be shown to be completely random or whether in some instances it appears to be correlated with other characters or other social factors, or further whether there is any biological feature influencing the scatter.[104]

The normal statistical method that Lidbetter thought might do was Udny Yule's coefficient of colligation, a variant of the coefficient of association.[105] Yule, like MacBride, had been Lidbetter's teacher at the Eugenics Society's course before the war.[106] Karl Pearson, when his opinion was asked, suggested his coefficient of contingency could be used to correlate measured characters and environment.[107]

The original technique of correlation had been designed to relate to quantities that could be measured on a continuous scale, like heights. Coefficients of association or contingency on the other hand could be used for nominal variables – those that could not be measured but only categorised, or were either present or absent. Association and contingency are closely related. The starting point for association is the proposition that there is *no* association between two attributes A and B. There will be the same proportion of As among the Bs as among the non-Bs. Yule's examples include one on the association in schoolchildren, of dullness of mind and visible developmental defects. Contingency expands the system to include more than two attributes, arranged in a series of rows [A1, A2, A3 ... An] and columns [B1, B2, B3 ... Bn] called by Pearson contingency tables.[108] Pearson and Yule argued, with a good deal of irritation, over the use of the two coefficients.[109] Pearson saw association as being based on the correlation of two hypothetical continuous bivariate normal distributions, that underlay the seeming discontinuity. Yule felt that in many cases, the discontinuities had to be regarded as real; for example, the categories, vaccinated and non-vaccinated versus survived an epidemic and died in it.[110]

Either of these methods might have been appropriate if the data had been organised with a view to using them. Yule, for example, had once collected data to show the association of pauperism with environmental factors such as crowding. But

Lidbetter wanted nothing more than to show the network of family relationships within the pauper family pedigrees.

It was clearly not easy for Lidbetter and the Committee to work together. He felt deeply possessive of the project.

Mrs Cartwright, his assistant, resigned in May 1925, and was replaced by a another young woman, Miss Martin.[111] A tactful letter of October 1925 from Cora Hodson tells her:

> Mr Lidbetter feels that he has a great deal, I think, which he will entrust to you tho' not to anyone else if you could get it from him from time to time.
>
> I am trying to persuade Mr Lidbetter to let us duplicate his index and each new bit of pedigree, keeping cards here so you can all refer to those indices and hand on to him any links that appear. I may not succeed, but if you see him and suggest it, I know it will save him much time and you all equally I fancy.[112]

Fisher's name does not appear in the minutes from the time of his criticisms of the work of October 1923 until November 1925, when a curious meeting took place with none of the usual Committee present. The Secretary, Cora Hodson, records that those present were Fisher, Julian Huxley and Ward Cutler, who was the chief protozoologist at Rothamsted Experimental Station and a colleague of Fisher's.[113] Cora Hodson wrote, and then crossed out, that no quorum was formed. Her rough pencil notes of the meeting say, 'Mr Fisher thinks our samples are not truly random. Cooptation of Prof. Huxley and Dr Cutler.'[114] An official resolution was then passed that Mr Lidbetter be asked to convene a subcommittee to consider the normal sample.

It is the first shot in Fisher's attack on Lidbetter and his research. The coopted members, Julian Huxley and Ward Cutler, were supposed to take over the Committee. But the attack failed; the minutes of the next meeting are crossed out and rewritten in several places and a note added in Lidbetter's hand:

> It was resolved that it be an instruction to the secretary not to take action except upon a resolution of the committee.

(Signed) E.J. Lidbetter, 16th December, 1925[115]

The account of this struggle for control that can be gathered from Cora Hodson's letters to Cyril Burt points to a contributing source of the Committee's difficulties. Burt was Chairman of the Research Committee, but he was frequently absent from its meetings, apologising for not answering Cora Hodson's letters, and explaining to her that he had not had time in Edinburgh to make use of the letters of introduction she had given him.[116] Although he was Chairman, he was not in control of either the Committee or the project. He had not been present at the meeting of 25 November; a note in the file tells Mrs Hodson that he will be late for that on 8 December, and that she really should accept his resignation after all. Cora Hodson's account of the meeting he missed is tactful but transparent:

> As you have seen Major Darwin recently, you will I feel sure understand the position, namely that some of the Officer's Committee desired to get more in touch with the research work, which is obviously much to be wished in view of its rapid growth.
> The last committee naturally somewhat resembled an 'overhauling' which is disturbing however much it may be useful. And I regret that Mr Lidbetter should have any added anxieties when his work is always a very difficult and delicate business.
> He wished me to assure you that none of his phrases should be construed as critical of any past work ... but only as stating the need for more careful organizing of the committee itself to cope with increasing business. He knows as well as our President that the progress of the work is due to your unfailing wise direction and ready help.[117]

On the same day, Cora Hodson wrote to Major Darwin that she had talked on the telephone with Burt, and that he suggested that Huxley should be named vice-chairman, standing in for Burt's frequent absences.[118]

But Fisher kept up his attack. Lidbetter's pedigrees were produced for the Committee's inspection and they gave Fisher plenty of ammunition. Pedigree no. 30, he stated, consisted of sixty-two persons, fifty-one of whom are named, with the occupations of four and no other information.[119] 'Mr Fisher criticised the work on the normal sample at some length, and Mr Lidbetter took exception to this', say the minutes; and several other critical and reformist resolutions were proposed by Fisher and seconded by other members of the Committee. The resolutions mainly concerned the importance of the ascertainment of environmental conditions in each case: occupational record and social status, the histories of individuals from school onwards, and that the proband, the original index case, be marked by a symbol in each family.

At the next meeting, according to the minutes,

> Mr Fisher stated that Dr Cutler had kindly offered his services as secretary to the committee, and that he, Mr Fisher, had arranged the matter with Major Darwin. ... The subcommittee's attention was drawn to the fact that Mr Lidbetter is secretary to the Research Committee being so appointed at the Committee's formation.[120]

It is the record of an attempted coup which was to have completed Fisher's victory over Lidbetter by the appointment of Fisher's colleague from Rothamsted in his place. But the project was Lidbetter's life's work and heart's blood and he hung on to his position – he is referred to as the Hon. Sec. in the subsequent meeting – and to his technique.

The Committee tried hard to quantify the pedigree technique, and bring it up to contemporary statistical standards. A grant application written probably by Ward Cutler in March 1926 restates the purpose of the project, and the method:

> The ultimate aim of the investigations undertaken by the Eugenics Education Society is the elucidation of the *causes of social failure.* The aspects of this problem which may be attacked by genealogical research, and upon which genealogical research alone appears capable of throwing light, may be listed as temperamental, occupational and racial. ... We believe that the full value of genealogical research can only be attained by overcoming the difficulty of assigning the normal man who is not conspicuously a failure or vicious [*sic*, altered to] either a failure or a success, a distinct status in the work scale, representing the aggregate of his exertions.[121]

Ward Cutler, who submitted this statement to the Committee for their approval, was a committed eugenist, and by no means a believer in the importance of the environment; he had written elsewhere:

the environment undoubtedly plays the main part in determining whether the capabilities of a man or woman are allowed to develop, but the environment alone will never create such capabilities. ... Modern research is doing more and more to show that to be 'well-born' is half the battle of life.[122]

But though he had no fundamental disagreement with the assumptions of the project, he was still not completely satisfied with the pedigree method. Soon after this, the Committee began trying to recast the pedigrees into a new form using a new 'statistical card'. One of these was to be filled up for each individual on the pedigree.[123] But it came too late. The only way to publish the material seemed to be as pedigrees interleaved with descriptive matter. It was not easy to see how it could be analysed further, and it was Lidbetter's suggestion simply to publish the pedigrees as they were.[124] Fisher was present at these discussions too, but he seems to have stopped trying to take over. The control group too was a source of difficulty. The committee had hoped to make it a 'vertical slice through the whole population from the poorest to the most aristocratic stocks'. It was supposed, according to the prospectus that described the project, to broaden and generalise the original investigation so that it would show:

a) the extent to which innate mental ability or outstanding social merit occurs in different strata of the community;
b) how far these qualities may be shown to be hereditary, i.e., whether they occur markedly within a family group taken through three or four generations or show a random scatter;
c) the extent to which certain prevalent disabilities such as feeblemindedness (&c) are distributed in the community as a whole;
d) how far any of these qualities and conditions may be correlated.

It is desired particularly to draw attention to d) as giving a fresh analysis of social data, and one which, without solving the well-worn problem of nature–nurture will at least reveal a few facts which will show whether there is any value in such a problem at all.[125]

With this new control study, the effort was no longer confined to a single, manageable parish, or a single class. It was as if Broadbalk field had been expanded to include the whole of Britain. The project that had been intended as a statistical nicety the better to show up the concentration of defectives in Lidbetter's pauper stocks had now become a 'vertical slice' of the entire British Isles, outgrowing its original purpose and evolving into a clumsily unmanageable project in its own right. But the method was still that of pedigree collection, and the 'fresh analysis' of section d) was never attempted.

The scale of the plan was far too large for the skimpy funding available. By March 1926, Miss Martin had stopped work in Bethnal Green because of lack of money.[126] The Henderson Trust had turned down the Society's request, which was for money for the control group study in Edinburgh using a 'normal working class population'.[127] This part of the study was reported in the Eugenics Review of 1926 in these sad words:

> It is impossible to speak of the 'result' of an investigation such as this after so short a period of work. The sum of money available was enough to provide an investigator for only a few months. ... Much useful work has been recorded and the outline of seven promising pedigrees prepared. In none of these however was it possible in the time available to prepare the work in such detail as to warrant publication.[128]

The Medical Research Council had been approached in 1923, and their response had been to ask for more details of the statistical treatment proposed.[129] Throughout the later twenties, the question of finance was almost all that was discussed. Fisher, Cutler and Lidbetter were constant attenders at these meetings, which went on until 1931, but there is no record of any further disagreement.

Over the decade of the twenties the problem of the environment and its influence was insistently present in the background. The Society's policy statements generally pointed out that theirs was the only society *not* concerned with social and environmental factors among the network of social activists to which they all belonged, but that that should not be taken to mean that they thought it was insignificant. It was just not their business. Leonard Darwin himself was aware of a new popular sensitivity.

Speaking to the Second International Eugenics Congress in 1922, he said,

> The first words I uttered as the president of my society ten years ago were that heredity should be its guiding star and in that opinion I have never faltered. A good deal of progress has been made since that date and now the man who calls himself well educated is as a rule beginning to have some dim idea that all human beings are the product of two factors, heredity and environment, and that consequently to both of them some attention should be paid. ... We personally should give our blessing to many reforms which eugenical societies do not help to promote. ... If eugenical societies confine their attention exclusively to heredity, it is only because so many other societies think only of environment.[130]

Lidbetter, writing in 1912, had made his statement in favour of heredity too: 'The believer in eugenics asserts that of the two factors heredity is the dominant partner.'[131] But the rest of his paper was full of examples of how environmental problems oppressed the poor, and contributed to their dependency. His original project had been, according to himself, to show that a large proportion of a given group of paupers had genealogies which connected them with many other paupers, the argument being that this gave a measure of the proportion of pauperism that was hereditary.[132]

Over the decade of the twenties, the Society's investigators were gradually persuaded that even though they themselves were sure that they knew the answer to the nature–nurture problem, they must appear to be leaving it open. A draft of the research prospectus from the mid-twenties put it like this:

> The well-worn problem of Nature–Nurture appears as insistent as ever for solution, and is a necessary basis to a wise treatment of social troubles. While this research is not primarily instituted for the settlement of this complex problem, the method of ascertaining data will at least give some of the facts which are so obviously necessary for the solution. Correlation of mental and physical imperfection with a bad environment has been abundantly proved; the grouping of definite stocks of disabilities of character of

138

temperament or of physique has not yet been sufficiently worked out, and the main problem is incapable of solution until such data are forthcoming.[133]

As long as the Society was content to lay aside the problem of the environment, and confine the study to a demonstration of pauper genealogies, the pedigree method was perfectly appropriate. But in the project's second period the need to consider the environment became more and more pressing, along with the demand for a quantitative analysis. The 'main problem', the relationship between environment and heredity, was incapable of solution by the genealogical method, the straightforward pedigree study. The relative importance of heredity among the 'causes of social failure' could not be shown by taking pedigrees alone. The study that Lidbetter was so deeply committed to had no relation to these new demands for controls and quantitation, or for the factoring-in, somehow, of the environment.

What means of quantitation could have been used? The now-traditional measurement of 'strength of heredity' was the correlation coefficient. As R.A. Fisher wrote in 1925,

No quantity is more characteristic of modern statistical work than the correlation coefficient. ... One of the earliest and most striking successes of the method of the study of correlation was in the biometrical study of inheritance ... it was possible by this method to measure its intensity.[134]

It had been used by Yule in 1895 to correlate pauperism with out-relief and with crowding, which he used as a measure of poverty; David Heron in 1906 had correlated, inversely, fertility with social class, also measured in terms of crowding. If the data were not in the form of two series of measurements, but were 'nominal variables' or categories rather than quantities, as was the case with Lidbetter's material, it was reasonable to suggest either Yule's coeffficient of association, or Pearson's contingency method. But it was Fisher who pointed out that there were in fact no data at all on environment with which pauperism could be either correlated or associated. His attempt to identify some environmental factors suggests that he had hoped to be able to use his factorial analysis technique just then being developed to deal with environmental factors in the yields of crops: Fisher seems to have been willing to see the residuum as a variety, with pauperism as its yield. But even this exquisitely ingenious transposition was impossible; the data on fertiliser were missing, and there were no comparable data from other parts of the field. But these were not the problems that Lidbetter felt were central to his research. For him, it was a matter of negative eugenics. These pedigrees demonstrated that defective stocks, as he called them, reproduced, and were

> supported as a class at the expense of the self-supporting community. This arises and continues with the passive consent of the average uninstructed citizen, whose social conceptions still derive from the teaching of earlier social economics. Those teachings were neglectful of the problems of original human quality, and in consequence social organization has proceeded upon the assumption that conditions can make any man.[135]

His reference is probably to the Booth studies on the Poor Law, and perhaps also to Udny Yule's calculation that pauperism was correlated with the amount of outdoor relief provided.

As things turned out, the best answer the Committee could find to the environmental problem was a completely non-quantitative one: a pair of contrasting pedigrees, showing two families who lived next door to each other in Bethnal Green. One of them was studded with paupers, the other had not a single one (Figure 3.5). It was the traditional *ad oculos* demonstration of the pedigree study, and the Society used it over and over again throughout the thirties, as part of their sterilisation campaign.

Lidbetter mentions the frequency of intermarriage among families with insanity.[136] He does not wish to say that defectiveness is a Mendelian recessive, yet 'defectiveness in recess' was very high, much higher, he thought, than would be expected. The transmission of defect through a normal member occurs with remarkable frequency. Ante-dating, the appearance of a defect earlier and earlier in each succeeding generation, was also a feature of his pedigrees, as it had been in 1912. Each of these problems had by the late twenties acquired a large body of *Vererbungsmathematik*, the mathematical Mendelism that had grown up mainly in the German literature on genetics and eugenics before and after the First World War.[137] Some of this would have worked on material in the form of pedigrees, but

ENVIRONMENT AND HEREDITY
TWO FAMILIES IN AN EAST LONDON AREA

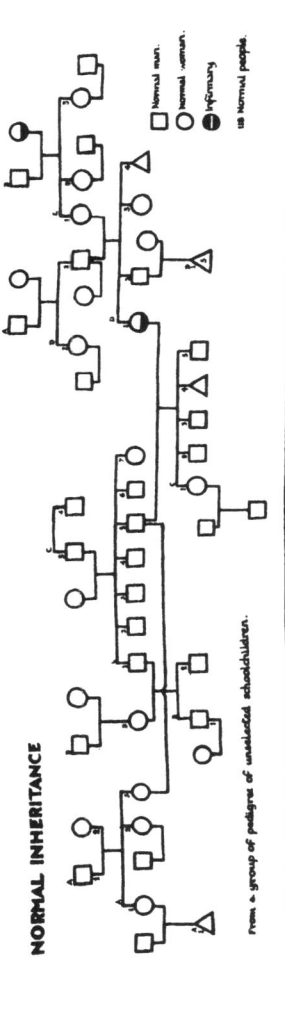

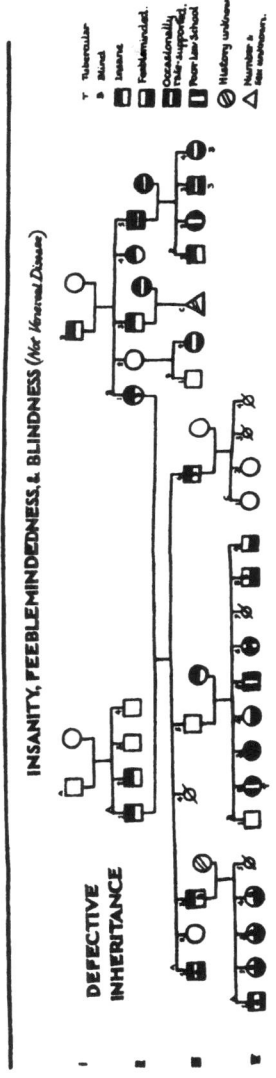

Figure 3.5 A Lidbetter pedigree showing two families living next door to one another, one studded with paupers, one with none. It seemed to be the best possible example of the preponderance of heredity over environment

Source: Poster used by the Society for exhibition purposes, Eugenics Society, Wellcome Institute, Contemporary Archive Collection, G.86

there seems to be no evidence that even Fisher, the professional statistician, knew of this literature. He never cites it, except perhaps on that one occasion when he complained that the probands were not being indicated on the pedigrees. Because of the Great War, the German eugenists had been out of touch with the British group since the time of the First International Congress in 1912. It is ironic that an exhibit by Otto Diem at that meeting would have provided at least a start on the problem of the statistical treatment of pedigree material.[138]

The pauper pedigree study came to publication at last in 1933, in a rather pitifully truncated form.[139] The book contained pedigrees only, with no attempt at any statistical treatment at all and no trace of any environmental investigations. Its material was essentially what it would have been if it had been published in 1913, twenty years earlier: a Ptolemaic survival in a Galilean world. It was optimistically labelled Volume I, and other volumes of analysis were supposed to follow, but none ever did. The committee remained faithful and had their names listed on the title page, and Major Darwin wrote a moving introduction.

The British Eugenics Society in the early twenties was passing through a period when its shifting ideology no longer seemed to fit comfortably with the methods at its disposal. The history of R.A. Fisher, the Cambridge Eugenics Society and the Research Committee's attempt to complete Lidbetter's pauper pedigree project are a case study in transition within the eugenics movement itself. Fisher was a deeply committed eugenist. He began by sharing the eugenists' conviction that the environment was a random disturbance that counted for very little in human life, but in the Rothamsted crop yield projects it was not possible for him to maintain this position. He had found it necessary to devise statistical methods to ensure this randomness mathematically, so as to leave the way clear for assessment of the effects of crop dressings, also, of course environmental. It may have been this experience that led him to try to fit the environment in somewhere in the pauper pedigree project. He hoped for a calculus that would assess the relative importance of heredity and environment as causes of pauperism, a variance divided between the two. The pedigree was not enough in itself to demonstrate heritability, since it could not be controlled or quantitated by biometrical methods. Fisher emphasises, and

Pearson and Udny Yule also advise, that some kind of correlation is the only method that can be used where no experiment is possible, only measurements of things as they are. Correlation coefficients are ideal for human studies. Before it came to be published, the pedigree study went through various attempts to adapt it to include environmental factors and to include some kind of statistical analysis. Almost everyone involved, from the Committee to the Medical Research Council, seems to have come to feel that pedigrees were not enough. Only Lidbetter felt that they expressed exactly what he needed. The change in emphasis from a demonstration that paupers were a genetic isolate – to use a later expression – to an investigation of the causes of human failure, even if the answer was already known to the eugenists, meant that environment had to be brought in somehow.

The assumptions of the eugenists were slowly breaking up, and with them the methodology that they could use. Confidence in pedigree studies had been unquestioned from 1900 until about 1923 when Fisher asked his questions of the Research Committee. By 1933, when Lidbetter's study came out, the Committee had been in difficulties for the past decade or so, over the problem of the part played by environment in social failure, and the problem of adapting the pedigree, essentially a visual method, an *ad oculos* demonstration of heritability, to statistical analysis. Both ideology and method were being questioned within the movement itself. They were soon to be attacked from outside, too.

The falling-apart of the study shows the crumbling of the consensus within the Society. The Research Committee appointed in 1923 was ambivalent about its goals. The statements it issued continued to emphasise heredity rather than environment, and to say that great insights were to be expected from the genealogical method, which it saw as a new contribution, peculiar to the Society itself. The discussions at the Committee's meetings, however, were mainly about the control group, the possible statistical methods, the problem of dealing with the environment and, of course, the insistent problem of funding. The suggested statistical methods were impossible to apply to the material in the form of pedigrees alone.

The personal problems grated continually during this second phase of the study. Lidbetter felt that it was his study and his life's work. He had spent all his free time and much of his own money on it for nearly twenty years, and he resented attempts to influence it. He had been trained by the Society itself in its own pre-war methods and he saw no need for change. His study was simply meant to show the genealogical network of the pauper families as proof that they were a circumscribed group that married and bred within itself. He was indifferent to both the question of the mechanism of inheritance and to the influence of environment. It did not help, either, that the Chairman, Cyril Burt, was often not present at meetings, and did not provide any leadership.

A further problem may have been the lack of institutionalisation of the eugenics movement in Britain. The Society itself had tried to remedy this lack by dropping the 'Education' part of its name. In 1924, it became the Eugenics Society, signifying that it considered original research, and not merely exposition and advocacy, to be a part of its mandate. The Research Committee was to embody this mandate, but it was no substitute for a full-time research group or a university department.

Although the British eugenics movement had the backing of so many individuals of the professional and academic classes, it had very little institutional support. In 1920, only two university courses included eugenics. Karl Pearson's Galton Chair in Eugenics at University College, London was endowed by Galton at his death in 1911, but did not become active until after the 1914–18 war; Imperial College, London, had E.W. MacBride's eugenics course included in its biology syllabus from 1914. By the early thirties, there were, in addition, some genetics courses: Reginald Ruggles Gates at King's College, London, was including genetics along with botany, and there may have been others who similarly touched on it. In 1930, Lancelot Hogben started work in the Chair of Social Biology at the London School of Economics, and in 1933, John Burdon Sanderson Haldane transferred from the John Innes Horticultural Institution at Cambridge to occupy the Chair of Genetics at University College, London. Neither Hogben nor Haldane were prepared to co-operate with the Society, though both were concerned with human genetics. Outside London, sympathetic departments included Alexander Carr-Saunders' School of Sociology in Liverpool, Frank A.E. Crew's Institute of Animal Breeding in Edinburgh, and the John Innes Institution, with R.C. Punnett.

There was no representation at all in the medical field, though Crewe had pointed out how much more effective an endowed medical school lectureship would have been for the Society's purposes than any number of what he called 'mother's meetings'.[140] R.A. Fisher, looking around in the mid-thirties for somewhere to send the Society's Darwin Scholar, could suggest only four centres in London and three outside it.[141]

Daniel Kevles, comparing British genetics of this period with genetics in America, pointed out the striking difference of scale.[142] The same difference of scale could be found in Germany during the twenties: Maria Günther lists twenty-five to thirty university courses in eugenics, and the first special purpose chair was founded there in 1923.[143] In Germany, eugenics was thoroughly institutionalised, with attachments to the field of social hygiene.

Along with a lack of institutional support, the British movement lacked outside contacts. The movement as a whole had been markedly international before the war, but many of the ties were broken in 1914. Though the Society had connections with the United States, little use seems to have been made of them. German eugenics and human genetics was vigorous and innovative during the twenties, but the British group had no knowledge of it until the end of the decade. Both the Eugenics Society and the Genetical Society, a group run by R.C. Punnett from the John Innes Institution, sent delegates to the Fifth International Genetics Congress in Berlin in 1927.[144] But even then, there seems to have been no interchange of ideas. It was not until the Society began its voluntary sterilisation campaign at the end of the decade, and under a new General Secretary, Charles P. Blacker, that efforts were made actively to seek German contacts, and to make use of the German literature.[145]

4

THE ATTACK FROM THE LEFT

Marxism and the new mathematical techniques

The period of the unchallenged dominance of the eugenists in human genetics came to an end in 1930. Up to this time, it is hard to find any evidence of British opposition to the eugenic platform: among British geneticists, only William Bateson seems to have disapproved of eugenics before 1930. But from 1930 onwards, the geneticists of the left combined to point out the ideologically determined assumptions on which the eugenists' science rested. From 1930 onwards, the left-wing attack on eugenics focused on the weakness of the eugenists' teaching on the influence of the environment. The link between the left and environmentalism was forged at this time; it represented a new alignment of method and ideology.

Before 1930, writers on eugenics in Britain had shown little self-consciousness about environmental influences. Many of them had been quite prepared to accept that heredity did not work alone in the creation of the finished product, the human being. The overlapping membership of the eugenists in the Society for the Study of Inebriety and the National Council for the Control of Venereal Disease shows that the 'race-poisons', alcohol and syphilis, were taken very seriously as cacogenic influences. Eugenists such as Tredgold had written about their fear of town life as a danger for the germ-plasm; MacBride had expressed his respect for the environment in classical Lamarckian terms. Frederick Mott, too, one of the most loyal supporters of Lidbetter's pauper pedigree project, was equally aware of the importance of environment:

> inherited tendencies of temperament or character may be more or less restrained by proper nurture, but given an

environment in which suggestion and imitation can play their part, e.g., temptation to drink, suggestion and imitation of evil companions and surrounding pauperism and unemployment, and the result will sooner or later be antisocial conduct in the form of insanity, crime or suicide. ...

Again, it is probable that as fast as nature eliminates degenerates, new tainted stocks are developed by the effects of environment. ...

Even some of the most ardent followers of Weismann and the nontransmission of acquired characters admit that environment may affect the germ-plasm and thus would account for variations.[1]

According to Mott, the environment could be *both* the cause of degenerate heredity *and* the opportunity for its expression.

In Germany, too, the social hygiene connection allowed for the environment to be considered side by side with heredity in the same literature. The *Handwörterbuch der sozialen Hygiene* of 1912 edited by Alfred Grotjahn, the leading social hygienist, contains articles on inheritance by the eugenist and statistician Wilhelm Weinberg, on degeneration by Grotjahn himself, and on family studies and genetics, side by side with items on dust control in factories, and old-age pensions.[2] Grotjahn, like the British writers, felt that the bad living conditions in industrial towns caused degeneration, and that hygienic reform was important for eugenic reasons.[3] And although he was a socialist by conviction, that did not appear to him to be any bar to an interest in heredity and eugenics:

concern with the problems of social causation of disease, and the influence of the surroundings on the body never made me overlook its polar opposite, the influence of heredity. Very early on I was convinced that social hygiene could not be carried on independently of the hygiene of human reproduction, or eugenics.[4]

The inclusion of eugenics and human genetics within university courses on hygiene was not an accident. The race/social/personal hygiene spectrum was systematically presented as a single unit. Even the hard-edged racist philosophy promoted by the Munich eugenists occupied merely a section of this spectrum, just as it did in the double course taught by Grotjahn and Eugen Fischer, social hygienist and race hygienist, in Berlin in 1932. The model curriculum published by Grotjahn in 1925 includes sections on population genetics and eugenics, and anthropometry as well as statistics, bacteriology and serology, public education, epidemic control and industrial hygiene.[5] As Max von Gruber, eugenist and Professor of Hygiene in Munich, put it: 'We do not inherit complete characteristics, only *Anlagen*. ... What is inherited is the seed corn, but the plant that sprouts from it, the phenotype, may be very different in different soil, climate, weather and cultivation.'[6] It was just the metaphor that R.A. Fisher was learning through experience to be literally true.

Nor did political writers at this time – before 1930, that is – see the problem in terms of a conflict between the principles of nature and nurture. As Loren Graham pointed out some time ago, the positions taken on eugenics by the political left and right during the twenties were very complex. Many on the left felt that social responsibility must include responsibility for the next generation. Eugenics was important to society.[7]

According to Graham, the first explicitly left-wing attack in eugenics came in 1927 from Hugo Iltis, author of a biography of Mendel. But it was the racism of the German eugenists, rather than eugenics itself that Iltis criticised.[8] The eugenics that he advocated included a touch of Lamarckianism, which by the mid-twenties was beginning to be associated with the geneticists of the left in Germany. In 1921, the right-wing eugenist Fritz Lenz remarked that the left clung to Lamarckianism because it was politically useful. By 1928, a full-scale Marxist attack on the German eugenics and race-hygiene movement had appeared in the Communist journal *Under the Banner of Marxism*.[9] But even here, the author did not wish to stamp out eugenics altogether. It was its racism and its bourgeois class-bias that he wanted to expunge, so that the purified remnant could become part of a future programme in which eugenics served the people as a whole.

Before 1930, there was no clear dichotomy between nature and nurture supporters either in Germany or in Britain. Emphasis on environment by left or right in both literatures often meant a Lamarckian tendency to blame the environment for damage to the germ-plasm leading to degenerate stocks, rather than for the production of a weedy phenotype. Nor was there a clear distinction between the political right and left on the question of eugenics. It was supported both by the social hygienist and socialist Grotjahn, and Nazi folkist Lenz. Attackers from the left felt that eugenics in itself, apart from its racist supporters, was an important part of social welfare.

In Britain, the explicit use of environment as a means of attacking eugenics began in 1931 with the work of Lancelot Hogben. Along with polemical environmentalism, Hogben brought in the mathematics of the German human geneticists; calculations of gene frequency based on the Mendelian *Vererbungsmathematik* introduced by Wilhelm Weinberg, tests for the Mendelian hypothesis and for consanguinity by Fritz Lenz, and finally the calculation of linkage based on the blood-group studies of Felix Bernstein – the apparatus of *Vererbungsmathematik* that had developed over the past two decades in Germany, and which had found its ideal material in the human blood groups.[10] In Germany, these methods had absolutely no implication of a left-wing critique of the class-bias of eugenics; blood-group studies in the twenties and thirties had contributed to *völkisch* anthropology or *Rassenphysiologie*.[11] But Hogben took up German mathematical Mendelism and the blood-group studies that went with it as a means of attacking British eugenics for its naïve procedures, its neglect of the environment and above all for its subservience to class interests. Only when these faults had been purged could human genetics work for the benefit of the human race. The attack from the left brought into the open the problem of the separation of the social from the biological in the human situation, a problem which had already troubled Fisher and the eugenists of the Society's Research Committee.

In the eyes of the opposition, the problem was political, but the solution lay in ethically neutral science. Lancelot Hogben, newly appointed Professor of Social Biology at the London School of Economics, criticised the eugenists not only for their over-emphasis on genetics in the determination of human behaviour, but also for bringing the problem into the political arena, with the result that 'social biology is full of terms that have no place in ethically neutral science'.[12] 'Eugenic social propaganda', he wrote,

has been dominated by an explicit social bias which in England can only serve to render the eugenic standpoint unpalatable to a section of the community which for good or evil seems to be assuming the role of a governing class.

The greatest obstacle to the spread of a sane eugenic point of view is the eugenists themselves. By recklessly antagonizing the leaders of thought among the working classes, the protagonists have done their best to make eugenics a matter of party politics with results which can only delay the acceptance of a national minimum of parenthood. [13]

Lancelot Hogben had been at Cambridge just before the First World War, at the same time as R.A. Fisher. He was one of the first group of boys to go up to Cambridge on a County Scholarship. Gary Werskey, who interviewed him towards the end of his life, felt that his hatred of the eugenists may have grown from the resentment he felt towards condescending upper-class colleagues. Hogben himself, in his autobiography, which was probably written at about the same time as the interview with Werskey, evinces nothing but scornful dismissal of the privileged youths who spent their time on rowing and beagling, and participated not at all in the intellectual life of the university. He felt himself, at least on looking back, to have belonged to an intellectual elite of scholarship winners.[14] He was enraged by the eugenists' arguments against the provision of scholarships for children from outside the professional classes, a rage which was still alive in 1938 when he picked out quotations on the harm done by scholarships, from Schuster, the Whethams and Major Darwin, to illustrate his attack on eugenics as a 'system of ingenious excuses for combating the amelioration of working class conditions'.[15] Instead of joining the Eugenics Society, like Fisher, he joined the Cambridge University Fabian Society, and in 1914 became its secretary. During Hogben's term of office the Fabian Society's politics moved sharply to the left.

Hogben's socialism was active and committed, a fact which he himself had lost sight of sixty years later, when he came to writing his autobiography. After leaving Cambridge, he wrote and lectured for the Independent Labour Party and the Plebs League, and helped to found and organise the National Union of Scientific Workers. During the First World War, he spoke out as a conscientious objector, and spent some time in gaol for it (see Chapter 5, pp. 221–4).[16] As early as 1918, he was writing the Independent Labour Party's *Socialist Review* against the confusion of evolutionary change with social progress. Social progress had its own motive forces, and they were economic rather than biological.[17] Hogben preferred socialism's economic determinism to the biological kind; he was a socialist before he was a biologist.

Hogben was a radical in science as well as in politics. Together with his young contemporaries, J.B.S. Haldane and Julian Huxley, and supported by the slightly more senior Frank A.E. Crew of the Edinburgh Animal Breeding Research Institute, the group decided to start a journal that would have a more up-to-date editorial policy than the existing biological journals, the Royal Society's journals, the *Quarterly Journal of Microscopical Science* and the *Journal of Physiology*. The young biologists wanted a medium for studies of evolution which would be based not upon the fossil record with all its gaps and defects, but upon comparative physiology as an experimental science. The new journal was funded by H.G. Wells, whom Hogben had met through Wells's son, a student in Hogben's department at Imperial College, London. The rest of the funding was given by Crew, out of his war wounds compensation. The *British Journal of Experimental Biology* began publication in 1923 with Crew as editor, and Julian Huxley, Hogben, the plant physiologist, Reginald Ruggles-Gates and the sociologist Alexander Carr-Saunders, all scientific progressives and eugenists, among the members of the editorial board. A few months later, the journal's editors evolved into the Society for Experimental Biology, devoted to making an exact experimental science of biology.[18]

As things were to turn out, each of them was to look to genetics as an expression of that exactness: Huxley took up genetics and evolution, Haldane genetics and population, Hogben social biology, and Crew, scientific animal breeding. Crew, Carr-Saunders amd Ruggles-Gates, as well as Huxley, were active members of the Eugenics Society, serving on its committees.[19] There was no sense in which the society was against eugenics. It was difficult to see genetics in the human species as anything other than a scientific eugenics.

Crew had joined the Eugenics Society in 1919, hoping to organise a branch society in Edinburgh University.[20] The branch did not work out, but Crew himself lectured for the society throughout the twenties to various northern groups – 'mother's meetings', Crew called them irritably. His own view was that it would have been much more effective as eugenic propaganda to have had a course taught to medical students. The Society would have been better to spend its money endowing a lectureship at the university.[21]

Besides the *Journal*, Crew and Hogben worked together on many other projects, both experimental and educational. Hogben was a diligent and productive writer. He did the first textbook in Crew and Ward Cutler's series of Biological Monographs, a work on the physiology of *The Pigmentary Effector System* (1924).[22] Crew himself wrote one on *Animal Genetics* (1925).[23] Julian Huxley, by then Professor of Zoology at King's College, London, also organised a series, and Hogben contributed to it a text on *Comparative Physiology* (1926).[24] Hogben by this time had left Edinburgh and was teaching at McGill, Montreal, but his textbook was based on his Edinburgh lectures.

One of the characteristics of the productions of this group of young biologists, besides the emphasis on the experimental laboratory, was the use of a very international literature as source material. The bibliography in Crew's *Animal Genetics* includes the German Wilhelm Weinberg on the inheritance of twinning, the Americans A.H. Sturtevant, C.B. Bridges and T.H. Morgan on linkage in *Drosophila* and the Dane W.L. Johannsen on pure lines, as well as J.B.S. Haldane's papers of 1919 on the calculation of linkage values. Crew's text itself did not make much use of the methods of *Vererbungsmathematik* but they were there to be found in his bibliography if a student was advanced enough to need them.

Hogben, too, was very aware of the international literature. Of the seventy-six references that made up the bibliography of his *Pigmentary Effector System*, thirty-three were in German, seven in French, and twenty-seven in English; the rest were to his own work. His super-reference was to a *Handbuch der vergleichende Physiologie* of 1914, which contained a 462-page bibliography.[25] Hogben's *Physiology*, the product of the course he gave to Edinburgh medical and honours science students, still referred to Winterstein's 'encyclopaedic pages'. Crew and Hogben knew and used the German (and American) literature on genetics, comparative physiology and endocrinology. Their textbooks were designed to introduce their students to it, and to emphasise its importance for a modern biologist. This is particularly true of Hogben's texts, which outbid all the rest in their citation of books and papers in German.[26] Hogben was later to say that he owed to Crew more than anyone the realisation of his ambition to become a man of science. The year in which he and Crew worked side by side in Crew's department was a formative one for him.[27]

Hogben's treatment of inheritance exemplifies this German-oriented approach. Mendel's method, he says, is the basis of all truly quantitative treatment of inheritance on experimental lines.[28] An immense variety of characteristics of plants and animals have been found to follow the rule of segregation, which he then explains in simple terms. However, 'factorial analysis as this method of investigation is sometimes called' is not often as simple as the case cited. In these textbooks, a detailed treatment of factorial analysis might at this date have seemed too difficult for students, but it was present, as it were, in the background.[29]

Another salient feature of Hogben's teaching was its thorough-going mechanistic conception of life, to borrow the phrase of one of his contemporaries, the German-American physiologist Jacques Loeb. Hogben's elementary textbook of animal biology of 1930 was again based on a course he had given, this time to the students at Cape Town University in South Africa. It was meant to supersede the biology teaching based on the type system introduced in the 1880s by Thomas Henry Huxley. Hogben designed his biology course to teach the habits of scientific thinking, just as T.H. Huxley had, and like Huxley's, his scientific thinking was a traditional robust positivism:

> At the outset the student should be made to realize that biological science ... differs from physics and chemistry only in its subject matter. Its method, the method of science, is identical. That is to say it treats of objects in the external world: it expresses the relation between them in the most economical way; and it makes no assumptions which involve *ethical* value. To interpret the phenomena of living matter in the most economical terms we are driven to ask whether the properties of living matter are not manifestations of the same general principles which have been established in the realm of inanimate nature.[30]

His emphatic positivism, however, had room for a cascade of mechanistic metaphors, which he probably did not think of as in the least metaphorical: his chapter headings include 'The machinery of response', 'The machinery of coordination', 'The machinery of inheritance'. Hogben's philosophy of science is a tough-minded mixture of positivism, reductionism and mechanism. Elsewhere he calls Darwinism an essentially dialectical construction.[31] 'Dialectical', he says, is 'not infrequently used as a term of abuse, implying suspicion towards undue reliance on mere verbalism.'[32] Two general methods have been used by men to gain knowledge. One is 'rationalized in its most rigid form in the philosophy of Hegel', the method of deduction, but 'the scientific method is irreconcilably opposed to the Hegelian method'. The Mendelian renaissance, he says, has formulated the problem of evolution in quantitative terms, and interpreted the hereditary mechanism in the light of experiment upon the machinery of inheritance.[33] Now that quantitative observation has superseded the qualitative and the dialectical, the real history of science has begun.

Hogben the reductionist, Hogben the mechanist, was an ideal candidate for the new Chair of Social Biology at the London School of Economics, set up as part of a package funded by the Rockefeller Foundation for the study of 'physical or natural bases of the social sciences', including Anthropology, Social Biology and 'Modern Social Conditions'.[34] According to Sir William Beveridge, the Director of the School, who conducted the negotiations with the Rockefeller Foundation, this area, in which he probably included eugenics, had always been an interest of his.[35] Though he was not a member of the Society, Beveridge spoke up publicly for the Society's policies.[36] The implicit invitation in these terms of reference to create a centre for such studies as race psychology does not seem to have alarmed him.

Hogben may have appeared to be the ideal man to reduce the social sciences to their physical bases, but he was willing to apply his reductionism only in a strictly limited way outside the bounds of laboratory biology. Human society, he felt, was not an essentially biological phenomenon:

> We cannot assume, without further evidence, that biological factors have exerted any significant influence on the history of civilization. Beyond the fact that man is *par excellence* a toolbearing animal, biology has very little to say which will throw light on the field of the historian.[37]

Hogben's acceptance of the social biology appointment focused his work directly onto the problem of the 'further evidence'. In a memorandum probably written early in 1931 on his plans for work connected with the new chair, he wrote:

> Under its terms of reference, the Chair of Social Biology in the University of London was primarily founded to encourage the study of biological aspects of population growth in the modern world and of human inheritance with special reference to the genetic basis of human behaviour. ... An examination of the more fundamental issues which a Department of Social Biology might usefully probe compels a recognition of dangers inherent in extending conclusions derived from the study of the lower animals to man himself.[38]

It was a danger which came very close to the purpose of his chair. In 1927, Hogben had already come out against eugenics for the positivistic reason that it was not ethically neutral science.

> What is the *good* of the race? What is a desirable social quality? What is a 'morally and mentally fit' person? These are matters of taste, not of science. For the scientist in the words of Poincaré: 'All that is objective is devoid of all quality, and is pure relation.' The experimental biologist is gradually elevating his subject to that plane: the eugenist is seeking to entangle it in the old ways.[39]

He repeated his attack in 1930, soon after his arrival in London, with the appearance of a collection of his essays. One of them is called 'The survival of the eugenist'. It starts off with a verse from the South African poet Roy Campbell, intended no doubt to express his view of the eugenist as a primitive survival:

> I am that ancient hunter of the plains
> That raked the shaggy flitches of the bison:
> Pass, World: I am the dreamer that remains
> The Man, clear-cut against the last horizon.[40]

This was a squib which he evidently liked, as he quoted it elsewhere, too. The difficulty in human social biology, he felt, was that biologists had always tended to overrate the importance of the biological.

Analogies from the animal kingdom have been pressed into ... service. ... Kropotkin's *Mutual Aid* was the *reductio ad absurdum* of that attitude to social problems. Kropotkin was neither more nor less scientific than the exponents of nature red in tooth and claw. Both were irrelevant. The same irrelevance has been evident wherever biologists have attempted to rationalize their political sentiments. The anti-feminist appeals to the fighting and protective male. The feminist can retort by invoking the worm *Bonellia* of which the male lives as a parasite in the generative passages of the female.[41]

Progress in the genetic analysis of social behaviour would be blocked until the problem could be formulated in *strictly* biological terms.

Very soon after taking up his appointment, Hogben became involved in the current problems of the genetic analysis of social behaviour. The Eugenics Society's Research Committee was trying to find funding for the publication of Lidbetter's pauper pedigree study. Sir William Beveridge had been approached in the hope that there might be some Rockefeller money available, and he had asked Hogben to look at the project. Charles Blacker, General Secretary of the Eugenics Society, also sounded Hogben out with a view to getting his help in putting a request for funding to the Rockefeller Foundation. Blacker told Lidbetter that he thought Hogben might sponsor the book with some amendments.

> His willingness to do this depends to a great extent upon your ability to discriminate between different kinds of pauperism, in particular between that which implies social inadequacy and that which implies misfortune without social inadequacy, He asked me if it was now too late to draw a distinction between these two essential groups. I told him, that, so far as I knew, the blocks had not been prepared.[42]

Indeed, in 1931, unemployment could hardly be regarded as due to hereditary social failure. But Lidbetter had in fact tried to exclude the new unemployed of the depression era. From 1921 onwards, the system of Poor Law relief had been changed so as to permit outdoor relief to be given, to meet the sudden increase in unemployment. The census of paupers in the East London Poor Law Area, upon which Lidbetter's report was to be based, excluded all those relieved under the new scheme as 'persons not normally reporting to the Poor Law'.[43]

Perhaps Lidbetter explained this to Hogben, and perhaps he explained also that there was a control group, based on a list of names of 100 schoolchildren from schools in the area, whose pedigrees were constructed in the same way as the paupers. But there was still no real statistical analysis of the pedigrees. Hogben reported to Sir William Beveridge that:

> There seems to be a great deal of sociologically instructive material embodied in them and I certainly think this should be made available. On the other hand, I think that it requires very careful scrutiny and preparation before the data can be interpreted without ambiguity. ... If the Rockefeller committee agree to subsidize the risk of publication I think that the School should be represented on the publication committee by at least two persons.[44]

Like Fisher, he felt that the pedigree method was weak and outdated, and that quantitative treatment must now replace the pedigree as the standard tool for research in human genetics. Like Fisher, too, he did not disapprove of the pauper pedigree study so whole-heartedly as to refuse to have anything whatever to do with it. He allowed Blacker to think that he was prepared to cooperate with the Research Committee in trying to make it suitable for publication. But in his memorandum of 1931 on his plan for the new department, he was a good deal more outspoken about the defects of the kind of work the Eugenics Society was doing:

> there is no prospect of further advance by adding to the numerous investigations of pedigrees displaying a family history of pauperism, crime and mental defect ... it is necessary to abandon the collection of isolated family pedigrees and to deal only with mass statistics ... with a view to quantitative treatment of the type which has been adopted in the blood groups.[45]

Hogben in 1930–31, then, was critical of the eugenist programme, as exemplified by the pauper pedigree project. He was sympathetic to the working class, and felt the need for new, more positivistic methods in research in human genetics. He was not against eugenics itself, as he was careful to say. But he felt that the existing methods of human genetics were simply unable to cope with the complexities of human biology and society; the gap between them had been stopped with middle-class propaganda. It was not until the middle of 1931 that both his working-class sympathies and the methodology of human genetics really came into bloom.

The year 1931 saw the Second International Congress on the History of Science, which met in London; the Soviet delegation which unexpectedly turned up at this Congress brought to Britain the startling new ideas of Marxist philosophy of science. Hogben and the biochemist Joseph Needham participated in the session on 'Historical and contemporary interrelationships of the physical and biological sciences'.[46] During this meeting, both Hogben and Needham and other left-wing British scientists were able to meet with the Russians personally, and to discuss both science and Marxism with them. N.I. Bukharin, the most senior member of the delegation, visited Hogben at home.

The meeting made a deep impression. Before this time the British group were politically left-wing, but not very aware of Marxism. After the meeting, and there is a great deal of evidence for this, Marxism came sharply into focus as a possible philosophy of science in Britain. Its influence can still be felt in the writing of later generations of British historians working on the social relations of science.

Hogben's struggle to accommodate dialectical materialism into his own system of thought is laid out at length in an article which appeared in October 1931. Hogben meant it as a sympathetic exposition of Bukharin's philosophy of science for an English audience, which would have been left behind by the foreignness of the Marxist terminology:

> Dialectical materialism, the official philosophy of the Communist movement, has now been forced upon our attention by the advent of a delegation of Russian scientists to the Second International Congress of the History of Science. ... It was disturbing to encounter an attitude which the communist speakers regarded as vitally significant to the organized development of science in modern society. ... No one previously unacquainted with their

terminology and its antecedents could have deduced the essentials of dialectical materialism from what they actually said.[47]

One of those who was disturbed but could not understand, was Hogben himself. Even the phrase 'dialectical materialism' seemed a contradiction to one who was sure he was a materialist, but who had taken 'dialectical' to mean 'merely verbal'. Bukharin had derived the Marxist dialectic from Hegel, who had always symbolised the enemy, the metaphysician, for Hogben, and Bukharin had also attacked Mach, who for Hogben was a materialist, and on our side. Hogben quotes Engels's definition of materialism:

> Those who declare that spirit existed before nature and who in the last analysis therefore assume ... that the world was created ... have formed the idealist camp. The others who regard nature as primary, belong to the various schools of materialism.[48]

Engels's Hegelian 'spirit' reminds Hogben of the arguments of forty years before, between Thomas Henry Huxley and the defenders of the religious views of the creation of the world.[49] For Hogben, the Marxist's materialism is indistinguishable from Huxley's; but it is difficult for him to accept that 'dialectical' is not the very opposite of materialist. He quotes Lenin again to show that this is a new, a positivist's dialectic, that the metaphysical is anti-dialectic. But he finds it hard to explain why the Russians seemed so anxious not to be called mechanists, which to Hogben was the essential viewpoint of the biological scientist; the Russians do not seem to have mentioned that the mechanist school had been officially condemned there in 1929.[50] The philosophers of communism told him that philosophy provided a framework that should guide studies of human society as well as the science of living matter. It is a statement of the position of the opponents of the Russian mechanists, who seemed for a while to be gaining the upper hand, but were eventually also condemned by Stalin as being idealists. The Stalinist version of dialectical materialism, in which the forces of production determine natural science, and are themselves influenced by it, had become the definitive version from January 1931.[51]

This aspect of dialectical materialism had been an important part of the paper 'Theory and practice' that Bukharin gave at the meeting, but it hardly figures at all in Hogben's explanation of what Bukharin said.[52] Hogben's Marxist philosophy of science is very much his own earlier mechanistic interpretation of life, reaffirmed by the feeling that now, with materialism the creed of a state, history is finally on our side:

> There has never been a generation when biologists as a whole entertained a more widespread and well-founded confidence in the continued application of physico-chemical methods to the analysis of animal behaviour. ... To be radical in religious matters was the prerogative of a small and privileged class confident of its security. In our generation the inbelief of Huxley and Tyndall has spread to all sections of society. ... Materialism is now the official creed of a hundred and sixty million human beings.[53]

It is the same nineteenth-century Huxleyan positivism that Hogben professed before the meeting, with a single exception. The exception originated not in Bukharin's speech, which he was supposedly interpreting, but in that of the biologist B.M. Zavadovskii. It was Zavadovskii's paper which came nearest to Hogben's own concerns, and it was actually Zavadovskii rather than Bukharin who had been concerned to 'disclaim identification with the mechanistic school'. It was Zavadovskii who gave Hogben a new tool to use in his own work; Zavadovskii's definition of dialectics included the 'law of the passing of quantity into quality'. He insisted that the point of scientific research was not 'the violent identification of the biological and physical' but the discovery of appropriate laws for each stage of development of matter; he attacked the 'bourgeois eugenists' who attempt to consider the *social* inequality of men as the direct result of biological inequality in their inherited characters. These class-bound scientists prove the socio-historical and class-determinateness of scientific theories.[54]

Hogben was already aware of the danger of reducing the social to the biological, and of looking for animal analogies for human behaviour. At this point he seems to have understood that Marxist philosophy of science was not simply a foreign form of positivism:

> With the holists and the exponents of 'emergent evolution', dialectical materialism is at one in recognizing that we

encounter different levels of complexity in the study of phenomena with laws of their own ... the philosophers of communism ... emphasize that dialectical materialism is something more than the mechanistic stand-point.[55]

Joseph Needham has pointed out that Hogben's was one of the first attempts to translate dialectical materialism into an English idiom. It was this same passage in Zavadovskii's speech that Needham too found profoundly significant: it formed a bridge between the organic and the inorganic, a solution to the problem of mechanism versus vitalism that was of particular importance to a biochemist, working in 'the most borderline of sciences', as Needham called it, and equally important on the other side of the border, to a social biologist.[56]

Hogben's thinking on the problems of social biology did not take a completely new direction following his contact with Marxism, but the Marxist analysis both sharpened his perception of the class-bound nature of the eugenic programme, and also provided a theoretical support for his campaign against the over-emphasis of the biological in human society. This last is the common factor in all the work he both produced himself and organised for his group during the thirties.

The book that he wrote during 1931 is built around the proposition that a science of social biology is possible, but only if its limits are carefully defined:

> *increasing complexity of cultural achievement may proceed in human society independently of any change in man's inborn equipment.* [Hogben's emphasis] ... Marx epitomizes the standpoint of economic determinism in the following words: 'The same men who establish social relations conformably with their material productivity produce also the ideas, the categories, conformable with their social relations'. ... German writers have stigmatized the standpoint of historical materialism as Lamarckian. This is a confusion of thought arising from the failure of genetically trained biologists to pay attention to the essentially human features of human activity.[57]

Marxism helped Hogben to define his problem, but it did not provide him with the tools with which to solve it. The tools came from the German mathematical geneticists Wilhelm Weinberg and Fritz Lenz, both leaders in the eugenics movement, and the mathematician Felix Bernstein. They consisted of the application of Mendel's laws in a new form to the analysis of human pedigrees, to the problems that the eugenists had been struggling with for so long.

It was Hogben's hope that it had now become possible for ethically neutral science to define the part played in human society by the biological, and to scrape away from human genetics the crust of class bias and tendentious assumptions that had stuck to it in the past. By comparing the observed with what would be expected on strictly Mendelian assumptions, he hoped to be able to sort out the traits which required particular environmental conditions for their expression from those which were able to manifest themselves under almost any conditions. It was a new statement of the old nature versus nurture controversy, in which the more rigorous new methods of the German mathematical Mendelism or *Vererbungsmathematik* would be the tool which allowed him to cut back the overemphasis on biological nature which human genetics had suffered from when its only method was to look at pedigrees – the studbook method, Hogben calls it somewhere.

Hogben's application of the new mathematics to human pedigree material appeared in the Cambridge-edited *Journal of Genetics* early in 1931.[58] His paper marks the irruption of the German methods into British genetics, and at the same time it is the first work on human material, other than the occasional anecdotal family history, typically accompanied by a pedigree, to appear in the *Journal of Genetics*. Hogben's source seems to have been a monograph on juvenile amaurotic idiocy by Torsten Sjögren, a geneticist from the Institute for Race Biology at Uppsala.[59] Sjögren collected and published pedigrees of fifty-nine families with 115 cases of the disease, all country people who seldom moved far from their birthplace. The cases clustered around twenty-three centres, and about 25 per cent of the marriages were consanguineous. Using the mathematical methods of Weinberg, Lenz and Bernstein, Sjögren calculated that juvenile amaurotic idiocy must depend on a single-gene recessive.[60,61,62] The contrast between Sjögren's methods and Lidbetter's could hardly be more striking.

Wilhelm Weinberg was one of the oldest members of the German eugenics movement, and leader of the Stuttgart group of the society, as we saw in Chapter 2 (p. 90).[63] Weinberg's statistical papers, beginning as far back as 1908, had formalised mathematically the implications of the Mendelian binomial in relation to the frequency of genes in a population. Mendel's own binomial had assumed random matings of equal numbers of his two alleles A and B:

$$AB \times AB = A^2 + 2AB + B^2$$

Weinberg incorporated the frequencies m and n of the two alleles as variables in the equation:

$$mA + nB = 100\%$$
$$m^2AA + 2mnAB = 100\%$$

an expression which he saw would hold good for every generation as long as there was random mating for the traits in question. The English mathematician W.B. Hardy proposed a similar equation at almost the same time, but Weinberg pushed his argument further.[64] He developed expressions for calculating the expected proportions of the two phenotypes among parents, siblings and children of the chosen probands. If a trait was really inherited according to the Mendelian laws, there should be a distinct difference in these values:

For a proband carrying an allele A:
Parents or children: $(1 + mn)A : n^2B$
Siblings: $[4(1 + mn) + mn^2]A : n^2(3 + n)B$

If the difference found between the values for parents or children and siblings conformed to expectations, that demonstrated that the trait was inherited according to Mendelian law. If there was no significant difference, Mendelian inheritance was ruled out. Sampling problems that arose from the fact that only affected families appeared in the samples could be corrected by the application of a method also provided by Weinberg.

Fritz Lenz, another prominent figure in the eugenics movement, and an enthusiastic promoter of Weinberg's painfully difficult mathematical methods, had proposed a method of testing whether a rare pathological condition was the result of homozygous recessive genes. His argument was based on the fact that the rarer the gene, the more frequently the parents of the homozygote will be cousins, both heterozygous for the gene in question.[65] Given the incidence of cousin marriages in the local community, and in the families of the patients, the conformity of observed and expected on the Mendelian hypothesis could be tested. Hogben saw that the method could be used to sort out conditions where the foetal or the social environment played a part in causation, for instance, in mental defect.

The Weinbergian *Vererbungsmathematik* could also be used to disentangle the type of Mendelian inheritance involved in a given trait, and the ABO blood groups seemed to be the ideal Mendelising traits. The blood groups had first been shown to be inherited by Ludwik Hirszfeld, who assumed that A and B were independent traits, determined by two independent chromosomal loci. Each locus carried one of a pair of alleles, A or a and B or b, which represented the presence or absence of the genetic factor, and at the same time, the reaction of the blood cells with the two test sera, anti-A and anti-B. Since this proposal accorded perfectly with the usual interpretation of Mendelian alleles as determining either the presence or the absecnse of a given trait, no one thought to question it for a generation. In 1924, however, Felix Bernstein, Director of the Institute for Mathematical Statistics at Göttingen, proposed another interpretation of the inheritance of the blood groups. Bernstein suggested that there were three alleles, determining presences of A, B and O, and all at the same locus. The frequencies of these genes, which he called p, q and r, added up to unity in any population, since they covered all possibilities:

$$p + q + r = 1$$

Using Weinberg's binomial, these frequencies could be calculated from the frequencies, written as A, B and O, of the blood groups themselves:

$$O + A = r^2 + 2pr + p^2 = (r + p)^2$$
$$O + B = r^2 + 2qr + q^2 = (r + q)^2$$
$$q = 1 - \sqrt{(O + A)}$$
$$p = 1 - \sqrt{(O + B)}$$
$$r = \sqrt{O}$$

Bernstein's three-allele system gave much better agreement to the observed figures than did Hirszfeld's, in all populations for which data were available, including those collected by Hirszfeld himself. But the test case was quite simple. According to Hirszfeld, an AB mother should be able to produce an O child: since an AB phenotype might be genotypically AA/BB, Aa/BB or Aa/Bb. This last could pass on an ab 'chromosome' to a child, which might, depending upon the genotype of its father, be phenotypically O. According to Bernstein, on the other hand, the AB phenotype represented an AB genotype. It could pass on A or B, but it had no O, and its children must receive either A or B. No matter who their other parent might be, they could not be group O. During the twenties, the problem was argued on both the grounds of population figures and of the existence or non-existence of the O children of AB mothers. As time went on, and the controversial data were examined more and more minutely, fewer and fewer O children of AB mothers appeared in the literature. Those that resisted re-testing began to be ascribed to illegitimacy or labelling mistakes, and hidden away. The last such case, sadly, was published by Hirszfeld himself. By about 1927, Bernstein had drawn ahead. This controversy drew attention to one very significant aspect of blood-group genetics: the blood-group material represented the first large-scale application of Mendelian inheritance to normal human populations.

Geneticists who wanted to work on human material had been hampered by the difficulty of collecting enough families showing the rare pathological conditions that were the only known examples of human Mendelian inheritance. Here, however, were figures on the scale of those on maize or fruit flies, the geneticist's preferred organisms. It was impossible in human genetics to produce the kind of controlled matings needed for an experimental genetics. But all normal families were a potential source of data for the blood groups, and any type of mating could be found in the masses of data that soon became available.[66]

Outside Britain, blood group immunology was already established as a significant area of investigation. The serologists already knew the work of Felix Bernstein on the ABO blood groups.[67] Blood-grouping had a fairly substantial literature in American journals: American workers such as Lawrence Snyder, and Karl Landsteiner's group at the Rockefeller Institute in New York were in touch with the German workers, and were using their methods. Snyder, for example, spoke at the

International Genetics Congress in 1927. He attacked Ludwik Hirszfeld's two-locus theory of inheritance, and supported Felix Bernstein's three-alleles-at-one-locus hypothesis, its rival. He was answered approvingly by Bernstein in person. But although there were many English geneticists present at the Congress, including Julian Huxley, J.B.S. Haldane, Ruggles Gates, Frank A.E. Crew and even E.J. Lidbetter himself, none of them seems to have been particularly stimulated by either Snyder's paper or Bernstein's own.[68] The enormous expansion of literature on blood-grouping and the expectations it had raised for the mathematical treatment of human Mendelian genetics had gone unnoticed in Britain. Neither the association with Mendelism, with mathematical genetics, nor with race-mapping, another important application of blood-group figures, had interested the British biologists, until they were introduced to the possibilities by Lancelot Hogben.

Hogben's first project on entering into his new Chair of Social Biology was to re-work old published material to demonstrate the application of the methods of *Vererbungsmathematik* or, as he called it, factorial analysis, to them. In some cases, his analysis of pedigrees in the new terms was very revealing. 'The value of human pedigrees', he wrote, 'lies in the fact that they can be used to decide whether the frequencies of observed traits conform to the quantitative requirements of the principle of segregation': using Weinberg's methods, no genetic hypothesis, for example, could be made to fit the pedigrees of deaf mutes in the *Treasury of Human Inheritance*. Hogben concluded, along Weinbergian lines, that deaf mutism could not be an inherited trait, a conclusion that removed from the eugenist's armamentarium a most persuasive example of a genetic cause of pauperism.[69] But the mathematical models available in early 1931 did not distinguish between the frequencies to be expected in cases determined by a single recessive gene and by two independent complementary dominants, and were still, therefore, incomplete. Hogben began work, attempting to extend the new methods to deal with the problem.

In the summer of 1931 Hogben came across another mathematical method which could be used to define the heritable in human families.

In 1931, Bernstein contributed a second important new idea, that of using the blood groups for the mapping of human chromosomes by means of linkage studies.[70] The *Drosophila* workers had managed to calculate the relative positions of loci on the chromosomes in terms of the proportion in which a particular combination of traits was transmitted intact from parent to offspring. Where a pair of traits tended to be transmitted together, they were assumed to lie near each other on the chromosome. But *Drosophila* had only four chromosomes, generation of thousands of offspring for each mating, and a large number of clearly Mendelising traits that could be seen and counted with a hand-lens. Bernstein suggested, and demonstrated mathematically, that human chromosomes might be mapped by using the blood groups as genetic markers.

Hogben seems to have already started work on his book, *Genetic Principles in Medicine and Social Science*, when he came across Bernstein's paper of 1931. The earlier part of the book was apparently written before seeing Bernstein's calculations, when Hogben was still very pessimistic about the chances of getting anywhere with human chromosome mapping. In the early chapter on single gene substitutions he wrote that as the number of human chromosomes is so large (it had recently been found to be forty-eight [*sic*] compared to the four of Drosophila), any knowledge of localisation of genes was going to be difficult to acquire.[71] 'The prospect of ascertaining in the immediate future how the hereditary genes are related in human inheritance is not very promising,' he wrote.[72] His book sets off from the material he had been publishing in the *Journal of Genetics* on the problem of disentangling the cases of true biological heredity from cases where a condition was familial but not genetically determined, as in deaf mutism.

When he comes to Bernstein's paper, he welcomes it with a whole chapter. He explains that the *Drosophila* workers had needed over a quarter of a million flies in order to locate the genes for *black* and *vestigial*. Only in the case of blood groups are data available on that scale for a human character. Snyder has said that nearly 4,000 families of 15,000 individuals have now been tested, providing statistical data for testing the Mendelian consequences of random mating in the human species. The importance of this is that 'human genetics may be made an exact science, and as an object lesson to those who are disposed to construct pretentious hypotheses on the basis of isolated pedigrees'.[73] Linkage to a blood group offered not only a means

167

of chromosome-mapping, but also a potential proof that a given trait was biologically determined, and independent of the environment. Conversely, in the future, it might be possible to demonstrate that a trait was *not* genetically determined, since it had no linkage.

Blood-group serology now provided the ideal stuff for Hogben's reform of human genetics. Blood groups were totally genetically determined: they were proof against environmental influence. Serology was laboratory-based, it was quantitative on a scale that no human biological data had ever yet been, and it was even German. Blood-group serology was the model human science.

Hogben's chapter on the blood groups starts at the beginning, since his English readers knew nothing about them. He explains the technique of serology, the four groups, A, B, O and AB, Hirszfeld's two-locus hypothesis of their inheritance, and its difficulties, and Bernstein's three alleles, with the test case of the O × AB matings. Blood-grouping has made transfusion safe and paternity testing possible. It has also provided a foundation for exploring the linkage relations of the pathological conditions caused by single-gene substitutions. Attempts to associate blood groups with diseases have so far been either negative or inconclusive; but linkage studies are just about to begin. Bernstein's paper adds to the existing methods of *Vererbungmathematik* a means of starting on this problem. New blood groups are now being found every year. Bernstein had used his method on only two independent systems, ABO and MN. When twenty-four independent systems have been found, one for each chromosome pair, there would be a marker on each of them. The single-gene substitutions could then be located in relation to this system of triangulation.

Bernstein's calculus for the mapping individual traits into linkage groups could be used to construct a network of relationships for each chromosome within which any given trait might be 'placed'.

Today the prospects of advancing Human Genetics as an exact science are much brighter than they appeared to be twenty years ago. New methods of mathematical analysis for testing the applicability of experimentally established hypotheses to human data have been elaborated. On the basis of such work as Bernstein's analysis of the blood groups it is now legitimate to entertain the possibility that the human chromosomes can be mapped.[74]

Hogben hoped that blood grouping would be both a sword and a ploughshare. He hoped that linkage to one or more genetic markers such as the blood groups would relate traits to a bedrock of 'ethically neutral' characters; the traits which could not be accommodated within this extension of the Mendelian Law of Segregation would be suspect, as being either wholly or partly environmental products, or simply products of the class bias of the observer. Bernstein's calculations would make human genetics an exact science at last: if the incidence of a trait did not conform with theory, the trait was not hereditary. And if it is actually linked to a blood group, it *must* be hereditary, since the blood groups are a simple direct product of the genes, unaffected by anything in the environment.

Hogben sent a copy of his book to the Director of the London School of Economics soon after it was finished, and followed it with a letter:

Now that I have completed an academic year at the school, I feel that the time has come for me to formulate more definitely a policy for the development of a Research Department of Social Biology, and to explore the prospects of carrying out such a policy successfully. First, let me say that the result of a year's work and thought in a field that was new to me has led me to entertain a very much more optimistic view than I adopted in my initial conversations with you in January, 1930.[75]

It was Bernstein's method for the calculation of linkage which had led him to entertain this new and more optimistic view.

Hogben's book was very widely reviewed in medical, scientific and lay journals.[76] It seems to have acted as a kind of explosive depth charge, bringing to the surface a latent hostility to the eugenists and their programme. The *British Medical Journal*'s reviewer was the most aware of its methodological newness: he felt that it marked 'the beginning of a new phase in human genetics'. Hogben's innovative statistical methods, which the reviewer noticed came from German and Scandinavian writers, would make it possible to get around the old problems of human genetics, the smallness of families and the length of their generation time.

The other reviewers, however, treated the book as an all-out attack on eugenics. The *Lancet*, in an obvious reference to the Society, wrote that 'the story of human genetics should be removed from the atmosphere of the drawing room to that of the laboratory, and that sincere scientific investigation should replace amateur political speculation'. The reviewer said that he was not surprised that Hogben objected to what he had called the eugenists' aristocratic bias, and he endorsed Hogben's opinion that they should be more sure of their facts before demanding political action.

The lay journals were even more trenchant. The *New Statesman and Nation*, well-known as a left-wing weekly, hit the Eugenics Society squarely on the jaw:

> When they assume a simple genetic character for such complicated combinations of heredity and environmental ingredients as produce feeble-mindedness, criminality and even pauperism, boldly confusing economic and biological factors to prove that the poor should be sterilized, the scientific mood has deserted them. Political bias, social prejudice and ethical predilections which have no connection with science have fathered assumptions about the rate and extent of selection which J.B.S. Haldane has shown by mathematical analysis to have no grounds. ... They have filled the bookshelves of the world with dead weight of hearsay, sham expert opinion and doubtful conclusions, based on sufficiently entertaining family histories illustrated by neat little genealogical trees.[77]

J.B.S. Haldane himself, reviewing for *Nature*, was much less hard-hitting. He suggested mildly that serious eugenists should read the book, and that if it provoked a reply on the same scientific level from a holder of the orthodox eugenic view, it would have done an immense service to the eugenics movement.

The eugenists seem to have found the reviews and the reaction to the book more disturbing – and surprising – than the book itself. Soon after the *New Statesman*'s attack came out, Carr-Saunders wrote anxiously to Charles Blacker, General Secretary of the Society:

Do you realize (a) what kind of influence Hogben's book is having and (b) how widespread that influence is? Does *he* realize it?

I have told you how much I genuinely admire the book. But (a) he has emphasized every point that tells against the importance of genetic differences and (b) has expressed some strong criticisms of eugenics.

The consequence is that the book is interpreted as undermining the eugenic position. ... As evidence of this see the reviews in the lay press. Also listen to those who read or look at the book. A man of some eminence ... told me that he understood that Hogben had knocked the bottom out of eugenics.

I have been very much impressed by the extent to which the book is exerting its influence. I am giving public lectures here on eugenics and several members of the audience have at least heard of the book. Tho' not all have seen it and few have read it they are somehow of the opinion that it has shown up eugenics.[78]

Carr-Saunders could not believe that this was what Hogben had really meant to do, and he hoped that Blacker would try to get him to put out some kind of denial.

Blacker, too, thought that Hogben had not really meant to attack eugenics; he saw the book as a correction stemming from within the movement. When Hogben said that eugenics had become associated with snobbery, anti-Semitism and so on, he meant, Blacker thought, that *true* eugenics did not imply anything of the kind. After all, he was in favour of selective breeding, though he wanted to call it 'genetic therapy'. Blacker told Carr-Saunders that he had shown Hogben the letter, and that Hogben denied that his book had given the *coup de grâce* to eugenics. He had pointed to the reviews in the *British Medical Journal*, and the *Medical Officer*, which he said were purely scientific and said nothing at all about eugenics.[79]

Hogben's attitude does seem to have been somewhat ambivalent. He had written that 'it might take years to purge the word "eugenics" of associations which are inimical to the thought of this generation', even though there were now men like C.P. Blacker among the younger leaders of the movement who were prepared to emphasise the medical rather that the political aspects.[80] He had said that it was difficult to see that any reasonable person could disagree with Galton's famous definition of eugenics as 'the study of agencies under social control which may improve or impair the racial qualities of future generations'. Negative eugenics was simply the adoption of the Webb's national minimum of parenthood, *en rapport* therefore with the social theory of the collectivist movement. But because of Galton's aristocratic bias at the start, the eugenic movement had become identified with a 'system of ingenious excuses for combating the amelioration of working class conditions'.[81]

The political aspect of eugenics he rejected completely. Its scientific aspect was defective, though with the new methods it could be improved. But to reject eugenics *as a whole* seemed to him to mean giving up hope of applying the findings of genetics to the human species, and of making practical use of them to improve the human race. In 1931, he still seems to have believed that this was the central tenet of eugenics, and that this at least must be retained. As time went on, and perhaps encouraged by the support of his reviewers, Hogben's belief in the future contributions of eugenics to the human race seems to have weakened. By 1933, in a collection of essays entitled *Nature and Nurture*, he could make the statement that hope for the future of mankind lay in changing not the genotype but the form of social organisation. Human genetics was a branch of medicine, and had nothing to offer as a means of preventing war or controlling unemployment.

Basing his argument on his dislike of the class aspect of the eugenic programme, he now began to focus on the environment problem. Very few human conditions were due to genetic differences that could manifest themselves indifferently in any environment. The eugenists had failed to separate genotype from phenotype, and this their failure as geneticists was political in origin.[82] It was a problem that undermined the credibility of the work of even the most respected of eugenists, R.A. Fisher and Karl Pearson, and was inherent in the mathematical method they used, the method of correlation.

The work on the correlation of the intelligence of twins gave Hogben his opportunity to look at the problem of nature and nurture in correlations between relatives, and to make a closely argued attack on Fisher's conclusion as to the factors contained in the variance. He noticed that, in the case of height, Fisher's conclusion depended on the assumption that environment is a randomly distributed variable, an assumption with obvious political content. Hogben's argument in essence is, that if the correlation coefficient r is written in the form

$$1 - r = \frac{V_p}{V}$$

where V is the variance for the whole population, and Vp is the variance within a single family, it is clear that r is greater or less according as differences *within* a family are large or small compared to differences *between* families, whether the difference is genetic or environmental. Hogben's argument rests on the controlled feeding experiments that had become the standard method of research in the physiology of nutrition: the variance between rats in the same cage was of a different order from that between rats in two different cages. The variance in growth between young rats in the same cage, the same distance from the light, and fed on the same supplemental diet, *might* be due to genetic make-up. But there could be no such conclusion if the rats were in different boxes, fed different diets and with different access to sunlight.[83]

Hogben knew, as everyone did, that there were striking differences in height between working-class and upper-class children at any given age. He felt that it was obvious that the environment of families belonging to the same social class was far more uniform than that of families belonging to different classes. Environment was *not* randomly distributed.

> That the study of fraternal correlations leads some students of human inheritance [sc., Fisher] to the conclusion that there is little or no indication of 'non-genetic causes' tending to produce differences of stature in human populations may throw more light upon the limitations of statistical technique and their method of interpretation than upon the physiology of human growth.

Hogben concludes:

> A much abused philosopher of the nineteenth century [sc., Marx, I presume] has remarked that, 'all the mysteries which seduce speculative thought into mysticism find their

solution in human practice and concepts of that practice'.
... The only practical significance which Fisher's analysis of
variability seems to admit is that if it were correct, we could
only reduce variance with respect to stature in a human
population by 5 per cent or less if the environment were
perfectly uniform.[84]

Under the aegis of the Chair of Social Biology, and with
the enthusiastic support of Sir William Beveridge, Hogben
organised a team to investigate the biological basis of human
society, directed consistently to the definition of the biological
and its separation from the social. The group in the London
School of Economics worked in three main fields: genetic
psychology, including the inheritance of intelligence; the physiology of human reproduction and its relation to demography,
by Enid Charles, then married to Hogben, with Robert René
Kuczynski and David V. Glass; and the work on mathematical
genetics and linkage, which was led by Hogben himself. In each
of these fields it was Hogben's intention to define the area of the
biological in human society, and to confine it within what
could be supported by rigorously scientific methods, freeing the
subject of social biology fron its penumbra of unfounded
assertions and class-bias.

It was Hogben's pride that *his* work could not be faulted for
class-bias. But his and his team's conclusions were certainly very
close to what he would have wished them to be. Their investigation of intelligence, class and educational opportunity in
London schoolchildren found that among all children of high
ability, one-half belonged to the most numerous class, that of
manual labourers, and only one-twentieth to the professional
class. But the educational opportunities they had were very
unequal: nineteen out of twenty children of the professional
class, with or without high ability, went on to higher education,
whereas among the unskilled, only one-fifth of even the most
able did so. The authors called those without high ability who
went to higher education 'wasters': one-third of the upper-class
children were wasters, but practically none of the labourers.[85]
Hogben sent his director a copy of a review of this work with a
thick marginal mark drawing attention to the place where the
reviewer had said: 'The work has evidently been done very
carefully, with every reasonable precaution against error and

prejudice. (The authors had, of course, no social, political, or educational axe to grind.)[86]

Hogben's own publications were mostly in the area of mathematical genetics, in both 'factorial analysis' and the search for linkage. That was clearly where he expected the most significant results. He lectured on it to medical schools and societies, and he managed to interest the Medical Research Council in setting up a Committee for Human Genetics with J.B.S. Haldane as Chairman.[87] The Committee helped him with funding for his linkage studies.[88]

The first of Hogben's projects to make use of the more rigorous methods of the new human genetics was his re-analysis of the old literature on alcaptonuria, which had been thought, by Archibald Garrod in 1902, to be due to a single recessive Mendelian factor. There was no means of doing a linkage study on this, as there was no blood-group material available on Garrod's families, but he was able to use the new method of factor analysis to confirm the old results.[89] David Slome, a young member of Hogben's team, did a similar analysis of cases of amaurotic family idiocy from the literature, using Hogben's method, based as before on Lenz's consanguinity calculation, as developed by Hogben himself.[90]

Their next investigation seems to have been the first in Britain to make use of blood grouping. Friedreich's ataxia is a degenerative condition of the spinal cord in which children appear to be normal at birth but begin to show the symptoms of ataxia in late childhood or youth. The team collected the names of Friedreich's families from hospitals in London and the provinces, and set out to visit them. The visitor was to take blood samples and test the family for the ability to taste phenyl-thio-carbamide, an ability just recently found to be inherited. The departmental 'leg man', Dr Ray Pollack, and sometimes her husband, drove from village to village in a hired car, staying in small hotels, tracing the relatives of the Friedreich's ataxia families, and of another family with brachydactyly. It is the first English account of a procedure that later became painfully familiar to everyone, including the author of this book, working on blood-group genetics.

The report on the project came out in 1935. No linkage had been found, As they remarked sadly, 'The yield of revelant information obtained in linkage studies confined to a few genes

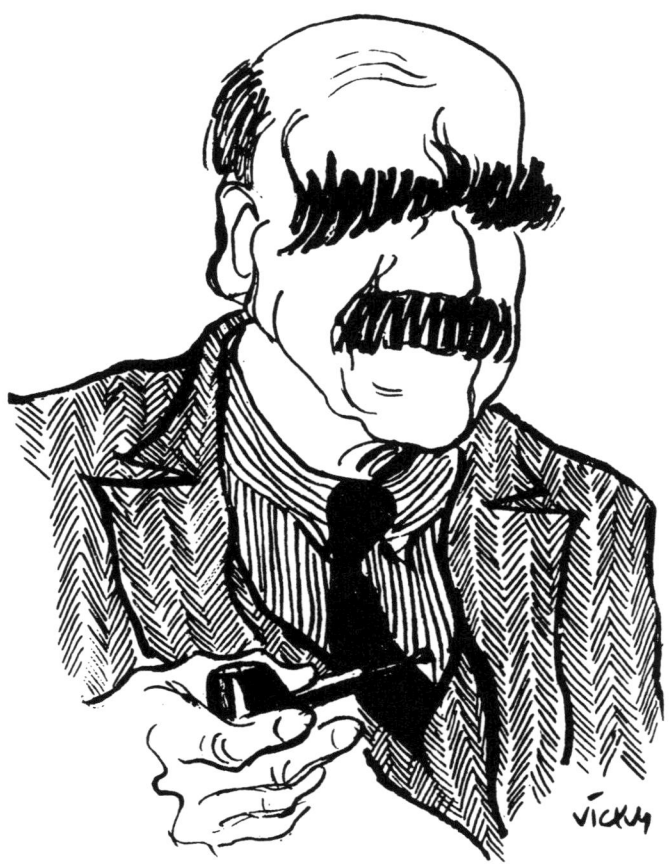

Figure 4.1 John Burdon Sanderson Haldane, a cartoon by Vicky
Source: New Statesman Profiles: Drawings by Vicky (1957), London: Phoenix House.
Courtesy of Library of Congress, Washington, D.C.

is very small.' R.A. Fisher later claimed that there had been a linkage hidden in their data but that they had missed it.[91] The study that Hogben's young South African colleague Zieve undertook with the blood group geneticist Alexander S. Wiener, a member of Landsteiner's group in New York, was as disappointing as Hogben's own. Wiener and Zieve found no linkage between allergic disease, blood groups amd eye colour, although again, it was later suggested that they might have missed it.[92]

In spite of the initial lack of success in finding a linkage, Hogben's new methods and his critique of eugenics attracted the attention of geneticists. One of the first to follow this lead was John Burdon Sanderson Haldane, who had known Hogben for many years and was his colleague in the Society for Experimental Biology and on the Medical Research Council's Human Genetics Committee. Like Hogben, Haldane was a mathematician, a geneticist and a leftist (see Figure 4.1). For him, as for Hogben, *Vererbungsmathematik* offered a means of purifying eugenics of its class-bias and of its amateurism. Human genetics might still contribute something to the human race, once it had lost its less desirable associations.

Haldane had been educated at Eton and St John's College, Cambridge. His father, John Sanderson Haldane, was Professor of Physiology at St John's College, Oxford; his father's brother, Viscount Haldane of Cloan, had been a Secretary of War who had reorganised the British army, and had twice been Lord Chancellor, once in the Labour Government of 1924. His grandmother, Mary Burdon Sanderson, was the sister of the Oxford physiologist John Burdon Sanderson. If Hogben's sense of the injustice of eugenics could be put down to lower-class resentment, or Nietzschean *ressentiment* at upper-class exclusiveness, Haldane's certainly could not. He himself felt that a distinguished ancestry helped to protect its possessors against the establishment. In fact, the Haldanes were a powerful part of the establishment and Haldane's own aristocratic self-confidence, and upper-class rudeness, are mentioned by several of his memorialists, and others who knew him.[93]

Haldane's interest in genetics dated from his childhood, when he and his sister Naomi, later Naomi Mitchison, carried out Mendelian breeding experiments with two guinea pigs named Bateson and Punnett.[94] Haldane had been a socialist since he was a student, but that had not prevented his mother, his sister and himself from being members of the Oxford branch of the Eugenics Society in 1913–14.[95] In 1923, after his war service, he transferred to Cambridge, to the Department of Biochemistry under Frederick Gowland Hopkins, to which he added, from 1927 onwards, the post of 'Officer-in-Charge of Genetic Investigations' at the John Innes Horticultural Research Station. In 1933, he became Professor of Genetics at University College, London, succeeding to one-third of Karl Pearson's chair. Of the

177

other two parts, the eugenics professorship was held by R.A. Fisher, and that of statistics by Egon Pearson, Karl Pearson's son.

In 1932, when Haldane first made a definite statement of his views of eugenics, he was not yet a Marxist. He called himself a 'lukewarm member of the Labour Party' and thought of himself as 'less interested in politics than most'.[96] His genetics and his politics, as well as his obvious pleasure in his own eccentricity, were the product of a mixed intuitive and scientific leaning towards the appreciation of diversity. It is a thread that can be followed throughout his political and scientific evolution. In 1932, diversity meant human inequality, of a kind that did not differ very much from that of the mainline eugenists. 'No doubt environment', he wrote, 'did count for something, but its field was limited; eugenics was the only way of improving the innate character of man'.[97] The year before, he had written an introduction to his wife Charlotte's translation of Johannes Lange's *Verbrechung als Schicksal* in which he welcomed Lang's demonstration that identical twins would usually have the same career in crime, if they were brought up in the same environment. The few cases recorded of identical twins brought up apart seemed to show that environment did count for something, so more work was needed, Haldane thought, to complete the experiment. His conclusion was that of biological determinism: there was no space left here to be filled up by free-will. Destiny was genetics plus environment.

Neither Charlotte Haldane, who was an enthusiastic leftist at this time, nor Haldane himself, had any difficulty in accepting Lange's thesis, however.[98] Genetic determinism, with a brief nod to the environment, was as typical of the left as of the right. It was the deterministic aspect that had attracted Haldane's interest. Two other well-known leftists, the Americans Eden and Cedar Paul, had also translated a German work; in their case the original was the famous genetics and eugenics textbook of Baur, Fischer and Lenz.[99] Environment had no particular significance for the Pauls either: the idea of 'scientific Calvinism' in which scientific laws had replaced humanistic anomie was attractive to the progress-oriented mind. Socialism and eugenics must go hand in hand, said Eden Paul in 1917.[100] As Haldane wrote in 1932, in a statement that can easily be interpreted as a general endorsement for eugenics, the progress of biology will force us to accept that men are innately unequal; the scientific state would make it its first business to investigate this inequality, and to tailor both education and vocational guidance to fit it. It is a statement which seems to accept class differences in intelligence, and to envisage class differences in education to match. But at the same time, he also recognised that eugenics as a practical programme was both scientifically and socially premature, and that it was steeped in class bias. Sterilisation, he said, had always been an instrument of class war.

In the classless society far-reaching eugenic measures could be enforced by the state with little injustice. Today this would not be possible. We do not know in most cases, how far social failure and success are due to heredity and how far to environment. And environment is the easiest of the two to improve.[101]

By the time he wrote this, Haldane had been preoccupied with the genetics of evolutionary change for the previous ten years. The heart of his science lay in genetic diversity and its mathematical relation to evolution. His 'mathematical theory of natural selection' appeared in instalments throughout the twenties, in dialogue with R.A. Fisher.[102] His first paper on it appeared in 1924, and dealt with the slow selection for a gene in a large population. It began with the model of a random-mating population composed of three genotypes in a ratio,

$$u^2 \, AA \; : \; 2u \, Aa \; : \; 1aa.$$

This is the Hardy-Weinberg ratio, which is reached after one generation of random mating. It remains in stable equilibrium unless it is unbalanced by selection pressures acting to shift the ratio to a new equilibrium, which will then be maintained as long as the selection pressure continues. Haldane calculated the changes in proportions under a variety of conditions: selection favouring a dominant, a recessive and a sex-linked gene. The effects of varying gene frequencies and selection pressures were worked out. The result of the calculations showed that the number of generations required for a given change in gene frequencies depended on the intensity of selection and on the gene frequency at the start. Selection for or against most genes, especially rare recessives, would be very slow indeed, requiring thousands of generations. If the selection was for a single

NATURAL SELECTION

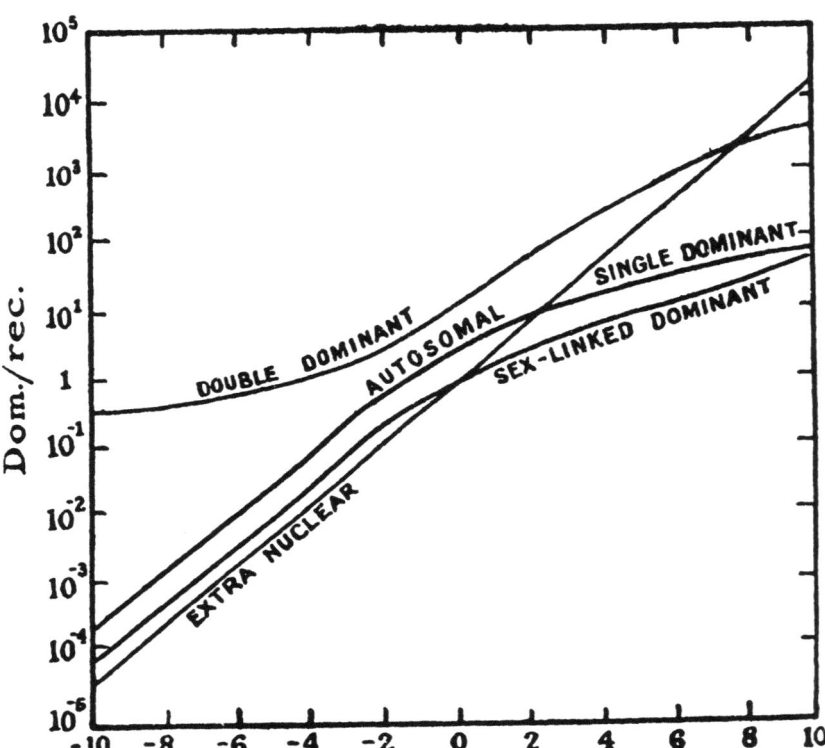

Theoretical results of selection on the composition of a population when dominants are favoured. Abscissa, number of generations multiplied by coefficient of selection. Ordinate, ratio of dominants to recessives. If the races do not interbreed the effect is the same as for an extra-nuclear factor. In the case of the double dominant, the genes are supposed to be present in equal numbers. If recessives are favoured, the sign of the abscissa is changed. For example, if $k = 0 \cdot 01$, it will be seen that about 400 generations are needed for the ratio of dominants to recessives to change from 1 to 10, if autosomal single dominants are favoured.

Figure 4.2 Haldane's calculation of the rates of genetic change to be expected in the case of different types of genetic determinant
Source: Haldane, *Causes of Evolution* (1932): 99

dominant gene, and 1,001 of its type survived to breed for every 1,000 without it, he calculated that it would take 11,739 generations to increase the number of dominants from $1:10^6$ to $1:2$. If the gene was a recessive, it would take 321,444 generations (Figure 4.2).[103]

Two things may be said about Haldane's mathematical model. Firstly, it is based on the Hardy-Weinberg equilibrium, and involves no correlation methods, unlike Fisher's paper of 1918: gene frequencies, not measured phenotypes, are the subject of selection in this model. It is the perfect example of what Ernst Mayr was later to call 'bean-bag genetics'.[104] The beans, or genes, leak gradually out of the bag by negative selection, and they may be dropped back in again by mutation. There is no suggestion of a real population, real defects or real data, even data from *Drosophila*, to test the results on. Real human data had to await the coming of the blood groups, the objective correlative, in T.S. Eliot's phrase, of the beans in human life. Weinberg had never been so bloodless.

Secondly, evolutionary change in Haldane's genetically diverse model populations was very, *very* slow indeed, unless selection pressure was unusually severe. The only type of gene that could spread in measurable time was a single dominant, and then only with very high selection pressure, since only with this type were all the genes, including those in heterozygotes, subject to the pressure.

Haldane's experience of actual organisms came from his work on the genetics of plants and their pigments at the John Innes Institution, and from his teaching on enzyme biochemistry while he was at Cambridge.[105] It was not difficult for him to find examples of all kinds of genetical diversity, or of the 'comparative biology of varieties' even though his own thinking in genetics took the form of simplified mathematical models.[106] The 'physiological point of view', as he called it, was that a gene determined a unit reaction, not a phenotype or even a unit-character. The direct product of the gene was a single enzyme. In maize, for example, there were eleven phenotypic varieties known that had no chlorophyll. There must therefore be at least eleven different pairs of genes involved in the chain of reactions leading to chlorophyll production. Similar conditions were known in animals and in man. Besides alcapatonuria, the original 'inborn error' of protein metabolism discovered by

Archibald Garrod in 1904, there was also phenlyketonuria, another hitch in protein breakdown found in 1934 by Fölling in Norway in some cases of mental defect. The two conditions were thought to be due to two different recessive genes, each determining the absence of a different oxidising enzyme in the metabolic pathway of protein breakdown. Other recently discovered (or recently popularised) forms of biochemical individuality were the blood groups of man and animals.[107]

This background in genetic theory was a major source of Haldane's views on eugenics. His 1934 answer to a claim by Dean Inge provides an example of that link. Inge had said in a lecture to the British Science Guild that no progress in the quality of the race could occur without evolution in human intelligence. Haldane answered that human progress and evolution took place along utterly different time scales, an insight that came from his calculations on the rates of evolution as well as from his belief that state and society could, and should, undergo rapid progressive change. Dean Inge's remarks only served to mark him as a conservative, a man who did not believe in social progress. Eugenic sterilisation of defectives would make little difference to the incidence of most abnormalities in any measurable length of time, and could never be carried out without class discrimination. It was always done on economic as well as genetic grounds.

Haldane argued that the phrase 'innate ability' was meaningless in all but a very few extreme cases, such as microcephalic idiocy. The eugenists had written a good deal on 'the so-called "social problem group"', men and women who were petty criminals, and unemployed even in prosperous times. He could accept that there was a genetic element there: they were, he said, quoting Lidbetter, 'on the whole endogamous'. But there was no proof at all that, given a different environment, they might not turn out to be quite different. His example of a variety and its performance in different environments came from stockbreeding. He felt that government action in applying the 'newer knowledge of nutrition' to providing a proper diet for poor children – subsidised milk in particular – would be the best way of preventing physical, and mental, defect. And he advocated a state medical service to take charge of preventive medicine for the poor, even though, as he said, the middle class would get more expert treatment from a capitalistic medical system.[108]

Here we can clearly see Haldane's association of leftist politics with concern for environment. He criticises Inge as 'conservative', he argues against what he sees as the interests of his own class, and he advocates a welfare state. His position on the politics of the environment has become clearer: but not only is Haldane moving to the left, the left itself is becoming associated with environmentalism and the conservative right with genetic remedies.

By 1939, Haldane had become even more outspoken, and more thoroughly political in his views on eugenics. He reiterates, as he did over and over again, that in our society the sterilisation of all certified defectives could not be anything but a class measure. The seeming frequency of certifiable feeble-minded children among the poor is not a sign of the innately low intelligence of their class, but of their inability to maintain a non-earning member. Sterilising such children, and turning them out of their institutions to face the economic struggle on their own, would relieve the better-off of the cost of maintaining them, but it would be a step backwards, morally. Haldane notes an American eugenist who says that she does not believe that care and pity by the strong for the weak have helped civilisation. He not only thinks otherwise, but associates this American view with eugenics as a whole. He ends what can only be called a polemic against eugenics by saying:

> I do not believe that any of these eugenical schemes are likely to be of much importance because I take the view that the economic changes which we may expect in the near future will be determined by causes much more powerful than the arguments that any biologist may bring forward; and it may be desirable that biologists should confine themselves to questions such as the heritance of well marked characteristics concerning which it is possible to arrive at some measure of agreement. If they do not, they may prejudice large sections of society against whole fields of biological research ... a consideration of human biology does not, in my opinion, justify the perpetuation of class distinctions.[109]

Eugenics, not biological research, had set the poor against the rich. Haldane echoes Hogben's fear that the increasingly influential working class will damn genetics altogether if it is always used against them.[110]

Haldane's new human genetics began to appear in the *Journal of Genetics* in 1932, soon after Hogben's. Like Hogben, he saw the history of his thought as beginning with *Drosophila*, and passing through Bernstein's blood-group *Vererbungsmathematik*, to linkage and chromosome mapping in the human species. With the right team of scientific workers on the job, he estimated that a sufficient background of normal genes could be assembled for between £3,000 to £4,000. Linkages would soon begin to fall into place.[111] But instead of going ahead with the use of blood-group markers for all chromosomes in the Bernstein manner, Haldane took up the problem of just one chromosome pair, that concerned with sex, and tried to map the genes associated with them. He argued that the sex chromosomes X and Y were unequal, X being longer than Y. Genes on the part of X that had no homology with Y would be completely sex-linked, as in haemophilia. If there were genes on the other, homologous, parts of the XY pair, they could be incompletely sex-linked, passed on from a father to most of his sons (linkage), and some of his daughters (crossing over), using sex as the genetic marker, rather than a blood group, which had been Hogben's plan. Haldane listed six pathological conditions that he thought might be 'partly sex-linked', and using a version of Bernstein's method, he calculated linkage distances and mapped them onto a human chromosome.[112]

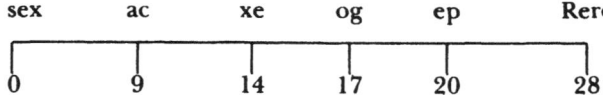

sex	ac	xe	og	ep	Rere
0	9	14	17	20	28

ac: *Achromatopsia:* total colour blindness, a recessive

xe: *Xeroderma pigmentosum:* severe light sensitivity, a recessive

og: Oguchi's Disease: night blindness with golden retinal pigmentation, a recessive

ep: *Epidermolysis bullosa dystrophia:* a severe blistering of the skin, a recessive

Rere: *Retinitis pigmentosa:* with deafness, a recessive; without deafness, a dominant

Figure 4.3   Haldane's map of the homologous part of human sex chromosomes
Source: 'Provisional map of a human chromosome' (1936), n. 112

Like Hogben, Haldane repeatedly says that he hopes that linkage studies and chromosome mapping will offer some hope of tracing deleterious genes in families known to carry particular recessives. It is here that what he calls a 'sane eugenic policy' may find application.[113] There is eugenics as proposed by the Eugenics Society – by men like the *moderate* eugenist Charles Blacker, whom Haldane quotes as saying that people who are below average in intelligence should be sterilised, even if they are not actually defectives – and then there is the 'sane eugenics policy' which could be constructed upon the results of 'good' biological research.[114]

The significance of the new genetics of the thirties was that it allowed for the repudiation of the old class-bound eugenics, which had represented, up to that time, all of human genetics. Thus the geneticists of the left could combine the explosion of polemics against eugenics with an acceptance of the idea that human genetics still had something to offer for the improvement of the human race. The product of this new rigorousness was Haldane's *New Paths in Human Genetics* of 1941. This was alone among Haldane's books in receiving reviews that were more than a polite appreciation of his talent for the general popularisation of science.[115] Unlike Hogben's, his polemics were never felt to have 'knocked the bottom out of eugenics'. The *Times Literary Supplement* said that he 'deals with matters of great importance for medicine and eugenics'. ... 'The range and power of modern genetical methods and ideas are abundantly illustrated in these pages. That they envisage a vast programme of future fruitful work is obvious. ...' A fellow geneticist, C.H. Waddington, wrote that the book was an account of some of the most important work to have been done in England in the past decade. English genetics as of 1942 was largely, he said, either Haldane's own, or carried out under his guidance and stimulus. There was no suggestion that he was attacking eugenics. The perception was rather that he was promoting human genetics.

As Loren Graham pointed out, there was no characteristically left-wing attitude at all on eugenics or environmentalism until about 1930, in Germany or in Russia, when the left began to insist on the part played by environment in human social biology, and to attack the eugenists for leaving it out of their calculations. A very similar change took place in Britain, where Hogben's book took the eugenists by surprise and suddenly brought the question of environment into political focus for them.

During the thirties, however, the idea of environment was changing. For the Lamarckian eugenists of the earlier period, it had been seen in terms of degeneration of the germ-plasm caused by 'race poisons', by drink, syphilis and town life. The *Drosophila* workers had been aware that otherwise innocuous factors such as humidity or wind speed could alter the effect of some of the mutations that they studied. But during the thirties the concept of environment in human life and growth began to acquire a new and more practical content.

Class-bound differences in height had been recognised since the *Fitzroy Report* on physical deterioration of 1904.[116] School meals schemes had started in a small way in 1906, under the permissive Provision of School Meals Act, but not all education authorities made use of the Act's permission (see Figure 1.1).[117] After the end of the 1914–18 war, work on nutrition began to gather speed, both in research and in practice. In 1919, the Medical Research Council's Committee on Accessory Food Factors brought out a report on vitamins and milk.[118] The new Ministry of Health, set up in 1919, and the Medical Research Council sponsored a controlled study of the effect of a daily pint of milk on children's growth. The effect was striking: in a single year the boys in the milk group put on twice as much weight and nearly twice as much height as the controls.[119] A Ministry of Health Committee began to pressure the education authorities to enlarge the scope of school feeding. They were backed by the dairy industry through its National Milk Publicity Council of 1922, and in 1924 a school milk scheme began, which in the thirties was expanded by the Milk Publicity Council to provide milk in factories, as well as in schools. From the Milk Council's point of view, it was a brilliant opportunity to increase milk consumption and absorb agricultural surplus. Research, government and industry were united in its promotion.

During the 1930s, official and semi-official interest in nutrition and growth went on expanding. The Medical Research Council produced a series of special reports, beginning with one on vitamins in 1932.[120] In 1933, the British Medical Association published its minimum nutrition scales. The most effective of these reports was that of John Boyd Orr, then Director of the Rowett Institute for Research in Animal Nutrition at Aberdeen.

Boyd Orr had already produced several milk studies, and had been speaking, writing and broadcasting on the need for a national food policy. His report on *Food Health and Income* of 1936 concluded that 'a diet completely adequate for health, according to modern standards, is reached at an income level above that of 50 per cent of the population'. A large part of the population lived on bread, jam, margarine, tea and sugar.

The report focused specifically on the relation of nutrition and height to income. Boyd Orr wrote,

> It is well known that stature is largely determined by heredity. The extent to which a child will attain the limit set by heredity is however, affected by diet. Certain deficiencies of the diet lead to a diminution in the rate of growth, with the result that the adult does not attain the full stature made possible by his inherited capacity.[121]

Measurements of boys from different classes of school showed the same orders of difference as they had done in the 1904 Fitzroy *Report*. In the early thirties, middle-class English boys of 17 were 3.8 inches taller than 'employed males', and boys from the highest income group were approximately 5 inches taller (Figure 4.4). Boyd Orr noted carefully that no diet, however good, would allow an individual to grow taller than the limit set by heredity. Short stature in the wealthier groups, he wrote, is mostly inherited.

Pressure for an explicit national food policy did come from the scientists of the left, but it was certainly not confined to the left alone.[122] Boyd Orr himself, who was instrumental in spreading the campaign for improved nutrition of children to the League of Nations, and finally to the post-Second World War Food and Agriculture Organisation, was no leftist. He sat in Parliament for a short time as an Independent, though his peerage was an award by the Labour Government of 1948.[123]

As interest in nutrition, and the links between class, height, nutrition and income became more widely publicised and accepted, the left wing's environmentalist attack on the old-line eugenists gained in persuasiveness. It began to persuade the eugenists themselves. Mary Karn, writing in the *Annals of Eugenics* under Fisher's editorship, recognised that the height differences she measured between groups of schoolchildren were probably mainly nutritional.[124] Insensitivity to environmental

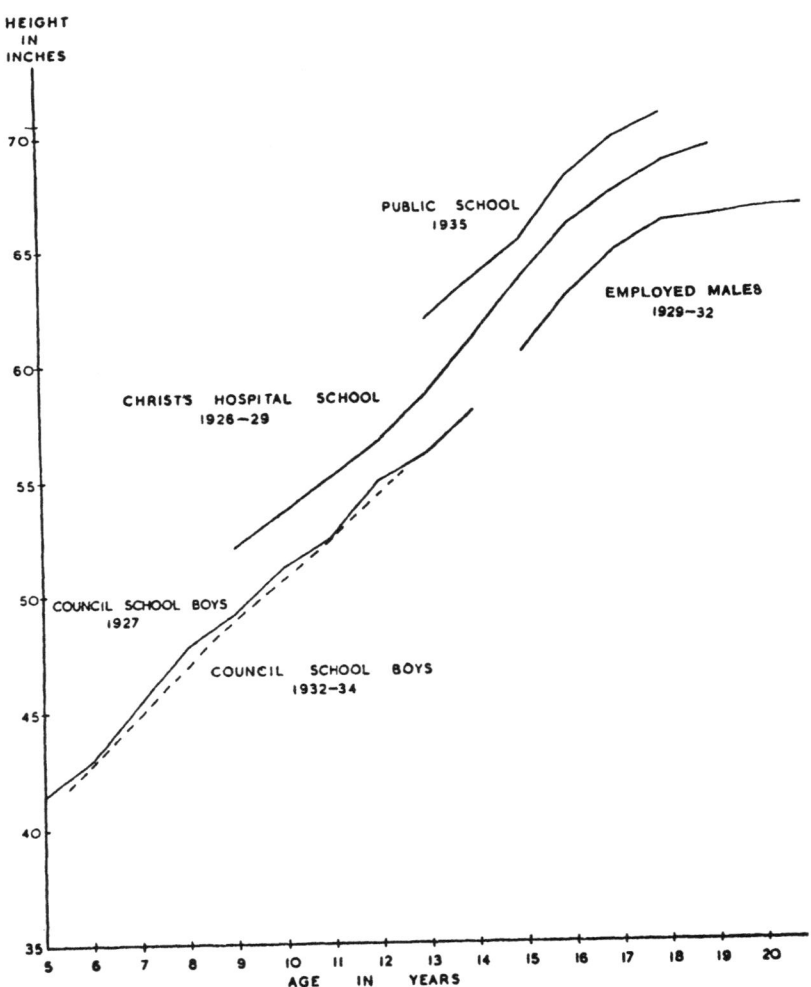

Figure 4.4 Heights of males by social groups
Source: Boyd Orr, *Food, Health and Income* (1936): 40

effects became synonymous with a stand against a very
generally accepted form of social progress, as Haldane and
Hogben were arguing. Milk programmes with their instant
benefits looked more promising than eugenic ones, at least until

the kind of inequality represented by class height differentials could be corrected.

Hogben had criticised Fisher's 1918 assumption that environment, by which Hogben had meant nutrition, had a random effect on height, and he had looked forward to a time when these class nutritional differences would be equalised. Haldane, in 1932, had argued that genetic inequality should be accepted and appropriate educational and vocational guidance provided, a tacit accommodation to class differences in intelligence. By 1938, his statement on the acceptance of genetic diversity had undergone a subtle change: now the state was seen as compensating for human differences in such a way as to produce a classless society. He rejected what he called the 'Jeffersonian doctrine of equality', the American liberal doctrine that all men were created equal, that is, identical, partly on the grounds of his own work on genetic variability, and partly on Marxist grounds.[125] '*From each according to his ability, to each according to his needs*', seemed to him to express an acceptance of human differences that matched his own theoretical genetics, with its emphasis on genetic diversity, and his sense of social justice.[126] The somewhat arrogant tone of his popular writing on this subject of 1932 gave way to his statement of 1938, when his Marxism had become more complete. Both statements were built upon Haldane's understanding of genetic diversity in animal and plant materials, and in mathematical models. But by 1938, he no longer expected biology to be linked to class. He now saw that the existing eugenics programme was an example of the impossibility of passing directly from biology to economics, which represented a new dialectical level.[127]

Neither Hogben nor Haldane ever felt that the repudiation of eugenics should include all of human genetics. Both thought that the eugenics programme was premature, that human genetics was not yet well enough developed to have anything to say about social policy. But they did not feel that it would always be so. The time *might* come when human genetics had gained and class differences had lost, and a eugenic programme might still be possible. To deny that completely would have meant denying the worth of their own field, and of their own work in it. Human genetics *was* eugenics, as it had been since 1900. It was impossible for geneticists who were interested in human material at all to distance themselves completely from the eugenic problematic, in spite of their disapproval of so much of the programme. It represented the practical utilisation of their own contributions to scientific knowledge.

It may seem paradoxical that the geneticists of the left still entertained some faint but persistent hope that their science was the longed-for 'agency under social control' that might benefit the human race, in some more perfect future time.[128] But human genetics had grown in sophistication and power. The introduction of the German methods during the thirties had re-made the science in a way that was to affect the thinking of both the left-wing critics and the eugenists themselves. It should be remembered that the source of the new methods was, for the most part, the German eugenics movement. Wilhelm Weinberg and Fritz Lenz were not only human geneticists, and leaders in *Vererbungsmathematik*, they were also leaders of German eugenics which was then, in the early thirties, reaching the apogee of its productivity and its political influence. There was no sense that the eugenics movement as a whole was in decline.

The lives of Hogben and Haldane have a curious complementarity, beginning from their entry from opposite ends of the social spectrum. Hogben's proposal of the method of linkage led to Haldane's discovery, if it was one, of human linkage and a map of a human chromosome. Hogben's Marxism and his radical leadership in social biology were followed by, though one can hardly say it led to, Haldane's 1937 conversion to Marxism. But by 1938 Hogben had abandoned both his Marxism and his Chair of Social Biology. During the thirties, Hogben's Marxism, and his belief in the practical benefits to society of science and scientific education, led him to write his two enormously successful 'self-educators', *Mathematics for the Million* and *Science for the Citizen*.[129] They were clearly Marxist in inspiration. *Science for the Citizen*, like J.G. Crowther's and J.D. Bernal's histories of science, was patterned after Boris Hessen's famous Marxist interpretation of Newton's work as a product of the practical needs of his day, one of the papers read at the 1931 Congress for the History of Science.[130,131] In 1936, Hogben's respect for Hessen, and for Crowther's *hessische* history of science, and for Soviet Communism, were firmly stated in a paper he wrote for the first volume of a new American Marxist journal, *Science and Society*:

> Soviet collectivism ... is planning the development of research on a scale unprecedented in the history of capitalism.

Inevitably, the younger scientific workers are forced to re-examine their orientation to the political struggle from which the Soviet Union has recently emerged. ... The vital issue is not whether the man of science should or should not be partisan. It is what form his partisanship should take. Part of his cultural task is to bring into being a new awareness of the scientific outlook. Part of his responsibility is to educate his fellow citizens to realize the potential of social welfare in the knowledge we possess.[132]

Science and education, and the potential of science for human welfare, were the theme of Hogben's writings through the middle and later thirties. In 1936, he put them in a context of Marxism, but they had an earlier connection with the Huxleyan positivism that had been his philosophy before 1931, and which had never disappeared from his thinking. But by 1939, less than a year after the appearance of *Science and the Citizen*, Hogben had suddenly rejected Soviet Communism altogether as being incapable of realising a 'planned economy of abundance'.[133]

The new creed that he adopted, which he called 'scientific humanism', put the responsibility of science to society at the centre, and dropped any further political implications:

The social contract of scientific humanism is the recognition that the sufficient basis for rational cooperation between citizens is scientific investigation of the common needs of mankind, a scientific inventory of resources available for satisfying them, and a realistic survey of how modern social institutions contribute to, or militate against the use of such resources for the satisfaction of fundamental needs.[134]

By the time he passed through Russia on the Trans-Siberian Railway in 1940, he was able to write of Russia in the tone of loathing and disgust that is sometimes found in English descriptions of conditions in Calcutta, describing the ugliness of its towns and villages, the sluttishness and disorderly habits of its people, their illiteracy and their inability to count.[135]

The last act of his Marxist years is the essay he wrote mourning Haldane's adoption of Marxism, and explaining his own rejection of it. In 1931, he had written as an English materialist trying to explain the philosophers of communism to an English audience. In 1940, he rejected Marxism for the same reasons that he had found it hard to accept and explain in 1931, and which had gone against the grain of his earlier training. 'Dialectic materialism' is a contradiction in terms, he wrote in 1940, returning to his old use of 'dialectical' to mean 'merely verbal'. His old dislike of Hegel reappears – the function of the dialectic is that of a myth which 'permeates the world of discourse with implicit conviction that progress can only be achieved through violence'. It is an ideology in which even its advocates cannot literally believe. 'This business of preparing for an Age of Plenty is so serious and compelling that we cannot afford to befuddle our brains with an unnecessary infusion of metaphors.'[136] 'Metaphors', he writes – but he means 'metaphysics': Hogben the positivist has reverted to what he has always known, that the dialectic is a form of metaphysics, and as such no more than a superstition.

In 1937, Hogben accepted a call to the University of Aberdeen, as Regius Professor of Natural History. The Department of Social Biology at the London School of Economy closed down, leaving only Kuczynski and Glass behind. There was no overt decision not to make a new appointment, but one was never made. The department came to an end.

The attack on the eugenics movement which was led by Hogben was directed against both its ideology and its methods. His criticism of its class-bias was paralleled by his criticism of the pedigree methodology. The new 'ethically neutral science' of factor analysis and linkage was to stop short at the boundary between the biological and the social. The use of the new methods was to be confined to distinct clinical and biological traits; the analysis of the inheritance of blood groups, of haemophilia and Friedreich's ataxia was to replace that of pauperism and the social problem group. But even the Society's enemies were constrained to engage with it in the problematic that it had constructed around human genetics. Hogben and Haldane, but especially Hogben, directed a part of their work to arguing against the eugenists on matters involving the classes and their supposedly inherited characteristics.

During the period 1931 to 1938 when Hogben was making this attack he was apparently a Marxist; but his Marxism does not seem to have been the only source of his thought. The outline of his thinking was already formed before he came across Marxism. His attack on the eugenists for their class-bias and their confusion of the biological and the social had already begun in 1930. Marxism provided him with useful arguments; it gave him a sense that there were powerful forces supporting his position. It seems to have reinforced his attitudes, but not created them.

The main elements of his criticism were a product not only of Marxism but also of the Huxleyan positivism that he professed before 1931. The emphasis on the social function of science which grew in his writing during the thirties and which he referred at the time to the example of Hessen, is equally consistent with the Huxleyan emphasis on the benefits of science as education, and it was to this line of thought that Hogben reverted after he abandoned Marxism. T.H. Huxley's statement of 1889 on the purpose of his life's work could have been written, *mutatis mutandis*, by Hogben:

> To promote the increase of natural knowledge and to forward the application of scientific methods of investigation to all the problems of life to the best of my ability, in the conviction – which has grown with my growth and strengthened with my strength, that there is no alleviation for the sufferings of mankind except veracity of thought and of action, and the resolute facing of the world as it is when the garment of make-believe, by which pious hands have hidden its uglier features, is stripped off. It is with this intent that I have subordinated any reasonable or unreasonable ambition for scientific fame which I may have permitted myself to entertain, to other ends; to the popularization of science; to the development and organization of scientific education; and to untiring opposition to that ecclesiastical spirit, which in England as everywhere else, and to whatever denomination it may belong, is the deadly enemy of science.[137]

Marxism reinforced Hogben's desire to 'forward the application of scientific methods of investigation'. He found support in the idea that materialism was now the philosophy of a state, a state dedicated to the promotion of science, scientific education and the social functions of science; but when his Marxism disappeared, his interest in the popularisation of scientific thinking remained. His hatred of the eugenists was expressed as a hatred of the looseness and lack of scientific rigour which allowed them to be influenced by a social bias which had no place in science. It is the positivist criticism which he expressed first in 1930. After 1931, the additions to his thought came not only from Marxism but also from the new methods of *Vererbungsmathematik*, which replaced the old, unrigorous pedigree method, and the method of correlation.

For Haldane, too, Marxism was a reinforcement of an already established position, although in Haldane's case the conversion was a good deal more thorough. During the period of the thirties when he and Hogben were reforming the methods of human genetics, Haldane was not an opponent of eugenics *per se*, but only of its more clearly class-biased manifestations, such as the teachings of the Dean of St Paul's.[138] Haldane, like Hogben in his Marxist phase, contrasted the ignorance of science among British politicians with the emphasis upon scientific education in Russia:

> What is needed in this country is that young men and women looking forward to a political career should study science seriously. I should like to see the students of Ruskin, for example, imitating the Communists in Sverdlov University in Moscow. ... I happened to go round the biological laboratories in which they worked. I could see at once that their practical work was quite as good as a great deal of the practical work which is done by those in this country who are taking science as a career.[139]

Haldane, the future Marxist, sounds very much like the Marxist Hogben, and even like Hogben, the ex-Marxist, in his belief in science and its methods as a personal philosophy. In both, Huxleyan scientism is reinforced not only by a Marxist philosophy of science, but also by a Communist emphasis on scientific education.

It was the Marxist scientists who forced the change in ideology and in methods in human genetics, but Marxism was not their only heuristic tool. The attack on eugenics was strongly ideologically motivated. The attackers were left-wing, radical and sharply sensitised to the part played by class in the eugenist problematic. They were Marxists but their critique of eugenics was not exclusively Marxist in nature: their heuristic principles were positivist, with Marxist support. The availability of the

German mathematical methods played as important a part in their critique as did their Marxism. This is not a conclusion that the author particularly enjoys; but ethical neutrality being what it is, it must be recorded. And if eugenics was confined to the medical scene, instead of being promoted as a social panacea for and by a single class, then there was nothing wrong with eugenics that could not be cleared up by the more rigorous methods of the new *Vererbungsmathematik*. Blood groups would be the guarantee of value-free science, and the 'newer knowledge of nutrition' would correct its insensitivity to the significance of environment.

5

HUMAN GENETICS AND THE EUGENICS PROBLEMATIC

During the decade of the thirties, the eugenics movement was battered by its critics, the geneticists of the left, and their supporters. But although the attack was furious, it could not aim at expunging the entire eugenics problematic, since that was so intimately interwoven with all current research in human genetics, in Britain as elsewhere. Both the eugenists and their critics were agreed that more research was needed, and both were roughly agreed on the questions that needed to be answered. There was even a broad consensus that, eventually, the knowledge gained might be used to upgrade the human race.[1] It was not until the 1950s, with the coming of the post-war Welfare State and the end of the Poor Law, that the eugenic problematic was finally to fall apart, leaving the field to a residual social biology that retained many of the eugenists' interests, but lacked the social activism that had been typical of the movement.

At the beginning of the thirties, the critics of eugenics were aggressively pointing out the weaknesses in the eugenists' methods of investigation, and the injustice of their class-bias. They felt that the current state of knowledge of genetics made any idea of upgrading humanity very remote, and that environmental improvement was more immediately within reach. The eugenists, on the other hand, kept up their propaganda with hopeful intensity, feeling that their support was growing and that Parliament would eventually pass the eugenic legislation for which they had been pressing so long. More research was needed, but its function was to provide more persuasive figures, rather than new knowledge.

As the criticisms of their methods were driven home with the help of the heavy weapons of mathematical genetics, the eugenists themselves began to show that they were listening to their critics. Men like R.A. Fisher, who had been active in the eugenics movement for decades, took up the new methods. Younger thinkers like Lionel Penrose, entering the field for the first time, found their stride at a time when pressure for change was coming from the critics of the left, and set their course accordingly.

The programme of research in human genetics, however, was still very close to traditional eugenics. Changes in method took place against a background of the old problems and the ongoing political initiatives. The central interests of both eugenists and non-eugenists were the inheritance of mental defect, the social problem group, which was the new name for the old residuum, and the negative eugenics or voluntary sterilisation campaign. The geneticists declared that their role was to investigate the truly scientific problems of human genetics, such as the ordering of genes on the chromosomes. But underlying the scientific search for linkage and genetic markers lay the old problems of negative eugenics.

The new human genetics of the thirties evolved in dialogue with the Society and its programmme. The Society's interests formed the thread upon which the geneticists' pearls were strung.

The thirties was a decade of large-scale official reports on the subject of feeble-mindedness. It began with the *Wood Report* of 1929, on the incidence of mental deficiency in the population, which was followed by the *Brock Report* of 1934 on sterilisation, and the *Colchester Survey* of 1938, Lionel S. Penrose's study of the genetics of feeble-mindedness. One further report that can be considered as belonging to this series on mental deficiency was to follow in 1957. It was that of the Royal Commission on the Law relating to Mental Illness and Mental Deficiency, whose chairman was Lord Percy.

The Eugenics Society was well represented on the Wood Committee.[2] The Committee's mandate, to find out the incidence of mental defect in the population, was a central part of the eugenics tradition. They could look back collectively to its predecessor, the Royal Commission on the Care and Control of the Feeble-Minded of 1906, which had been one of the factors in the foundation of the Eugenics Education Society, as it then was. In fact, A.F. Tredgold, one of the members of the Committee, had appeared before the Royal Commission as an expert witness, and had later represented the Society on a joint committee with the National Association for the Care and Protection of the Feeble-Minded. This committee had drafted the Bill for compulsory detention, which was the forerunner of the Mental Deficiency Act of 1914.[3]

The Wood Committee engaged an investigator to organise a survey of the numbers of the mental defectives in representative communities up and down the country. Their man was E.O. Lewis, an inspector from the Board of Control.[4]

Lewis surveyed six different areas, a careful balance of rural and urban populations, and found that, on average, 8.57 per 1,000 of the population were feeble-minded. Though family histories had not been a focus of the inquiry, he included a few pedigrees in his report, to show the usual mixture of economic and social problems (Figure 5.1).[5] Lewis's conclusions reflected Tredgold's guiding hand.[6] They were that feeble-mindedness was of two distinct types, primary and secondary. The common primary type often amounted to no more than dullness of mind. It was frequently found in families, families that clustered in a single class, with a very low standard of living. The severe or secondary type did not seem to him to be familial at all; the very low-grade cases of idiocy and imbecility were sporadic, scattered evenly through the population in all classes and all kinds of home.

Using Lewis's findings, the Committee reported that mental deficiency was both a genetic and a social problem. Social and economic failure were primarily due to poor mental endowment, but low mentality and poor environment formed a vicious circle. Primary amentia, the commonest type of feeble-mindedness, was often the end result of degeneration.

The report defined the lowest 10 per cent on the social scale as the social problem group. As a group, it was associated not only with feeble-mindedness, but also with insanity, epilepsy, pauperism, crime, unemployability and alcoholism. Only about 10 per cent of this group could actually be certified under present laws, but the Committee thought the others were probably carriers of defect. The science of eugenics was doing valuable service in focusing scientific thought and public opinion

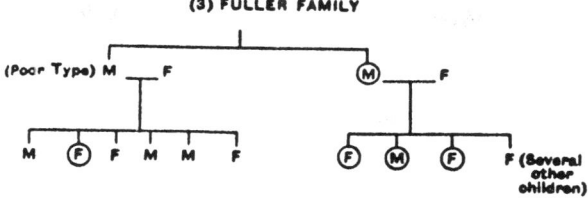

(3) FULLER FAMILY

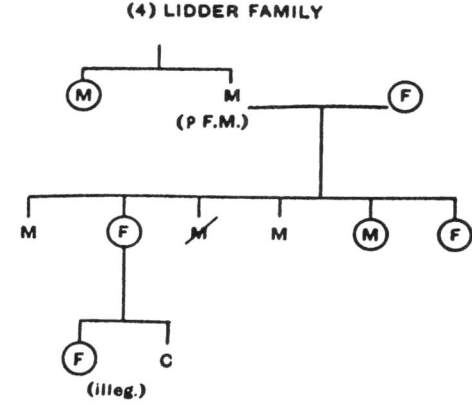

(4) LIDDER FAMILY

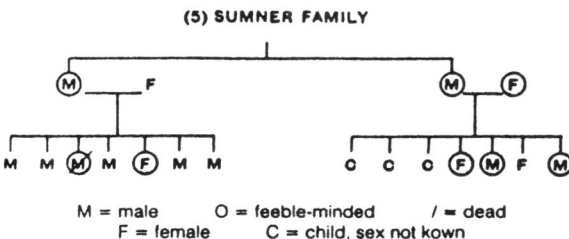

(5) SUMNER FAMILY

M = male   O = feeble-minded   / = dead
F = female   C = child, sex not kown

Figure 5.1 Pedigrees contributed by E.O. Lewis, showing the eugenists'
usual mixture of familial, economic, social and possibly genetic
problems
Source: Wood Report (1929), n. 4, Part IV: 136–7

upon the racial, social and economic problems that the subnormal group represented.

The report did not endorse sterilisation as the solution to the
problem, however. That would not help the social problem

group in their economic struggle, nor would it be any help with the type of very severe amentia that they had called sporadic, since it did not seem to run in families or to have any association with a class. Instead, the Committee's recommendation was for segregation: the lowest 10 per cent must be protected from themselves, and society must be protected from their excessive fertility. This conclusion essentially repeated that of the Royal Commission of twenty-six years before and reiterated the position of the Central Association for Mental Welfare upon the ineffectiveness of sterilisation.[7]

The Wood Committee's *Report* in some ways did what the Eugenics Society's Research Committee had been wanting to do throughout the twenties. Indeed, there was some overlap in the composition of the two committees: Cyril Burt, the absentee chairman of the Research Committee, was a member of the Wood Committee too. The Wood Committee's investigator, E.O. Lewis, and his assistant had quartered the whole country, comparing urban with rural communities and ascertaining the general incidence of feeble-mindedness just as the Society's Research Committee had wanted to do. He had tied feeble-mindedness to pauperism and economic failure and to the class for which the Wood Committee had invented the phrase 'social problem group', but which the eugenists had for many years called 'the residuum'. Lewis's pedigrees were in the traditional eugenists' style. If the Society's Research Committee had had the money, they might have produced the *Wood Report* as a supplement to Lidbetter's pauper pedigrees.

In contrast, the Report of the Vagrancy Committee of the following year showed no influence of the eugenists at all. The Committee, appointed by a Labour Minister of Health, the former economics lecturer Arthur Greenwood, included not one member of the Society, nor did the Society offer a brief in evidence. E.O. Lewis was again invited to do the survey: this time, of the mental level of a sample of vagrants. He found that 15 per cent of them were feeble-minded, 5.4 per cent insane, and 5.7 per cent psychotic. This committee, however, did not think that social failure was mainly genetically determined. Their list of causes of failure buried feeble-mindedness among many others. They cited senility, diseases such as chronic bronchitis, tuberculosis and heart failure, as well as mental infirmity and feeble-mindedness. And they pointedly included a second group of causes, the environmental:

The great part played by environment in all social problems makes it imperative that anyone who wishes to study human failure should have an intimate knowledge of the difficulties the poor have to overcome if they are to steer clear of economic and social disaster.[8]

The eugenists' position was not, therefore, the only one possible for the time. By this time, it was rejected by the left, and particularly, as we shall see below, by organised labour.

The eugenists' position was also rejected by the British Medical Association, whose Mental Deficiency Committee was set up in 1930, and reported in 1932.[9] Five of its twenty-one members were members of the Eugenics Society, including A.F. Tredgold, who was on the British Medical Association's committee, the Wood Committee of 1929, and then on the Brock Committee of 1934. He had also, as we saw above, been an expert witness in 1906, before the Royal Commission on the Care and Control of the Feeble-Minded, and had been involved in the preparation of the Mental Deficiency Act of 1914. Tredgold's was the essential expert opinion in any discussion of feeble-mindedness. But the BMA's Committee also included a number of people soon to become well known as anti-eugenists, such as Letitia Fairfield, a Catholic and Honorary Medical Secretary of the Central Association for Mental Welfare, and Frank Douglas Turner, Medical Superintendent of the Royal Eastern Counties Institution at Colchester who had also served on the Wood Committee, and was to be instrumental in organising the *Colchester Survey*.

The preamble to the BMA's *Report* says that it had been impossible to secure unanimity, which was not surprising in view of the membership of its committee. But the gist of the *Report* is not favourable to the eugenists. A certain amount of valuable work had been done on the study of human pedigrees, the Committee stated, but it had not been sufficiently analysed, for lack of funds – a reference, probably, to the Lidbetter project. More research was needed before any strong claims could be made about the exact type of inheritance of mental defect. The Committee felt that medical practitioners were in a good position to collect pedigree data, and they recommended the Eugenic Society's pamphlet, 'How to prepare a family pedigree', for general use. But the section of the *Report* that dealt with heredity was very short, and essentially went no further than asking for more data. The section on environmental causes was longer and more detailed, and covered conditions such as the injuries and infections which medical people already knew and understood, unlike the laws of heredity, which most of them found difficult and unfamiliar.

The *Report* also pointed out that though there was a 'high correlation between scholastic and social incapacity, nevertheless the two are not identical'. Children who were simply doing badly at school should not be certified; that would only burden them with an additional stigma later on. Such 'defectives' often turned out to be quite capable socially and needed no special care. This common-sense statement from the physicians, with its sceptically anti-eugenic tone, looks forward to the *Colchester Survey* of 1938. It might have been suggested by Douglas Turner, who certainly held those views.[10]

The section on 'Social considerations' took the same position. The problem of undesirable social behaviour was not the same as the problem of mental deficiency. The Report stated in emphatic italics that '*There is a continuous curve of variability in mental power and social capacity and behaviour from the idiot to the normal person*'. The idiot and low-grade imbecile were devoid of all social behaviour. Beyond them, the distinction was not so much the actual social behaviour exhibited, as the capacity for developing any social behaviour at all. It must never be forgotten, they wrote, that 'bad living conditions often produce the same kind of results that bad genes do'. The authorities cited for these statements were Lancelot Hogben, and the American anti-eugenist, Herbert Spencer Jennings. There seemed to be a tendency with certain writers, and perhaps among the professional classes generally, the BMA's *Report* stated, to speak of those who were able to do only simple routine tasks as 'unfit' or 'socially inefficient'. They were not. They were needed by society, even if technically feeble-minded, and must be regarded and treated as effective units in the social machinery. Anti-social conduct was not a necessary, or even a common characteristic, of the mentally defective. Nor did the *Report* find that the feeble-minded were more prolific than the norm.

The section on the prevention of mental deficiency must have caused the Committee a good deal of difficulty, since on this problem its members obviously had irreconcilably different positions. The final statement shows that the eugenists had been voted down. The *carriers* of defect could never be sterilised as a class, since they appear to be quite normal; if certified defectives only were sterilised, the Committee stated, the incidence of mental deficiency would not be appreciably reduced. Sterilisation, therefore, could make no difference to the number of defectives for many generations. The Committee did admit that there was a small number of defectives whose propagation was dangerous. These *might* be sterilised, under safeguards. But no indication was given as to who they were. They could not have been those whom the eugenists saw as the chief danger, the merely dull-at-school, since the physicians saw these people as normal.

The eugenists had failed to persuade the British Medical Association to share their worries. The dangers to the next generation of the feeble-minded and the social problem group, their exuberant and frightening fertility, and the remedy of sterilisation had been discussed, and effectively dismissed. Sir Henry Brackenbury, the Chairman of Council of the British Medical Association, who had been on its Mental Deficiency Committee, took a very outspoken position on the futility of trying to reduce the incidence of mental defect by a sterilisation programme.[11] The eugenists protested at what they called his 'regrettable dogmatic pessimism'.[12] But they had lost the battle for the sympathy of the medical profession, in striking contrast to the position in Germany.

The Wood Committee's *Report* of 1929 was pivotal in the history and politics of human genetics through the thirties. It had recommended a general eugenic policy as a solution to the 'social problem' of feeble-mindedness, even though it had not been in favour of sterilisation, and its findings set the stage for the decade. The Wood Committee's successor, the Brock Committee, began its investigation into the genetics of feeble-mindedness, and the use of sterilisation as a preventive, in late 1932, and reported in 1934. The Medical Research Council's survey of the genetics of feeble-mindedness, carried out by Lionel Sharples Penrose at the Royal Eastern Counties Institution at Colchester, began in 1930 and was reported in 1938. These two reports, the *Brock Report* and the *Colchester Survey*, were linked in turn with the Eugenics Society's campaign to legalise voluntary sterilisation, and with the outpouring of closely argued papers by L.S. Penrose based on the Colchester material, which grew more and more sophisticated throughout the thirties. Both Charles Blacker, General Secretary of the Eugenics Society, and Lionel Penrose were influenced by the ongoing criticisms from the geneticists of the left, and, in their different ways, by the quantitative work of the German eugenists.

The Eugenics Society's campaign for the legalisation of voluntary sterilisation began in 1929.[13] Early in 1930, an initiative by R.A. Fisher, Julian Huxley, E.J. Lidbetter, Charles Blacker and a physician, John A. Ryle, resulted in the formation of the Society's Committee for Legalising Sterilisation, and in the production of the first of a series of propaganda pamphlets in the Committee's name.[14] It was in connection with the updating of the first pamphlet, which gave figures on the transmission of feeble-mindedness, that the Society first made contact with Ernst Rüdin, head of the Genealogical Department of the Deutsche Forschungsanstalt für Psychiatrie in Munich, and a leading German eugenist.

Rüdin's interest in the genetics of psychiatric conditions dated back to 1911, when he produced a long and rather ponderous paper intended to explain Mendelian inheritance to his fellow psychiatrists. It was followed in 1916 by a monograph on the inheritance of *Dementia praecox*, in which he made use of the mathematical methods recently introduced by Wilhelm Weinberg to analyse its transmission.[15] This monograph made Rüdin's reputation: it impressed Emil Kraepelin, doyen of German psychiatry, who had himself claimed that 70 per cent of the cases that he called *Dementia praecox* had some kind of 'hereditary taint' in the family.[16] Kraepelin appointed Rüdin to lead the department of Genealogy and Demography at the Forschungsanstalt then in process of foundation in Munich.[17]

In the course of the twenties, however, Rüdin's interests shifted from the Weinbergian *Vererbungsmathematik* to a new, more empirical type of quantification. Rüdin and his group came to look back on the early attempts to use the Weinbergian method as more or less artificial attempts to force the figures into a Mendelian mould. Psychiatric diagnoses were not clear-cut; the families of *propositi* often contained members who were not strictly psychotic, but were not quite normal either. Rüdin proposed to slash through the difficulties by simply collecting data on the families of psychotics, and recording all abnormalities.

The method required the collection of very large amounts of data on affected families and on normal populations to act as controls. It gave figures which quantified the 'genetic danger' posed by an individual: the data on the children of schizophrenics, for example, showed that only 37 per cent were completely normal, though not all the abnormals could be diagnosed as schizophrenic. Rüdin and his large and well-funded group aimed to collect enough data to build up a 'prognostic canon' that would cover all psychoses, and could be used for the purpose of predicting the quality of the descendants of any individual. They called the method *empirische Erbprognose*, empirical hereditary prognosis.[18] Its practical result was to be the selection of diagnostic categories that would require sterilisation for the elimination of pathological genes from the population. The very large proportion of more-or-less abnormals in the affected families gave a much more alarming picture of the inheritance of defect than did the numbers obtained when a strictly Mendelian model was used. The eugenists at the Munich Forschungsanstalt found the raw data of empirical prognosis satisfyingly appropriate for backing a demand for legislation. It not only magnified the apparent danger, but was far easier for both psychiatrist and politician to understand than the complex arguments of *Vererbungsmathematik*.

In 1930, needing more data to support its sterilisation campaign, the British Society turned to Rüdin. Cora Hodson, the Society's Education Secretary, sent him a copy of the Society's pamphlet. The effect of sterilisation on the numbers of the feeble-minded, she said, had been worked out by R.A. Fisher using figures from the pedigrees collected by H.H. Goddard, in which one or both parents were feeble-minded.[19] Cora Hodson told Rüdin that they proposed to revise the study, and as 'one or two of our people have some prejudice against American work (largely discounted in this country)', she had been asked to beg him to send them whatever data he could.[20]

Rüdin replied with five foolscap pages of detailed references on work by his group and by others in Germany on the inheritance of feeble-mindedness, its incidence in different populations and on the fertility of the feeble-minded, together with four reprints of his own work. Among these was an essay on 'Psychiatric indications for sterilisation', in which Rüdin described the basis of his division's plan of work:

I very much hope to be able eventually to determine the empirical prognosis of descent in definite types of insanity. My procedure is to ascertain the number of psychopaths a) in affected families, b) in families carefully selected as stocks in which neither the 'probandus', nor his brethren, parents, uncles, aunts or grandparents show any morbidity c) a sample of the average population, which usually includes a sprinkling of diseased stocks. This contrasts with investigations which have already been made on a considerable scale of the pedigrees of affected families; in such researches results will show that if a certain individual occurring in the pedigree had been prevented from procreation, a given number of insane or criminal persons would not have been born. However useful these family studies may be, they do not give us the definite numerical prognosis which we require.[21]

Contacts with the German eugenists and their methods, through Rüdin, were thus bringing the Society the same message that they were to hear from the British geneticists of the left. The simple pedigree methodology that the Society had relied upon for so long was now outdated. But this was not the *Vererbungsmathematik* that was attracting the attention of the British geneticists. Rüdin's group did not work with mathematical models. Instead, they collected survey data. Their intention was to build up on this empirical base a means of giving a genetical prognosis for relatives of all degrees, irrespective of the detailed genetics of the conditions in question. There was no need for mathematical models with this empirical approach.

The mandate of the Departmental Committee on Sterilisation, chaired by Sir Lawrence Brock, Chairman of the Board of Control, was to inquire into the information available on hereditary transmission and other causes of mental disorder and deficiency, and within that category, into E.O. Lewis's primary type, the high-grade mental defect that he had found running in the families of the social problem group. The inquiry was not concerned with other forms of mental disability: the psychoses made their appearance only in the form of quotations from the German literature.[22]

When Brock contacted Blacker in 1932, inviting the Society to present a brief, and to summarise for the Committee the research on the inheritance of mental defect, Blacker wrote at once to Rüdin, quoting Brock's letter at length. Brock had asked for answers to three questions: what research on the heredity of mental defect had been done abroad, granted that feeble-mindedness is hereditary, what is the pattern of inheritance; and why, in the USA, with legislation already in place, had there been so little actual sterilisation done? Blacker passed Brock's questions on verbatim to Rüdin.[23]

Rüdin answered enthusiastically that Blacker's enquiry had made him very happy, as he could see that the British government was going into the matter of the scientific grounds for sterilisation very carefully, and that the Eugenics Society was clearly playing an important role as the government's scientific informant. His ten-foolscap-page letter dealt with each of Blacker's points in turn, citing and explaining the relevant Munich literature. Data had been collected on the incidence of abnormality in the children of psychotics of different types, of epileptics, hysterics, sufferers from Huntington's chorea, alcoholics and addicts. He listed papers on the incidence of abnormality in nieces and nephews of abnormals, including the feeble-minded, in cousins, in siblings and in parents, and in cross-sections of different populations. Only by comparison of the relatives of patients with that in the general population could the role of inheritance in mental disease become clear, he said.[24] It was the position that had guided Rüdin's programme for his division in the past, and that he was to go on promoting in the future, after the Nazi accession.[25] He emphasised to Blacker that though there were lacunae in the existing research, it was important to get on with legislation on the basis of what information we already had. He sent Blacker a copy of the Proceedings of the Prussian *Landesgesundheitsrat* announcing that eugenic sterilisation was to be permitted there upon a voluntary basis.[26] This pre-Nazi legislation was the first step towards the compulsory sterilisation law, the *Gesetz zur Verhütung erbkranken Nachwuchses*, that was to be passed in July 1933, almost immediately after the Nazi accession.[27] Rüdin is said to have had it already prepared in his desk drawer.[28]

The German work covered a very wide range of mental problems, but the main emphasis lay in the area of the psychoses, especially schizophrenia, and it was for the psychoses that Rüdin particularly advocated sterilisation.[29] Less work, he says, has been done on the genetics of the feeble-minded and their ilk, but they should probably be sterilised too, if only from an environmental point of view. 'Occupational inefficiency, distaste for life, suicidal tendencies, cruelty, sex perversions and criminal tendencies' are no more than marginal indications, but these people traditionally set low standards for their children, which are transmitted for generations to come. This is just his personal opinion, though, and not the result of research, he says. The eventual German sterilisation law, in fact, covered all groups of abnormality, the social as well as the pathological. The 1933 *Gesetz zur Verhütung erbkranken Nachwuchses* listed schizo-phrenia, manic-depression, epilepsy, chorea minor, inherited blindness and deafness and physical defect, as well as the feeble-mindedness of the more non-specific type that interested the British eugenists. In Britain, the eugenists had traditionally had little interest in the truly *Erbkrank*. It was the borderline feeble-minded of the social problem group, who were regarded as normal by physicians, whose fertility constituted the danger to the race, not helpless idiots or schizophrenics. As C.P. Blacker wrote to R.A. Fisher, who was a member of the Brock Committee, the Society was less interested in legalising the sterilisation of mental defectives than in 'extending the principle of voluntary sterilisation to the social problem group'.[30]

The departmental bibliography that Rüdin sent to Blacker in 1933 listed 153 items.[31] Blacker chose to use only three of them, plus a fourth one from outside Rüdin's department, to summar-ise and comment on for the Brock Committee. He also cited three more from America and one from Denmark, all eight of them on the families of those Lewis had called the 'primary aments'. Each author gave figures for percentages of affected parents, siblings, nieces and nephews, aunts and uncles, of his feeble-minded *propositi*, who were mostly inmates of institutions. They did not deal with the cases with specific pathology, such as amaurotic family idiocy, mongolism and cretinism, which Lewis had found to have no relation to class.

The figures from this international literature were difficult to compare with one another. Blacker read them carefully, follow-ing up Rüdin's explanations with letters to the individual members of the German group, asking for clarification as to the meaning of their numbers. Carl Brugger, for example, had stated in his paper that if both parents were feeble-minded,

93.15 per cent of their offspring were also feeble-minded. That seemed clear; but his 205 *propositi* had between them 105 affected parents; he did not say how many of the parents were both feeble-minded, or how many of the *propositi* were siblings. From these figures, complained Blacker, one could not answer the question invariably asked in Britain; namely, that if all the feeble-minded of the last generation had been sterilised, what would have been the reduction in the numbers of the feeble-minded today?[32]

It was not possible to reduce the heterogeneous international literature to a neat table of comparable figures. The problem was the same in each case, but none of the authors had recorded exactly the same measurement. Blacker was finally forced simply to list them with a comment on each, rather in the style of Rüdin's letters.[33] To add to the difficulty, it was not of course the cases with a clearly defined Mendelian pattern such as Huntington's chorea and juvenile amaurotic idiocy that he wished to propose for voluntary sterilisation, but the social problem group with all its ambiguities. In Blacker's hands, Rüdin's scientific programme appeared in a much weakened form. It focused on the kind of cases that Rüdin himself had seen as 'no more than marginal indications'. The *Report* of the Brock Committee came out in full support of the Eugenics Society's work. Sir Lawrence Brock himself thought that Fisher's contribution, an analysis of the children of known defectives, was new and significant, and that it put 'many of the much-quoted continental investigations absolutely in the shade', in terms of its range and magnitude.[34] Fisher's figures, like E.O. Lewis's incidence data, had been collected from local authorities all over Britain, while Rüdin's, as Brock was proudly pointing out, were only from single institutions. The Munich group's work, however, had probably been the model for Fisher's contribution; unlike the Society's usual Lidbetter-style approach to the inheritance of feeble-mindedness, it contained no pedigrees at all.[35]

The Society's sterilisation campaign received a good deal of encouragement from the *Brock Report*'s whole-hearted support. One result was the formation of the Joint Committee on Voluntary Sterilisation, a grouping of interested societies which included representatives of the Central Association for Mental Welfare, the Mental Hospitals Association, the National Council for Mental Hygiene, and the Eugenics Society.[36] The Eugenics Society dissolved its own Committee for Legalising Sterilisation, and turned to providing funding and office space for the wider group. For six years, from 1934 to 1940, the Joint Committee campaigned for the legal enactment of the *Brock Report*'s recommendations, in the form of a Bill which the Committee drafted. The Campaign was taken to the country as well, in the form of meetings held up and down the land, persuading any organised body whose interests might be affected to pass a resolution of support. Those that did included the Royal Colleges of Physicians and Surgeons, the Royal College of Nursing, two groups of Medical Officers of Health (but not the British Medical Association), many societies for the welfare of the blind, and the British Social Hygiene Council, which was being run by Sybil Neville Rolfe, the erstwhile Mrs Gotto, founder of the Eugenics Education Society. About half the groups voting their support for Eugenic Society's resolution were women's organisations, probably as a result of the Society's specially targeting these groups. The women's groups were both left- and right-wing politically. They included the National Conference of Labour Women, the Conservative Women's Reform Association, the National Council of Women, and about eighty women's co-operative guilds.

Blacker was very conscious of the importance of trying to correct the Society's right-wing image by reaching out to organised labour. But given the eugenists' programme, it was not easy to do. He felt that he would be able to convince the Labour Party's membership that voluntary sterilisation was in the interest of the poor, if only the arguments could be presented to them by one of their own.[37] He needed first to persuade a Labour leader to cooperate with the Society.

It was difficult to get anyone suitable. After a good deal of effort, he found Caroline Maule, an American physician living in England, who seemed like someone who might be able to carry eugenics into the Labour movement. She was fairly successful in collecting some prominent Labour women – Mrs Harold Laski was one of them – and in forming a 'Worker's Committee to Legalise Voluntary Sterilisation'. It was, in Blacker's words, subsidised under the table by the Eugenics Society.[38] But he had a forceful opponent in George Gibson, of the Mental Hospital and Institution Workers' Union, who proposed, and carried, an anti-sterilisation motion at the Trades Union Congress of 1934. Gibson argued that legalisation would put too much power in the hands of the experts, the doctors. He felt that it would amount to setting up a 'medical dynasty' whose opinion would be law. So far as the poor person was concerned, sterilisation could never be voluntary.[39] The seconder of Gibson's resolution before the Trades Union Congress explicitly linked sterilisation to the economic and class status of its likely subjects. If the 'eugenic extremists' had their way, it might well be that prolonged unemployment would come to be considered unfitness:

> It is quite within the bounds of human possibility that those who want the modern industrial evils under the capitalist system to continue, may see in sterilisation an expedient, degrading though it may be, to exterminate the victims of the capitalist system, rather than change the system that largely produces them.[40]

The political ideology of the eugenists' interest in the social problem group was not hidden from the trades unionists. The English eugenists, as the evidence shows, were equally aware that the opposition to their movement now came largely from the political left. In fact, to R.A. Fisher, at least, it seemed as if *all* the opposition to eugenics in this century had come from what he called 'communists and fellow-travellers'.[41] Both the scientific counterblasts of Hogben and Haldane and the more directly political opposition of Gibson, and even the milder criticisms of the British Medical Association, were rooted in the perception that the eugenists' programme was directed against its promoters' class enemies.

The left was not the only institutionalised opposition, however. As the promoters of the *Brock Report* discovered, their resolution was also absolutely unacceptable to Catholics.[42] The Catholics frequently quoted 'Dr Fairfield's book' as the source of their arguments against sterilisation.[43] But their primary source was the papal encyclical on Christian marriage of 31 December 1930, known from its *incipit* as *Casti connubii*. Two following decrees, of 18 and 21 March 1931, condemned both positive and negative eugenics, and at the end of the decade, two more, of 21 and 24 February 1940, explicitly condemned sterilisation in particular.[44]

The Catholic position was that the interests of man's spirit had to be placed before those of the race. Catholic thought, according to the Canadian commentator Father Hervé Blais, did not condemn the entire eugenic programme outright, but subordinated it to man's proper purpose upon earth. Eugenic advice might be offered at the level of individual pastoral counselling, but the Holy See condemned absolutely civil law that originated in contempt for the biologically inferior. A great soul might inhabit a miserable body, and it was the interests of the soul that must come first. Eugenics was a materialistic code more suited to the breeding of animals than of men, whose soul had been directly created by God. The 'statism' that put the state before the individual was an insult to the fundamental human right to home and family.[45] In many ways, this position on eugenics paralleled that of its left-wing critics. Blacker had written of 'the artificial alliance subsisting between the Catholics and the Labour Party in this matter'.[46] It was no artificial alliance, however. Both had understood the sterilisation campaign to imply a contempt for the individual who was seen as a failure in the material sense.

The sterilisation campaign entailed a further spin-off for the Society. By tradition, the Society's policy had been oriented towards legislative solutions to the socio-biologic problem of human failure. But in its efforts to publicise the sterilisation campaign and perhaps to counterbalance the British Medical Association's negative report, the Society turned to a new group of potential supporters, the physicians. C.P. Blacker, as General Secretary, edited a collection of essays entitled *The Chances of Morbid Inheritance*, which appeared in 1934.[47] It was edited by Blacker, but, as usual with the Society's projects, it was the product of a collective. The chairman of the group was J.A. Ryle, who had been among the founders of the sterilisation campaign. His committee included three other physicians, E.A. Cockayne, R.D. Gillespie and E.A. Mapother, two neurologists, Sir Russell Brain and Reginald Langdon Down (not the eponymous author of Down's syndrome, who wrote in 1866, but a descendant, who was born that year)[48] and a geneticist, Reginald Ruggles-Gates. A number of physicians, most of them distinguished names in clinical medicine, contributed papers and were temporarily coopted as members of the Society's Consultative Council. The introductory essay on 'Eugenics and medicine' was provided by Sir Humphrey Rolleston, President of the Society and himself a physician. The book, he said, was an attempt to draw the medical profession into the eugenics movement:

> There are two groups of people whose fertility should on biological grounds be restricted; the first is the 'Social Problem Group', a term employed by the Wood Committee to describe the lowest stratum of mentally retarded and socially parasitic members of the community. The second group, with which this book deals, comprises the subjects of defects and diseases of a hereditary nature. ... Much could be done by [means of clinician's] ... cooperation in the collection and analysis of information, and one of the chief objects which the Eugenics Society has in presenting this book is to bring about this much needed collaboration of the medical profession.[49]

The papers in the collection dealt with hereditary conditions within the province of the new audience, the physicians. They covered such conditions as the haemorrhagic diatheses such as haemophilia; *Erythroblastosis foetalis* and the haemolytic anaemias; asthma, eczema and migraine; skeletal defects, cardiovascular diseases and tubercle.

Most of the papers were written by hospital clinicians who dealt with these diseases in their practice, and they were mainly non-quantitative, clinical descriptions of disease. In most cases, no attempt was made to go beyond a simple statement that the disease in question was inherited, usually as a dominant, the type of inheritance most easily appreciated in the clinical setting. Only one of the contributors, Aubrey Lewis, of the Maudsley Psychiatric Hospital, was a member of the Society. Lewis's paper on the inheritance of mental disorders is remarkable for its total admiration for the German work and workers:

> during the last twenty years painstaking work has wiped away the reproach from genetic psychiatry, that it was bad psychiatry and bad genetics. This has been due to a few men, the foremost of whom is Rüdin; his studies have been the starting point and model for almost all of value that has been done so far in the field.[50]

Lewis's references are heavily weighted with German literature:

the English, American and French between them get twelve citations; the Germans get twenty-one, all but three of which could have come from the Munich group's bibliography that Rüdin had sent over to Blacker in 1933. It was obviously Rüdin's work that inspired him, and which he wished to present to the English clinicians as the new movement in clinical genetics. His paper is quantitative in the sense that, like Rüdin's surveys, it gives percentages of affected relatives in the different types of mental disorder. It does not make use of the mathematical models typical of *Vererbungsmathematik*.

The mathematical models do appear in this clinically oriented book however, in an appendix on 'The analysis of pedigrees' by Lancelot Hogben. Hogben lays out a textbook explanation of the statistical laws based on the principle of random mating; that is, on the Weinberg formula. The method he gives for identifying recessive inheritance through an excess of consanguineous marriages is the one suggested by Fritz Lenz in 1919.[51]

No other contributor had made any use of the new (to Britain) *Vererbungsmathematik*. Of course, this was not a theoretically oriented research collection, but a clinical guide, and these mathematical methods were not of much use to clinicians. Hogben's paper was placed apart from the others, as an appendix: it looks as if Blacker had invited him as a token geneticist, or perhaps as an attempt to disarm the critics of the left by including the most critical in his book.

Unlike the other contributors, however, Hogben did not join the Society's Consultative Council. Blacker and his colleagues continued to regard him as an enemy. R.A. Fisher, from his position on the Brock Committee, wrote to Blacker about Hogben's appearance before it in extremely hostile terms:

> Hogben gave evidence on Monday and made a complete ass of himself. He quite forgot he was there to offer information to the Committee, and was thinking all the time that they were there to find fault with *him*. Our Chairman has an excellent manner and is most tactful, so Hogben's reply 'Well, what's wrong with that ?', with the air of a rather peevish victim of the Inquisition gave a tone to the whole sitting.
>
> I say this as I should like you to treat the Committee as open-minded, anxious to consider all reasonable and

well-founded opinions, and not on any account to give your time to developing an attack on an imaginary antagonist.[52]

Blacker replied:

You may have heard that at a recent meeting of the Rationalist Press Association Hogben read a chapter of a book he is about to publish which contains a vitriolic attack upon the Society, based upon extracts from recent numbers of the Eugenics Review.[53]

If it was, in fact, published as a book, the book must presumably have been Hogben's *Nature and Nurture*. It does not contain any 'vitriolic attack upon the Society', however. The final chapter is a critique of Fisher's paper on the 'Correlation between relatives on the supposition of Mendelian inheritance' of 1918, in which Fisher had calculated that only 5 per cent of the correlation was due to environment. Hogben ends the chapter with a warning that behind a façade of flawless algebra there might be concealed assumptions that have no factual basis – an observation that is pointed, rather than vitriolic.[54] It was no more than Fisher could have expected, in view of his own review of Hogben's *Genetic Principles*.[55]

At this point in the early thirties, with the tide of left-wing criticism setting against it, but feeling the fair wind of the sterilisation campaign in its sails, the eugenists felt themselves to be the focus of all that was vigorous in human biology. Their traditions and their problems were still at the centre of modern thought, even for those who were most determined in attacking the movement.

Lionel Penrose was one of these attackers.[56] Entering the field of subnormality in 1930 as Research Medical Officer to the Royal Eastern Counties Institution, he was plunged immediately into the world of the *Wood Report*, of E.O. Lewis's social problem group and his primary and secondary amentias.[57] Penrose was set to examining the institution's mental defectives from physical, mental and genetic points of view, to attempt to find the parts played in causation by heredity and other possible factors.[58] Penrose's research post was funded jointly by the Institution itself, the Medical Research Council and the Darwin Trust, a fund administered by the Society. He was to work under Dr F. Douglas Turner, Superintendent of the Institution, who had been a member of the Wood Committee and of the British Medical Association's committee. Turner was among the mental deficiency experts known to be opposed to sterilisation as a solution to the problem of mental defect.[59] Penrose, therefore, from the beginning of his career was immersed in the Eugenics Society's problematic, though he was sheltered by his association with Turner from the pressure to endorse the eugenists' solutions.

Soon after beginning his work at Colchester, Penrose was contacted by C.P. Blacker with a request to contribute to the Society's new project on its usual target, now called the social problem group.[60] Blacker wrote that E.O. Lewis had found his primary aments clustered together with epileptics, inebriates, recidivists and prostitutes in that group. The question to be answered now was whether the *relatives* of all these deviants, like those of the aments, were part of the social problem group too. Were the families from which all these people sprang 'appreciably below the normal social average' as E.O. Lewis had supposed? Lewis himself, wrote Blacker, was not available; would Penrose contribute a section on mental disease and defect to the Society's new study?[61] Penrose declined the invitation: 'I certainly think that Lewis' "social problem group" should be investigated, particularly as I am not at all certain as to whether his hypothesis is correct that there exists such a group.' He went on to say that people in Lewis's group would have to be found by going through schools and taking the families of duller children there, rather than those of the institutionalised cases, who were more severely affected. He could not do this himself: he had all he could manage within the institution. In addition, he said, the relatives of these higher-grade cases were becoming less and less amenable to visits from social workers, because they had had so much of it. Some of them had got wind up about sterilisation, and now preferred to conceal their family histories if they could.[62]

Penrose's letter is very diplomatic, but quite firm. He offers 'all the help I can', but refuses to take part in the project. He questions the basic hypothesis: to the eugenists, the social problem group was not a hypothesis at all, but simply a new name for their old residuum. And he speaks for the people who were the subjects of the research, in saying that they are tired of being interviewed, and apprehensive that they would be sterilised. At the time of writing to Blacker, Penrose had been working at Colchester only nine months. But already his position seems clear.

Penrose's first research results came very quickly. His characteristic large-scale surveys of mental defectives and their families, with his very ingenious statistical analyses, began to appear within a year of his appointment at Colchester.[63] By 1932 he had produced the first of his important papers on mongolism and maternal age, in which he introduced the idea of arranging the environmental influence, the maternal age, in order of intensity, so as to look for genetic effects where they should be easiest to find; namely, where the environmental effect was at its most intense. Finding that the incidence of mongolism was greatest where the mother was over 40, he selected 'partial fraternities' containing at least one mongol child, and counting only siblings who had been born after the mother reached the age of 40. To test whether the resulting sibships conformed to a recognisable genetic pattern, he used a mathematical model, derived ultimately from Fritz Lenz, by way of Torsten Sjögren and Lancelot Hogben. The expression gives the expected number of affected offspring:

$$e = \frac{s n_s p}{1 - (1 - p)^s}$$

e = expected affected children
n = fraternities with at least
  one affected child
s = size of fraternity
p = ratio of
  affected : total children

The ratio p depended theoretically on the type of inheritance: it would be 1/4 for traits determined by a single recessive gene or two complementary but independent dominants, and 1/16 for two independent recessives. Tables of the outcome with different values of p, and examples of its use in disentangling the inheritance of different kinds of dwarfism had been given by Hogben.[64] Penrose used both the mathematical model and the model procedure. Penrose's Buckston Browne Prize Essay of 1933, entitled 'The influence of heredity on disease', gives an organised exposition of the whole spectrum of new methods available to human geneticists. His stance is immediately clear from his listing of the heroes of the new methodology:

> an enormous literature on pedigree studies of diseases has come into being. The interpretation of these data, by the use of the theoretical methods elaborated by such writers as Weinberg, Lenz, Dahlberg, Bernstein, Snyder, Haldane and Hogben has now proceeded far enough to lay the foundation of a science of human genetics.[65]

Penrose's prize essay is a presentation of *Vererbungsmathematik* directed mainly to a medical audience, whom he thinks have difficulty in understanding the primary sources, the papers by these writers themselves. The appeal to the medical profession recalls Blacker's *Chances of Morbid Inheritance*, which appeared in the same year, 1934. But except for Hogben's appendix to Blacker's book, the two have very little in common. Blacker's contributors make no use of 'factorial analysis' while Penrose's essay consists of nothing but, or at least, on its application to the practical situation. Penrose's references to the Eugenics Society's favourites, both concepts and people, are all negative. Forel's *Blastophthoria*, Mott's 'law of anticipation', Goddard's view that feeble-mindedness is inherited as a unit Mendelian character, and Fisher's, that less than 5 per cent of the variance of stature is due to causes not heritable, are all dumped as forthrightly as is consistent with politeness.[66] The final chapter, 'Medicine and eugenics', is equally plain-spoken: 'one of the chief aims of human genetics is to identify as many as possible of the Mendelian unit characters in man and to allocate the positions of these characters on the chromosomes'.[67]

Linkage and chromosome mapping are the important issues. He emphasises the use of the blood groups in the search for linkage, using Bernstein's model, in line with Hogben's programme of research. And it is unwise, he thinks, to be 'unduly optimistic' about the results of eugenic measures in medicine. Sterilisation would be quantitatively ineffective in controlling anything but dominant or sex-linked characters that cause severe disease. Here at least eugenic measures would work. But that is not what the eugenists are interested in. Eugenics is not about eliminating specific genetic diseases, but about breeding the best possible race. Here, he says, we leave the realm of practical science and enter into philosophy, and the philosophies

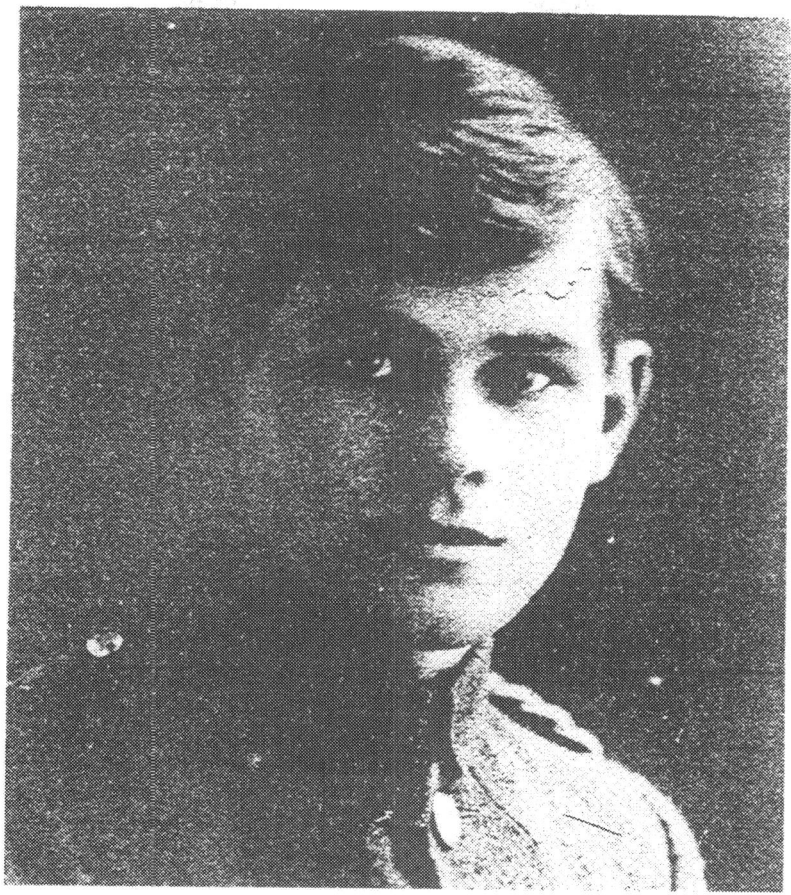

Plate III Lionel Sharples Penrose
Source: Identity card for the Friends' Ambulance Unit. Courtesy of Friends'
House, London

of medicine and eugenics sooner or later diverge. Perfecting the
race may be against the interests of the imperfect individual. It is
rapid *environmental* change which has benefited both individual
and race. The eugenic programme that would be the most in
line with medical philosophy, he says, would be to encourage the
breeding of those who are best at coping with a changing
environment. It is not a serious suggestion.

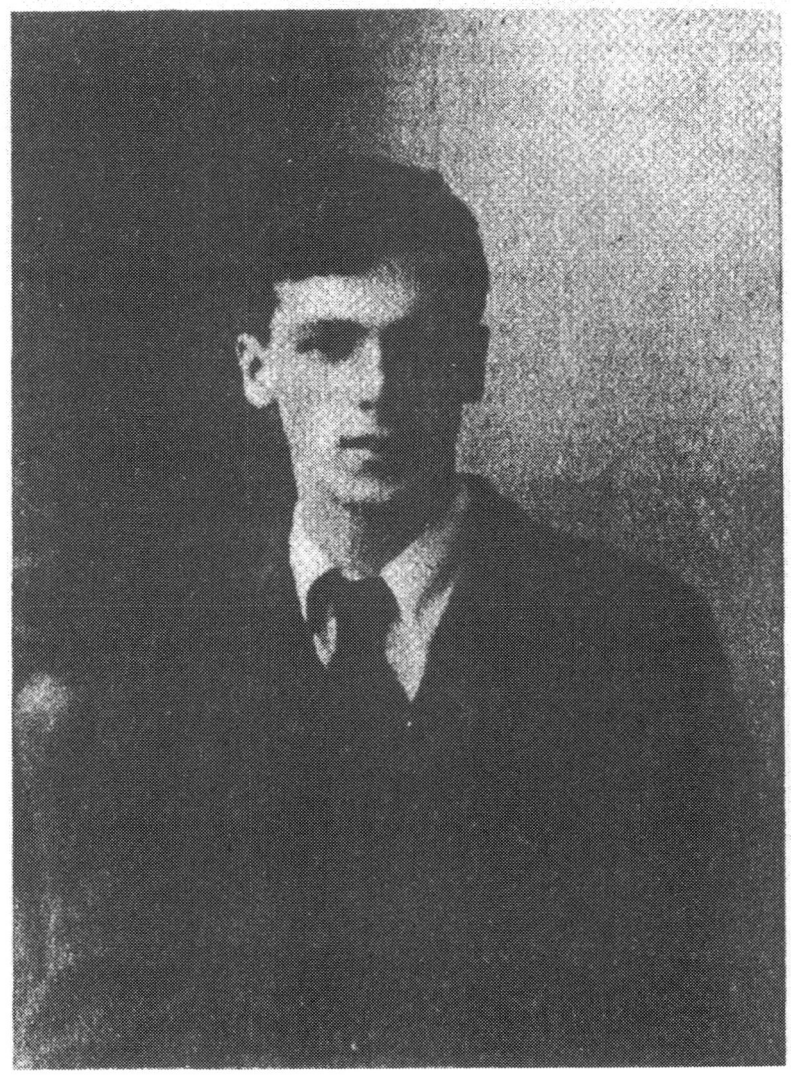

Plate IV Lancelot Hogben
Source: Identity card for the Friends' Ambulance Unit. Courtesy of Friends'
House, London

In Penrose's essay, it is Hogben's influence that first strikes the reader. The largest number of his references, nine, are to Hogben, and all are positive. The next largest group, eight, are to Karl Pearson; of these, all but two place him as an antique forerunner whose work has been 'discredited'.[68] To Fisher and Haldane he refers five times each. Fisher is 'important': right twice and wrong three times; but Haldane is right every time, in Penrose's estimation.

What was Hogben to make of this outspoken admiration? Penrose was not a Marxist. His ideology was formed from his Quaker background, and it came often into the foreground of his life.[69] His service in the Friends' Ambulance Train of the Red Cross during the 1914–18 war, and his work for the Psychologists' Peace Society in the 1930s, and the Medical Association for the Prevention of War in the 1950s, are all evidence of the importance of his ethical stance (see Plate III). During the war, Hogben had served in the Friends' Ambulance Train, too, but had then withdrawn from it and spent the rest of the war as a conscientious objector in Wormwood Scrubs Prison (Plate IV).[70] He must have found Penrose very sympathetic, although Penrose's objection to the eugenics programme was on the spiritual grounds of sympathy with the individual, rather than disgust at the eugenists' class position, as in Hogben's case. It was another example of what Blacker had seen as the unnatural alliance of religion and the left, and as such, is worth a short detour.

One of the most significant of the links between religion and the left during the first half of the twentieth century was the peace movement. Before the First World War, organised socialism had stood for the international solidarity of the working class, and had rejected national sentiment, national boundaries and war. But the International with its strong German component did not survive the outbreak of war. The Bureau of the Socialist International meeting in Brussels a few months before the declaration came out against war, but also stated that socialist parties could if they wished take part in national defence. In Britain, the Independent Labour Party took the view that the quarrel was a diplomatic one, between the ruling classes of Europe, and that the workers should play no part in it. The Party's National Council issued a manifesto with these words: 'Out of the darkness and the depth we hail our working-class comrades of every land. Across the roar of guns, we send sympathy and greeting to the German Socialists. ... They are no enemies of ours, but faithful friends.'[71] The appeal was fruitless. The International collapsed, and was not restored until 1923.

The Independent Labour Party in England, of which Hogben was a member, took a strongly anti-war line. Fenner Brockway, one of its leaders, has written that in retrospect the English group tended to become 'bourgeois pacifists, rather than working class socialists'.[72] But it was the ILP that faced the overwhelming power of popular patriotism and anti-German feeling, and organised the No-Conscription Fellowship for the support of conscientious objectors to military service.

They were joined in their campaign by the Quakers. Quakers had a long tradition of opposition to war, but the decision as to whether or not to accede to the tradition was respected as a matter for the individual conscience.[73] During the 1914–18 war, many young Quakers did join up, or took a half-way position by performing some non-combatant or humanitarian service connected with the war. The Society of Friends was not the only religious group to object to fighting. The apocalyptic churches such as the Plymouth Brethren, the Christadelphians and Jehovah's Witnesses, the Pentecostal churches with their fundamentalist interpretation of scripture, as well as some Methodists and Wesleyans, together provided a fairly large proportion of the conscientious objectors of the First World War.[74] The organisation of resistance to military service, however, was provided by the Society of Friends and the Independent Labour Party through the No-Conscription Fellowship. The Fellowship was supported by the Friends' Service Committee, who recommended that no exemption from military service should be acceptable to Quakers whose grounds were not available to Quakers and non-Quakers alike. Many in both groups stood for absolute exemption from any form of war-related activity at all, even so-called alternative service, which might be either non-combatant military duty or 'work of national importance'.

The Friends' Ambulance Unit, to which both Hogben and Penrose belonged during the war, was one of these forms of alternative service (see Plates III and IV).[75] Set up unofficially by a group of Quakers, it was never fully approved by the Meeting for Sufferings, to which other Quaker relief schemes were responsible. The Ambulance Units saved lives and reduced the suffering of both military and civilian wounded, on both sides. But the work was seen as too close to patching up casualties to go back and fight again, or to relieving the military, who might otherwise be fighting, of responsibility for the wounded. The Friends' Service Committee advised Quakers to refuse absolutely to take part in any alternative service at all. When it became known that leaders of the Unit had been asked by the War Office to provide 'alternative service of national importance' for all Quakers coming before the conscientious objectors' tribunals, the Friends' Service Committee distanced itself from the Ambulance Unit. Many members of the Unit resigned and came home to trial and imprisonment. Penrose stayed with the Ambulance Train; Hogben, with his more radical temperament, came home and was imprisoned.[76]

Quakers were deeply involved in the No-Conscription Fellowship. It had been set up by Lilla and Fenner Brockway of the Independent Labour Party, but its Treasurer was the Quaker Edward Grubb, and about one third of its committee were also Quakers.[77] Like the Friends' Service Committee, the No-Conscription Fellowship called for absolute exemption for all conscientious objectors. After conscription began in May 1916, if they had not been granted exemption, many of these men were arrested, court-martialled and sent to jail for what sometimes turned out to be a series of sentences of hard labour following one after another. Fenner Brockway and the No-Conscription Fellowship's chairman Clifford Allen were among those who spent long periods in jail, and who like Hogben refused to accept alternative service. The Friends even rejected the efforts being made to prevent the ill-treatment of conscientious objectors in prison, feeling that these lobbying efforts reduced the significance of their witness for peace.[78]

All the men and women who were involved in the peace movement during the First World War and after had the experience of standing alone as dissenters against a majority that regarded them with contempt as 'Hun-lovers', 'the save-their-skins brigade', and the 'won't-fight-funks', in Fenner Brockway's words.[79] Although both Quakers and Independent Labour Party members had the support of their own group, their stance was that of a critical minority, determined to bear witness, reviled and despised, and suffering physically if necessary, for what they knew was right.

Lancelot Hogben was not born into a Quaker family, but he had joined a Quaker meeting while he was in Cambridge, and transferred his membership to a London meeting when he came down from Cambridge. The record shows that he remained a member for some time after the war in London.[80] During the war, he had adopted the most radical of the Quaker positions. He had first refused to fight, then refused even to serve with the Ambulance Unit, and had gone to jail for his conscience's sake. His commitment to the left had begun with the ILP, also while he was at Cambridge, and was later to go progressively further leftwards. The born Quaker Lionel Penrose had joined the Ambulance Train in spite of 'official' Quaker disapproval of this service.

The two men's criticism of eugenics had in both cases something about it of the stance of the conscientious objector. Their relationship in the scientific controversy in which they were involved was that of old comrades-in-arms who recognised and understood each other. Hogben's position on eugenics was that of class war. The Quaker convert and member of the 'slightly bourgeois' ILP had become, if only temporarily, the committed Marxist. Penrose's position was that of the Quaker who respected the individual's personal worth and personal experience, and hence the equal rights of individuals. Although their points of origin were different, they had much in common in their attitude to the eugenists' programme, as they had to the cause of peace. Penrose's prize essay is the distillation of this period in the early thirties when, under Hogben's influence, he worked with the eugenists' problems, but refused both their methods and their fellowship. His statement, that 'the sub-cultural group [of mental defectives] is not to be confused with the so-called 'social problem group' ... not all sub-cultural mental defectives behave anti-socially', is a statement that attacks the Society's theory and practice at its very root.[81] Elsewhere, in his monograph on *Mental Defect* of 1933, he wrote that 'pedigree studies may give suggestive facts, but unless the simple Mendelian ratios are found on analysis of affected families, this kind of inheritance can only be established with some difficulty'.[82] The way to examine for these ratios is to use the 'factorial method'. He recommends the Sjögren-Hogben formula for families with at least one affected member, and Lenz's development of 'mathematical Mendelism', the formula for calculating the incidence of cousin marriages. The use of correlation coefficients is less suitable for the kind of material collected in work on mental deficiency, where only families with at least one affected member can be counted, giving a non-random sample of the population. However, correlations can be used to test for sex-linked inheritance. Absolute values may be unreliable, but comparison of coefficients between father–son and father–daughter pairs could give good results. Each of these suggestions had been introduced into the English literature on genetics by Hogben, though only the last was his own contribution.

Penrose had pointed to the environment effects in the form of maternal ageing as the source of the clustering of cases of mongolism in the offspring of women over 40. In *Mental Defect*, however, he also drew on the kind of environmental influence cited by the critics from the left – that is, on poverty and deprivation – as a possible factor in mental defect, much as Hogben had done in his criticism of the eugenists' overweighting of the importance of heredity in the nature and nurture controversy. In Penrose's critique, his earlier studies of Freudian psychology weigh in on the same side of the balance.[83]

> It is not usually believed by those who study mental deficiency that the retardation observed can be due to psychological causes. In view of the recent work of psychologists who have stressed the exceptional importance of the first few years of life in the formation of character, it is well to reconsider this belief. ... Those persons who have been brought up in well-ordered homes with kindly parents find it difficult to realize the possible mental state of a young child in a family where, say, the mother is feeble-minded and the father a drunkard or epileptic. ...
> It is hardly necessary to point out that the educational opportunities of different children vary with social class. Lack of such opportunity may, later on, cause failure in mental tests of a scholastic nature.[84]

Penrose criticises the simple pedigree methodology trusted by his predecessors. He cites a pedigree for a patient with microcephalic idiocy, with many different pathological conditions appearing over several generations – it is just this kind of pedigree which would have seemed a perfect demonstration of the inheritance of a neuropathic constitution. But, he says, such an interpretation would be quite out of line with modern genetics. This pedigree gives little information that could be used to establish the presence of Mendelian factors.[85] Among the enemies whom he smites hip and thigh are E.J. Lidbetter, and the authors of the *Wood Report*, whose description of the 'social problem group' lists the lowest 10 per cent on the social scale as including a much larger proportion of insane, paupers, criminals, unemployables, prostitutes, inebriates and habitual slum dwellers than any group of families *not* containing mental defectives:

> This terrible indictment is coupled with the totally un-proved assertion that the mental defectives concerned are of the primary (hereditary) type. That mental defect may be to some extent due to criminal parents dwelling 'habitually' in slums seems to have been overlooked. ... There is a distinct correlation between the intelligence of school children and their environment, whether measured by the economic position of the parents, by the care taken of the home or by the clothing of the child.[86]

Penrose's *Mental Defect* was published as the first in a series of textbooks on social biology edited by Hogben. Its endorsement of Hogben's point of view could hardly have been more pointed.

Penrose's main preoccupation throughout the thirties was the *Colchester Survey*, the massive project that assembled and analysed data on 1,280 patients in the Colchester institution, their 6,629 siblings, 2,560 parents and 127 children. The finished survey appeared in January 1938.[87] The *Colchester Survey* is the last grand manifestation of the eugenist problematic in its most traditonal form. It also marks the beginning of its end. The emphasis in the preface on its origin in the *Wood Report* of 1929, its reference to mental defect as an important social problem, and its association with destitution and the Poor Law, all place it within the well-known eugenic framework. The Preface states that

'Mental deficiency is a social problem of major importance.' This was the conclusion arrived at in 1929 by the ... Wood

Committee. ... It is only in recent years that students of social problems have come to recognise the importance and significance of mental deficiency. The reasons for this are obvious ... administratively, the mentally defective individual was simply one of a large number of destitute persons for whom the Poor Law Authorities had to cater ... the Medical Research Council have been aware of the importance of mental defect as a social problem. ... They have recognised that lack of knowledge may be a main limiting factor in combating this evil, and that such knowledge can come only by means of skilfully directed research.[88]

The *Colchester Survey* was the last of the group of four reports on mental deficiency. The first one, the *Wood Report* of 1929, had dealt with ascertainment and had introduced the idea of the social problem group; the second, the British Medical Association's *Report* of 1932, had come out strongly against sterilisation as a means of controlling numbers of the feeble-minded. The third, the *Brock Report* of 1934, had enthusiastically endorsed *voluntary* sterilisation, though it could not accept that it might be made compulsory. The *Colchester Survey* dealt specifically with the causes of mental deficiency.

Penrose's plan was to try to separate different types of mental defect as far as he could by clinical examination, by estimation of mental capacity of the patients and their families, and by assessment of their social status, and then to use the new methods of statistical analysis on each group of cases separately. His own statement of aims of his survey repeats what he had said in his Prize Essay of 1934, and contrasts rather oddly with the statements of the Preface:

It is the aim of modern research in human genetics to examine the behaviour of individual genes, to determine the topographical relationship of one gene to another and to ascertain precisely how genetic effects interact with one another and with environment. The recognition of genes which are incompletely dominant is of much interest biologically and has great importance in the prophylaxis of hereditary disease. Some evidence has been brought forward in this survey that some severe cases of defect which appear to have recessive determination are due to genes which underlie milder conditions in heterozygous relatives. The examination from this point of view of families with parental consanguinity has given particularly suggestive results.[89]

He emphasises that the causes of defect are multiple, that more than one may operate at a time, and that a 'facile classification' (like Lewis') into primary and secondary amentias would have led only to a 'fictitious simplification of the real problems inherent in the data'.[90]

The first part of the *Survey* follows the pattern of empirical enquiry laid down by the Rüdin group in Munich. Penrose himself commented on that, and on his own improvements on the Munich methods, in a paper that he sent to the *Eugenics Review* just after the *Survey* was published:

> Luxenburger [a statistician, and a member of the Rüdin group] has made extensive calculations to estimate the probabilities of the occurrence of all types of mental disease among relatives of patients and in the general population. His results, based upon a large amount of empirical data, are somewhat difficult to apply because of the variety of grades. ... Brugger's [another member of the same group] material, in which grades of defect are separated, could be adapted for use in this country if the criteria for mental grade were more standardised. The data collected in my recent report may be of service from this point of view, because they consist of a large number of sibships selected on account of the presence of at least one defective child.[91]

In Penrose's report, the family of every case has been visited, and information collected about parents, siblings living and dead, children, cousins, aunts and uncles, grandparents, and nephews and nieces. Assessments of intelligence were made on a six-point scale: superior, normal, dull, simple, idiot and imbecile. Overall, 7.6 per cent of the parents of patients were defective. The proportion was highest where the patients were in the simple (M_1) grade, where it reached 12.1 per cent, and lowest in the idiot (M_3) grade, where it was only 2.7 per cent. The number of defectives in the *Survey* who had children of their own was very small: there were only 67 fertile women, who had had 124 children between them. Only 54 had lived long enough to be tested: about half of them turned out to be defectives. This proportion was far higher than the proportion of patients' parents who were defective, which was under 10 per cent.

The figures that Penrose was collecting here were the central stuff of the voluntary sterilisation campaign, which occupied the Society and its sympathisers throughout the thirties. As Blacker had written to Carl Brugger, the question 'invariably' asked in Britain was that if all the feeble-minded of the last generation had been sterilised, what would have been the reduction in numbers of feeble-minded today. It was from figures like Penrose's, and Brugger's, and the series collected by R.A. Fisher for the *Brock Report* of 1934, that the eugenists hoped to get an answer that they could use persuasively in their sterilisation campaign.[92] Neither Penrose nor Turner, however, would help them personally.[93]

The next group of figures in the *Survey* compare with those collected by Lewis for the *Wood Report* of 1929. Lewis had said that only high-grade feeble-mindedness was familial; low-grade imbecility and idiocy were 'sporadic' or secondary, and since he found so few families with more than one low-grade case among them, he thought that there was no evidence that the defect was inherited. High-grade cases came from typical 'social problem' homes, whereas the low-grades were evenly scattered. He cited a few telling pedigrees to make his point.[94]

Here Penrose's newer methodology allowed him to take Lewis's work a step further. His material had very similar characteristics but his conclusions were different. Like Lewis, he found that idiots and imbeciles had few affected sibs. Those who were affected were low-grade like themselves, and the others quite normal: the sibs of idiots, said Penrose, were more intelligent than the sibs of patients who were merely dull or simple.

The second part of the *Colchester Report*, the clinical classification of cases, helped to explain this paradox, which had led Lewis to think that very low-grade defect was not inherited at all. Penrose separated out cases that were clinically similar and assessed their inheritance. He had two cases of phenylketonuria: one of them had one affected sib and the parents of the other were consanguineous, pointing, as in Sjögren's cases of amaurotic idiocy, to a recessive pattern of inheritance. In microcephaly, he found occasional affected sibs, including a pair of identical twins, and in one case, parental consanguinity. Other anomalies of head shape including one of hypertelorism, also had consanguineous parents. One patient with an abnormal head had a sibling, an uncle and a cousin with spina bifida. Penrose suggested that there might be a 'partially dominant genetic influence' in this and some other types of case, in which relatives affected in a slightly different way from the patient *propositi* might be heterozygous, and the patients themselves homozygous. A few clinical types, such as epiloia, and Huntington's chorea appeared to be simple dominants, with direct parent-to-child transmission.

After all these recognisable types had been subtracted, as well as the cases in which there was a clear history of injury or infection, Penrose was left with what he called, in an echo of the old eugenists' terminology, the 'residual group' of non-specific, 'subcultural aments'. Typically, they graded as simpletons; very few were lower than grade M_1. There were relatively few of them in the Institution – only 308 out of 1,280. The families of this group differed strikingly from those of the more clinically recognisable types. They were clustered at the bottom of the social scale, normal parents and sibs were fewer and defectives commoner. There was generally a close resemblance between the patients and their families. Penrose's suggestion here was that in the 'residual group' the factors making for mental defect were 'more dominant' than in other groups. Here Penrose repeated his earlier suggestion that this type of amentia was probably the product of multifactorial inheritance of the kind proposed by Fisher for height in 1918. Since the condition was so common, consanguinity was irrelevant, as Lenz had pointed out, but the correlation between the grade of mothers and fathers, and between grandmothers and grandfathers, pointed to strongly assortative mating for intelligence.[95]

The official report on the *Colchester Survey* represents only the tip of the iceberg of Penrose's thought on the subject of the causes of mental defect. In the report itself, he avoids the display of mathematical methods other than the simplest correlations, but his references within the text point the reader to Penrose publications, mostly in the genetics journals, where the mathematical arguments are shown in full. He published several papers on mongolism and maternal age.[96] There were also a number on the other specific forms of defect, on the inheritance of phenylketonuria and epiloia.[97,98] He made calculations of mutation rates in man, one paper written jointly with J.B.S. Haldane.[99] There was also one paper on the sib-pair method for the calculation of linkage, based on Bernstein's method as modified by Hogben so as to use pairs of siblings, rather than parent–child pairs as Bernstein himself had done, to look for crossing-over between blood groups and other alleles.[100] Penrose and his wife, Margaret, had investigated blood-group distributions in mongols and in the local normal population, and shown that the blood of mongolian idiots was not at all like that of the inhabitants of Mongolia.[101] Bernstein's contribution was deeply embedded in Penrose's thought: the problem of the ordering of genes along the chromosome was the goal of genetics of the future. These carefully argued papers underlie the simple statements of the report.

During the early thirties, the biologists of the left had set up a vigorous opposition to the eugenics movement. They attacked it for its class bias, and its concomitant underrating of the effects of environment, and also for its reliance on the outdated method of pedigree study. But as we have seen, during the twenties R.A. Fisher was already aware of these weaknesses in the programme of the Research Committee of the Eugenics Society, and he was already looking for a way to strengthen his methodology. The pitying review of E.J. Lidbetter's book by J.L. Gray, a member of Hogben's group at the London School of Economics, actually expressed very much what Fisher probably felt about it:

At present genetical science only permits us to detect the existence of defects or metrical characters which can be observed to conform to the statistical requirements of Mendel's laws. Many of the diseases and so forth which Mr Lidbetter includes as defects are not unambiguous clinical entities. If chargeability to the rates is a metrical character, to which of the categories of genetical analysis does it belong? . . . Is 'living in sin' a sign even of the inheritance of 'neuropathic constitution'?

Mr Lidbetter . . . does not accept the assumptions of modern genetical science.[102]

The opposition to Lidbetter's thinking was coming to some extent from within the Society, as well as from the biologists of the left. If that seems surprising, it is because one tends to assume that the political left belong to a social group which has little in common with the political right. In this case, that assumption would be a historian's artefact, no more than a convenient analytical tool, a means of disentangling the strands of thought which made up the history of human genetics during this period. If one widens the social frame of reference, it is clear that the members of the two groups were not so far apart that they could not interact. They were not located in different cultures, although their attitudes were deeply marked by their sympathies: to see them as living in separate compartments is one of the weaknesses of the use of conflicts of ideology as a tool for historical analysis. Hogben, Haldane and Fisher, as an internalist historian of the ideas of genetics would point out, were all involved in the same *kind* of genetics, that of the mathematical analysis of human population data. From this point of view, W.B. Provine is quite right in isolating the substance of their ideas from its social context: ideologically motivated they may well have been, but they were speaking to one another. The criticisms of the left are actually heard by the right, and responded to – Hogben, Haldane, and Fisher read one another's publications.

Furthermore, all three of them were members of the same small group, the scientific intelligentsia. In Britain at this time, the biological scientists were intimately linked over several generations. Francis Galton was Charles Darwin's cousin.[103] Thomas Henry Huxley had called himself 'Darwin's bulldog'.[104] Julian Huxley, his grandson, was a eugenist, though a somewhat uncertain one.[105] The Huxleys and the Haldanes at Oxford, and the Darwins at Cambridge, all knew one another very well. J.B.S. Haldane had been Julian Huxley's fag at Eton, and later they were colleagues at New College, Oxford. Fisher, at Cambridge, knew the sons of Charles Darwin: he and they were equally interested in eugenics. The Cambridge biologists R.C. Punnett and A.C. Seward, along with Fisher and the Darwins, were founding members of the Cambridge Eugenics Society. Only William Bateson, although he was interested in their problems, never liked the eugenists themselves. As I mentioned above, the Haldane children, J.B.S. and his sister Naomi, had a pair of guinea pigs called Bateson and Punnett, with which they used to do breeding experiments on Mendelian lines.[106] J.B.S. Haldane and Naomi Haldane (Mitchison) had been members of the Oxford Eugenics Society. Haldane, like R.A. Fisher in Cambridge, was an undergraduate member of its Committee.[107] Haldane, left-wing as he was, was not opposed to trying to improve the human race genetically, even as late as 1938, though he reviled eugenics as a movement and felt that economic change was a more important part of social reform, and far more likely to be effective. It was the class-centredness of the eugenists that disgusted him.[108] Hogben, alone, perhaps, of all the biologists, may have felt himself to be an outsider in this group of upper-class intellectuals; but even he had been a Cambridge undergraduate. Although there are no records of his having any contact with Fisher or the eugenists there, one of his earliest publications was a paper which appeared in the *Eugenics Review* in 1924.[109] It was done while he was working with the eugenist F.A.E. Crew of the Animal Breeding Research Department of Edinburgh University. It was hardly possible for a member of the biological sciences intelligentsia to escape all contact with eugenists. In 1933, R.A. Fisher succeeded Karl Pearson as Galton Professor and head of the Department of Eugenics at University College. Along with the Chair, he inherited the editorship of the Galton Laboratory house journal, *Annals of Eugenics*, which henceforth also became an organ of the Eugenics Society. In addition, he took his seat as a member of the Medical Research Council's Committee on Human Genetics, whose chairman was J.B.S. Haldane. Haldane, too, in 1933, had accepted a Chair at University College, at first the Chair of Genetics, and later, also in succession to Pearson, who had held Chairs in both Eugenics and Biometry, the Chair of Biometry.[110]

One of the earliest contributions accepted by Fisher for the *Annals* was an enormous paper by Haldane which appeared in the first issue for 1934, in which Haldane took up Hogben's introduction of Bernstein's method of searching for linkages and went on to refine it further and increase its power.[111] Fisher printed it with an accompanying paper of his own, in which he improved on Haldane's algebra.[112] This was followed in 1935 by a series of papers by Fisher on the mathematical detection of linkage in man, in the cases of dominant and of recessive abnormalities, and another by Haldane on the detection of sex linkage.[113,114] This time, too, Fisher followed Haldane's paper by a commentary of his own, which appeared in the next issue:

> The paper by Haldane published in the last issue of *Annals of Eugenics* is of importance to the future of human genetics ... never before has any considerable body of data bearing on the detection of linkage in man been assembled. ... Haldane makes the point, and it is one with which I most strongly agree, that quite apart from any linkages that may be discovered, an examination of actual data is of immediate importance in the present state of our knowledge, for the experience it provides of sources of error to which this use of pedigree material is necessarily exposed. It must be clearly recognized that the collectors of pedigrees had in the past no knowledge of many of the purposes to which the result of their labours is now being put. Many facts of which we now recognize the value, such, for example, as the sex of normal children, have often been omitted. Worse still, they may have been recorded inaccurately. In particular, the great importance of putting fully and accurately on record the method of ascertainment or the procedure of enquiry by which pedigrees of defect were brought to light, and of indicating the particular defective individual in each pedigree who first came to the investigator's knowledge, has been overlooked.[115]

Here, then, is Mr Lidbetter's obituary notice: it is clearly he whom Fisher means by the collector who did not know what he was doing, who left out all the important information, who had not recorded which defective individual was the original *propositus*, a feature of the first importance for the new mathematical Mendelism. Fisher had been critical of the looseness of Lidbetter's methods in 1924, but at that time he had not been able to suggest anything better than simply tightening up the accuracy and completeness of the data. The statisticians whom the Research Committee had consulted had proposed different varieties of correlation to deal with the material mathematically, but in the end no mathematical analysis was attempted in the final publication.

It was this need, which Fisher had felt ten years earlier, that was now filled by Haldane's analysis of human pedigrees. But where Hogben had seen in the new mathematical method of analysis of human material a weapon with which to beat the eugenists, Fisher planned to use it in their interests, and he applied to the Rockefeller Foundation, which was already funding Hogben's unit at the London School of Economics, for financial support.

Starting in 1923, the Rockefeller Foundation had been collaborating with the Medical Research Council in giving fellowships to young medical graduates from all over the world, to help them spend some time abroad studying the 'primary sciences of medicine' before starting on a career of teaching and research. At first the fellowships were only to be used for study in Canada or the States, but this restriction was later dropped. In the years between 1923 and 1935, seventy young British men and women had had Rockefeller Fellowships, and according to the Medical Research Council in 1935, they had been well chosen: twelve had become university professors, thirty-six held whole-time and sixteen part-time research positions.[116] The fellowships thus represented a major influence in the medical sciences in Britain.

In 1934, however, a change of policy at the Foundation brought this programme, temporarily, to an end.[117] Under the new policy the Foundation was to continue its support for research in the 'primary medical sciences', through the Medical Research Council as before, but it was to concentrate it in certain fields which had been chosen for special attention. These fields were 'neurology, psychiatry and related subjects', which came to include human genetics, especially the inheritance of mental defect. Among the fifteen or so groups which received support under the new programme was the Deutsche Forschungsanstalt in Munich.[118]

The Medical Research Council had been actively supporting projects of this kind for some years. They had contributed to the *Colchester Survey*, which in fact was published directly by the Council itself. They were also funding studies in mental hospitals in London and Birmingham, and in Cardiff, where J.H. Quastel was investigating the biochemistry of mental disorders. In 1934 the Council set up a new committee to look after research on mental disease, citing as its reason for doing so the large, and increasing, numbers of mental defectives in the country:

The Council have long regarded the subject of mental disorders as one demanding most active investigation: they could indeed hold no other view when the number of mental defectives in England and Wales alone is of the order of a quarter of a million when the proportion of defectives alive today is generally believed to be larger than it was a generation ago. To enable them better to discharge their responsibilities in this respect they have in the past year appointed, in consultation with the Board of Control, a new committee to advise and assist them in promoting research into mental disorders. The membership of this ... committee ... includes respresentatives not only of psychiatry, medical deficiency, but also of neurology, physiology, biochemistry pathology and genetics.

... [T]he Council have had referred to them by the Board of Control certain recommendations of the Departmental Committee on Sterilization, as contained in the report published last year.[119]

The Medical Research Council's sense of the importance and the urgency of studies of mental defect takes its place in the context of the two *Reports*, the *Wood* of 1929, and the *Brock* of 1934. The organisation of their committee on mental disorder was 'in consultation with the Board of Control', whose powers were in part a result of the earliest Eugenics Society campaign, which had resulted in the Royal Commission on the Care and Control of the Feeble-Minded, and the Mental Deficiency Act of 1913.[120] The initial request was that the Council would advise on the physiological and psychological effects of vasectomy.

Thus the Medical Research Council's Committee on Human Genetics, which Hogben claimed to have been instrumental in setting up, and which included Haldane, Penrose and Fisher among its members, was responsive to the suggestions of both eugenists and anti-eugenists alike in its support of research programmes in human genetics. The Medical Research Council took the Wood Committee's findings on the increasing numbers of feeble-minded extremely seriously; and it arranged investigations into the biological effects of sterilisation, as requested by the Brock Committee. It also funded L.S. Penrose in his study of mental defect: and Penrose in 1933 had passionately denounced the inhumanity of the Wood Committee's remarks on the social problem group, as well as their assertion that the mental deficiency they found in it so commonly was of the primary or hereditary type.[121]

The Rockefeller Foundation, too, funded the research of both groups. The request made to the Foundation in 1924 by the Director of the London School of Economics, Sir William Beveridge, was for grants for 'the study of the physical or natural bases of the social sciences'.[122] This direction of research was approved in 1927 by the granting agency, the Laura Spelman Rockefeller Memorial, and its director, Beardsley Ruml. Hogben's Chair of Social Biology had been the result.

The Rockefeller Foundation's new policy of support for research programmes leading to 'psychobiological knowledge' was intended to produce new data that would 'help in interpreting as well as guiding the behaviour of man'.[123] In 1934, funding was being given to fifteen programmes of this kind, in addition to the social biology group at the London School of Economics. None of the other Rockefeller psychobiology projects at this time were specifically for human genetics.[124]

In July 1934, the Foundation's Assistant Director for Medical Sciences, Daniel P. O'Brien, visited University College, London, and discussed with R.A. Fisher his plan for future research. The Foundation must have been very favourably impressed, as appears from a letter dated November 1934 from W.E. Tisdale, the Rockefeller Assistant Director for Natural Sciences, to his Director, Warren Weaver:

> I am attaching here a memorandum ... concerning a project in GENETICS, which DPO'B and I feel should be presented when further matured by NS MS and if they agree SS [sc., the natural sciences, medical sciences and social sciences sections of the Foundation] because it has so many pure Genetics phases and so many purely medical phases, and the possibility of sociological phases, that we ought all to be together in supporting it, if it is to be supported.
>
> There are but two geneticists with real possibilities in Europe today and those are R.A. Fisher and J.B.S. Haldane.[125]

Soon after O'Brien's visit, Fisher wrote to him setting out the plan and purpose of the project he wanted the Foundation to support, the formation of a research unit for blood-group genetics. Fisher felt, he said, that this was the next important step forward in human genetics, one which 'presented a great opportunity for giving to the subject a solidly objective foundation under strict statistical control'.[126] The most obvious use of this serological research, as O'Brien explained to his Director, was its application to pedigree studies of mental defectives. Genes responsible for anomalies might be detected serologically, even if the anomaly itself was not detectable; or they might be detected through linkage with other genes on the same chromosome.[127]

After some uncertainty, the Foundation approved a grant of £1,575 a year for five years, with the funding coming through the Medical Research Council. It was a substantial amount: the Department of Eugenics had had a total annual budget up to that time of £3,825. The project was considered to fall within the special interests of the Foundation in psychiatry. The role played by inheritance in the causation of mental disease and defect was one of four possible approaches to psychiatry, the others being the effect of infections on the nervous system, the bearing of bodily changes mental activity, and the effect of psychogenic difficulties. A research grant towards a similar pedigree study of mental disease had already been made to the Medical Research Council, and it was suggested that the two might share each other's material.[128]

The very direct relationship of Fisher's new blood-group project and his eugenics is implicit in his correspondence with the Rockefeller Foundation, since, of course, he was Galton Professor of Eugenics, and head of the Department of Eugenics. But it is expressed still more clearly in a speech which he made at the Eugenics Society's Annual General Meeting in May 1935, just as the project was about to start.[129] In this speech, he states that it is the technique of linkage which is likely to revolutionise the methods of individual prognosis in the future. Besides blood-group antigens, he was planning to record other small normal variants, such as the form of ear lobes, the presence of hairs on the second joints of fingers, hair colour and eye colour, and to work these into pedigrees which were to be examined for linkage.

Fisher's example of an inherited disease which might be prevented by timely eugenic advice was Huntington's chorea, a progressive dementia which did not become detectable until middle age, when most carriers of the gene had already had their children. If the linkage to a blood group or other common normal factor could be found, those members of an affected family who had inherited the Huntington's gene could be distinguished from those who had not, even if they had not yet reached the age of onset of the disease, and still seemed to be quite well. They could be advised not to have children, and offered voluntary sterilisation. The technique of linkage might be the answer to the eugenists' problem of the normal carrier of a hidden defect. It was the theme of Fisher's talk to the Society that such 'academic' eugenics should be united with the 'practical', that is:

> practical action in the legislative sphere, based on and prepared by educational propaganda appealing directly to the eugenic conscience of the nation. Only by framing legislative proposals, as in the advocacy of voluntary sterilization, and by preparing ourselves to mobilize our political influence, can the Society, I believe, achieve aims which deserve to be called practical.[130]

Fisher's programme reflects the discussions and conclusions of the Brock Committee on sterilisation, of which he was a member. The *Brock Report* had pointed out that Huntington's chorea is the only mental disorder so far found to be transmitted in a recognisably Mendelian pattern. It was a Mendelian dominant, transmitted directly from an affected parent to half of the children.[131] Environment seemed to play no part in its development, which made it a good subject for both genetical investigation, that is, 'academic' eugenics, and also 'practical' eugenics, or sterilisation. The serology unit which Fisher set up at the Galton Laboratory in 1935 was exactly like the team which Hogben had said in 1931 was what was needed for the human genetics of the future.[132] It included a serologist and an assistant serologist, George L. Taylor and Robert R. Race, who were both physicians; a geneticist, who was Fisher himself, and an anthropologist and a statistician. Fisher, like Hogben, believed that the time for solo projects in human genetics was over. Effective research needed an organised team.[133]

The unit's first project was very much like Hogben's linkage study.[134] Huntington's chorea, like the Friedreich's ataxia that

Hogben had investigated, was a progressive dementia rather than an amentia, as Tredgold would have called it. But it could stand for any heritable feeble-mindedness.[135] Like Ray Pollock, Robbie Race searched out the families of the known cases; they had been traced in the first place by another group of workers, who also had a grant from the Rockefeller Foundation.[136]

Race went from address to address, interviewing the families, taking family histories and samples of blood and saliva, and recording the results of any genetic tests that he could do on the spot. The data he collected included the blood groups ABO, MN and P, the secretion of blood-group substance in the saliva, the ability to taste phenyl-thiocarbamide, the colour of eyes and hair, and the presence or absence of freckles, attached ear lobes, hair on the second phalanx of the fingers, right- or left-handedness, and any other genetic peculiarity that he noticed while talking to the family. Sometimes the results were difficult to decide upon. There was the case of a Mr T., whom Race put down as left-handed. He wrote with his right hand, but, he said, when he played cricket he bowled and threw left-handed, though he batted with his right. He had wanted to bat left-handed, he said, but had had to change over, as 'otherwise he would have had to stand on the curb while batting against a lamp post'.[137] But the data that Race collected from the Huntington's chorea families was never published. There were no linkages to be found between any of the markers and the disease itself. It did not seem to be worth publishing; better examples were sure to be found.

Another project that was very like the first, did, however, get through to publication. Acholuric jaundice, a disease in which the red cells are unusually fragile, was thought to be transmitted as a Mendelian dominant.[138] It had been claimed that the red-cell fragility was part of the so-called haemolytic diathesis, in which it was associated with a long list of more than twenty miscellaneous abnormalities of development. Race quoted one German constitutionalist who called it a 'link in the chain of general hereditary degeneration', though other Continental writers thought that these 'associations' were only coincidence, and that the abnormalities were even more common in the normal population of south Germany than in the series of cases of haemolytic anaemia.[139] Race himself, who by this time had experience of examining a very large number of families, was sceptical about the abnormalities. He brushed off the two most popular, attached ear lobes and hyperextensible joints, with Fisherian 2×2 contingency tables that showed them to be no more likely to be found in affected cases than they were in the normal.[140] His linkage method was also Fisherian in origin, updated by Fisher's student the statistician D.J. Finney.[141,142]

Although he found no linkages between the disease, the blood groups or the family markers, this time the data were worth publishing for the curious pattern of inheritance, a variable penetrance that made it seem in many cases as if the disease was acquired rather than inherited, according to Race. If it was indeed a dominant condition, there were too few affected siblings in his families. Race suggested that the most severe cases were lost as miscarriages, and that perhaps some might have been homozygotes. But the gene, he thought, was probably not present in equilibrium in this population. Within the previous ten years the operation of splenectomy had been found to cure all the symptoms of what had been a serious disability. Natural selection, said Race, must now be distinctly more lenient with the carriers of the gene.

Although Race said nothing about eugenics as such in his paper, it must have been clear to him that environmental change had bypassed the eugenists' attempts at genetic amelioration. The search for a linked marker had been intended as a means of pinpointing the hidden carriers, with a view to offering them sterilisation. Now, with the disease reduced by surgery to an innocuous anomaly, like attached ear lobes, the failure to find a linkage was unimportant in practice, and sterilisation was unnecessary. The Galton serology unit, like Hogben's, in fact, found no linkages during the 1930s. In spite of the high hopes in both laboratories, blood groups and linkage at this time were to contribute nothing to the understanding of the inheritance of mental deficiency. Linkage was still the focus of the serological unit's projects, but its successes — that is, those of Fisher and Race and their colleagues — lay in the field of research into the serology and genetics of the blood groups themselves. They were made when the eugenic aspect of this line of research had been pushed aside by the demands of the Second World War, and the serology unit had been evacuated from London to work on the large-scale production of blood-grouping sera for the Emergency Blood Transfusion Service.[143]

The search for linkage-based on blood-group genetics continued to be a major interest of the Galton Laboratory, which outlasted even Fisher's tenure of the Galton Chair. Lionel Penrose, succeeding him in 1945, was still able to say in 1949 that one of the aims of the laboratory was to build up a large amount of material for linkage studies.[144] Annual Reports on the work of the laboratory put the search for linkage first on the list of its projects, and Penrose's lectures on human genetics always included the blood groups and their 'derived theorems', as he called them, the *Vererbungsmathematik* that gave blood grouping its significance.[145] The search for linkage in fact outlasted the study of eugenics at the Galton Laboratory.

While Lionel Penrose was working on the Colchester material, and attempting to disentangle the genetics of mental defect, the Society was following up another aspect of the *Wood Report*. The *Report* had postulated the existence of the so-called social problem group, a social class consisting mainly, or even entirely, of people who were subnormal in various ways, which it described as the lowest 10 per cent in any society. Here there collected the social inefficients, the paupers, inebriates, habitual criminals and slum dwellers, the prostitutes, unemployables and casual labourers. According to the *Report*, the majority of the members of this class were of a very low-grade mentality, though they might not be quite low enough for certification.

The concept of the social problem group was perfectly in tune with the eugenic problematic: here was a class that was defined by biologically determined social failure. It was the Society's old residuum or pauper class under an updated name. The investigation of this class was quickly adopted as the Society's 'next task', in the words of its President, Sir Bernard Mallet.[146]

The Society took it as its mission to bring before the public the idea of a social problem group, which would widen and generalise the Lidbetter study of the pauper families of East London, which was at that point almost ready for publication. On Friday, 31 July 1932, the Society held a preliminary meeting to set up a Social Problem Investigation Committee, which was to have nine subcommittees, one for each of the categories of delinquent listed in the *Wood Report* as making up the class in question. The categories were:

1 Public assistance
2 Mental disease and defect
3 Epileptics
4 Criminals
5 Slum dwellers

6 Unemployment
7 Prostitution
8 Inebriates
9 Casuals

The question before the Committee was whether the families from which the persons in these categories tended to come, were 'conspicuously below the general social average' – that is to say, belonged to the bottom 10 per cent, and could be defined as members of a class.[147] A secondary question was the part played by Category 2, mental disease and defect, in all eight of the other categories. It was this suggestion that Penrose had called a 'terrible indictment' of the mentally defective. He refused Blacker's request to take part in the Society's investigation.

The Society's last achievement of the thirties, before the outbreak of the Second World War stopped all activity for the duration, was the publication of the collection of essays that resulted from the work of the Social Problem Investigation Committee, entitled *A Social Problem Group?*. The question mark represents Charles Blacker's realisation that it was not at all easy in practice to obtain this kind of information about the *Wood Report*'s categories, and that it was even possible that the group itself was no more than a statistical artefact. Well-to-do people could arrange for themselves to look after a member of their family who was epileptic, feeble-minded or alcoholic. It was only those who were already in poor circumstances who came to the attention of the authorities, who ever became a 'case' to be included in some investigation. The preponderance of these cases in a sample must create a bias that 'threw a bad light', in Blacker's words, on all the members of the category, and downgraded the aggregate class of the sample.[148]

Blacker was explicitly aware that these fundamental weaknesses in the data raised doubts about the very existence of the social problem group as a class, and many of his contributors shared his doubts. One of them was Eliot Slater of the Maudsley Hospital, who, like his colleague Aubrey Lewis, was in touch with Kraepelinian psychiatric research in Germany. Slater cited data collected by Hans Luxenburger from the psychiatric clinics in Munich, clinics which, unlike those in Britain, served all classes, rich and poor. Luxenburger had divided his patients into four classes. If the social problem group had had a higher incidence of mental abnormality than the others, class IV, which covered the bottom 20 per cent, should have shown it. But none of the conditions listed by Luxenburger was concentrated in class IV; manic-depression, on the other hand, was notably over-represented in class I. However, Slater's own collection of cases, approached from the point of view of having been on relief for at least two years, did show a fairly high proportion of 'neuras-thenics', substantiating, though rather feebly, the Society's hopes.[149]

One man who might have been expected to be able to contribute to the problem of the definition of a class was David Caradog Jones. He was a social statistician from the University of Liverpool, who had worked on the voluminous *Social Survey of Merseyside*, which appeared in 1934, along with Alexander Carr-Saunders, and had collaborated again with Carr-Saunders on the *Social Structure of England and Wales* of 1937. Both of these surveys, especially the Merseyside one, dealt with the relation-ships of class, income and subnormality of various kinds.[150] Both were extensively reported in the *Eugenics Review*, in terms that were perfectly in accord with the Society's point of view.[151] It was Jones who provided the summing-up for Blacker's collection.

Jones agreed that simple poverty might cause some of the conditions in question; it certainly aggravated most of them. But he thought that poverty was not the fundamental feature that the families had in common. He picked out quotations from several of the essays tending to show that many of the families investigated showed more than one of the categorical conditions. He cited the essay on epilepsy as an example, followed by Sybil Neville Rolfe (Gotto) on prostitution, and the Lidbetter pauper pedigrees, all mentioning the multiple problems presented by the problem families. The fundamental feature that united the families whose members appeared in these multiple categories was a biological one. It was intelligence.

Intelligence is the supreme gift which raises man above the level of the beasts, and when this is defective ... the resulting lack of balance or judgement may declare itself in more than one form. Intelligence, moreover, is the quality most essential if men are to get on together as members of any social group; those who fail to reach a certain standard of intelligence are liable to become a social problem group. ... Consequently, it is not surprising that the term 'social problem group' should first call to mind the symptoms and not the source of the disability, and that this may have caused some mental confusion among students of social science. If the above theory be correct, it would be more appropriate to think of such a group in terms of biology than in terms of economics.

Jones's words harked back to the earliest days of the Society's Research Committee, to the investigation of the biological cause of pauperism that had begun in 1910. The able-bodied pauper of those days had 'come into the world with his mainspring broken', in the the words of James Slaughter and the Society's Poor Law Committee.[152] In 1937, the Society was still trying to find the data that would persuade public opinion of the appropriateness of this metaphor.

When the war started in 1939, most of the Society's activities were suspended for the duration. Charles Blacker was in uniform, serving as Regimental Medical Officer of an infantry unit. As his war-time letters show, he had no opportunity to do anything for the Society until the war was almost over.

The climate of thought after the war was not, however, favourable to a point of view based on the attempt to define a class, biologically or otherwise. Following the *Beveridge Report* of 1942, with its grand dramatisation of the 'five giants', Disease, Ignorance, Squalor, Idleness and Want, that lay in wait for all citizens on their road through life, it had become very difficult to pin these same features upon a single class.[153] Beveridge's plan was for the abolition of want. He had evidence that five-sixths of it, he said, was due to interruption of earning power, and the rest to the needs of a large family outrunning income. By redistribution of income and children's allowances, these problems *could* have been overcome before the war. After it, they *must* be overcome. The plan covered social insurance, national assistance, allowances for children, health and rehabilitation services, and maintenance of employment.

As part of post-war reconstruction, the series of Acts passed between 1944 and 1948 radically reorganised health and welfare services, and abolished the Poor Law. The Poor Law had made a separate class of those that that needed its help, and labelled its clients paupers. It had given way to the fully developed Welfare State, whose benefits were available to all, without loss of status or distinction of income group. A contemporary commented that administrative divisions were now arranged according to the service offered, such as hospital treatment, sheltered employment or financial assistance, rather than according to the persons served.[154] No one became a pauper by making use of the National Health Service; the state medical service was no longer to be referred to as 'medical relief'.

The sociological theories that emerged during this post-war period reflected these changes in public feeling on the subject of class. The Marxist model of two classes defined by ownership of the means of production, and separated by profoundly conflicting interests, was seen as applying, if at all, to the newly industrialised nineteenth century rather than to the present day. New theories claimed that the age of ideology was over, and that class barriers had given way under the pressure of increased social mobility.[155] The rigidity of the old class system, and its political expression, seemed outdated. From 1951 onwards, a succession of Conservative governments assured voters, in Prime Minister Harold Macmillan's words, that they had 'never had it so good', and as members of a newly affluent society, they believed it. Richard Titmuss, Professor of Social Administration at the London School of Economics, in an effort to bring Labour voters to their senses, referred in a Fabian pamphlet of 1959 to the 'Welfare State Myth':

> The last decade has also witnessed a demonstration of the effectiveness of myth as a motive force in British political beliefs and behaviour. ... Reinforced by the ideologies of enterprise and opportunity it has led to the assumption that most – if not all – of our social problems have been – or soon will be – solved. Those few that remain will, it is thought, be automatically remedied by rising incomes and minor adjustments of one kind or another. In short, it is coming to be assumed that there is little to divide the nation on home affairs except the dreary *minutiae* of social reform, the patronage of the arts, the parking of cars, and the effectiveness of corporal punishment.[156]

In the egalitarian climate of the years after the war, it had become increasingly unacceptable to take a standpoint that inferred that any class was less valuable than the others – or indeed to mention class at all. Blacker's Galton Lecture, given in February 1945, tries to make the Society's post-war policy acceptable in terms of the new *mentalité*. He was aware, he said, that the attack from the left led by Lancelot Hogben in the early thirties had had its effect on the public image of the movement. Antipathy to eugenics had been grafted on to political sentiments, with the result that eugenics had come to be regarded as an expression of political reaction, as class prejudice camouflaged as science.

Blacker's solution was to try as far as he could to detach the expression of eugenic policy from any class implication. The post-war programme was to give a new importance to the environment, as the critics of the thirties had demanded, but in a peculiarly eugenist manner. Blacker argued that in an environment where philoprogenitiveness entailed economic hardship, the prudent, who were the eugenically desirable type, would not have many children. That would be left to the feckless. His argument incorporates the pleas of pre-war days for a 'eugenically sound' system of family allowances, in which the allowance was *directly*, not inversely, proportional to income. This approach, he said (in 'Eugenics in retrospect and prospect'),

> avoids the thorny question of social class. There are eugenically valuable people in all social classes, though it is possible that they may be proportionately more numerous in some classes and occupations than others.

Blacker had tried hard to accommodate his critics. Indeed, he claimed in his Galton Lecture to have learnt a lot from Hogben and Haldane. But his ingenious argument betrayed itself. It was impossible for him to re-think eugenics so as to do without social class as an indicator of social worth.

Soon after the war ended, the Society was again pursuing its old object, the social problem group. The committee had changed its name, however, and was now to be known as the Problem Families Committee, a reflection of its sensitivity to criticisms that the problem families did not constitute a group or class at all. By November 1947, the Committee had designed a project to investigate that point.

According to the Committee's mandate, families were to be

defined as 'problem' if they met four criteria: intractable ineducability, instability or infirmity of character, multiple social problems and a squalid home. As an illustration of this last and most characteristic feature, the Committee quoted a graphically disgusting description of squalidity by R.C. Wofinden, Deputy Medical Officer of Health at Bristol, and which Wofinden himself was to quote over and over again. Families of this description were to be traced in six different areas, through the administrative authorities running the social services in each area. These included the health visitors, sanitary inspectors, probation officers, social workers from child guidance clinics and mental hospitals, and officials from labour exchanges and housing authorities, as well as the Charity Organisation Society, now called the Family Welfare Association.

Families ascertained from the lists of clients of any of these were to be visited by a field worker, who was to weed out all those who were dependent by reason of injury or chronic disease, who 'fell outside the spirit of the description'. A supplementary inquiry by Caradog Jones was to cover the measured intelligence of a sample of the families, to tie this multiple failure to a biologically based mental defect. A card index was prepared of the genuine problem families of each area.[157]

Once again, E.O. Lewis's paragraph from the *Wood Report*, on the criminal and anti-social tendencies of the mentally defective, was quoted. The object of the inquiry was still, as it had been before the war, to confirm his suggestion that these squalid and feckless families did indeed constitute a group, a class that could be marked out from the rest of the population by its many different problems and its demands upon many different social services.

It had been fairly simple, before the war, to list the numbers of paupers on relief on a given day, as Lidbetter had done. The contemporary equivalent of the pauper class, the problem families, was to consist of the families whose names came up again and again on the lists supplied by a series of different welfare agencies. Although the welfare services were now available to all citizens with no stigma following their use, the Society's investigators expected to find that the pauper class still existed, and that it could be defined under the new conditions by the multiplicity of its needs and failures.

The project, as had often happened with the Society's projects, did not come to the full fruition that had been planned. Its most enthusiastic supporter was R.C. Wofinden of Bristol, but even his findings were not very clear from the Society's point of view.[158] Unlike Lidbetter, Wofinden failed to find an extensive network of intermarriages between the Bristol families on his list. Compared with the number of children expected for working-class families, these problem families were often large: if dead, absent or grown-up children were included, the figure was 5.8 per family, as against a working-class average of 2.5. Wofinden's social worker, Sister Comer of the Health Department, assessed a large percentage of both parents and children as being of subnormal intelligence, but her assessments were not based on formal intelligence tests. Wofinden said he could find only a weak indication that problem conditions 'ran in families'. In addition, the numbers ascertained turned out to be much smaller than expected. In Bristol, there were no more than 155 families with a total of 1,036 members in a population of 425,596, a proportion of 0.24 per cent, far less than Lewis's postulated 10 per cent of the population.[159]

The collection of data from the six areas was intended to be a pilot study for a more extensive, country-wide survey of problem families. In Wofinden's opinion, however, the method of data collection was not a success. Many families were not discovered by his initial circularisation of the welfare authorities. When he circularised them a second time with a list of names collected from all agencies, he was told in many cases that the family in question had been a problem, but that now the problem was solved. Wofinden's recommendations for dealing with the families centred mainly on their medical and economic needs, and the possibility of helping them in practical ways to learn the techniques of housekeeping and child-rearing. He had found them both pathetic and disgusting, but he had little to say about sterilisation, and nothing about the danger to society of the families' high birth rate.

Blacker had put a great deal of effort into organising the project, and had expected that the result would have been important enough to support the call for an official inquiry into problem families. But the results were patchy and incomplete; the various Medical Officers of Health who worked on it had neither enough time nor enough funding. E.O. Lewis himself, the originator of the social problem group as a concept, felt embarrassed by the standard of the work, and perhaps even by the fact that it had been done at all. He wrote to Blacker:

> On the whole, I think it would be advisable to withhold it at present. ... It is as well to bear in mind that the subject of problem families and its cognate The Social Problem Group is becoming a favourite 'Aunt Sally' with a group of scientists of a certain political hue.[160]

Blacker scribbled in the margin of the letter that 'Lewis seems ... unduly scared of this'. The opposition of the left-wing scientists was something that Blacker was quite used to.

The *Percy Report* of the Royal Commission on the Law Relating to Mental Illness and Mental Deficiency, which sat from 1954 to 1957, exemplified the post-war reluctance to see social problems in terms of a class. The *Percy Report* stated that the new system of administration had divided up the responsibilities of the Poor Law into a whole range of different services. Instead of poor persons receiving everything from a single authority, particular authorities provided particular forms of service for people whose needs arose from a variety of different causes. The new system, in the words of the *Report*, had 'broken away from the idea of dividing people into categories with labels which may be regarded as derogatory and as putting them in a class apart from the rest of society'.[161] The *Report* made a special point of saying that the labelling and segregation of the feeble-minded was unnecessary. The majority of those now classified as feeble-minded were capable of mixing and working with other people, and should not be sent to mental deficiency hospitals where they would be cut off from all normal company. Most of them could manage to live in their own families, with the help of the welfare services. The *Percy Report* led to the passage of the new Mental Health Act which came into force in 1960.

The turn away from the eugenic tradition was obvious, too, in the evidence submitted to the Royal Commission by the professional societies, the Royal College of Physicians, the Royal Medico-Psychological Society and the British Psychological Society. The statements of all three included some contribution from Lionel Penrose.[162] The British Psychological Society, for instance, a group with 1,200 members at that date, presented a memorandum put together by a committee which included M.I. Dunsdon, of the Burdon Mental Research Department at Stoke

Park Hospital, Bristol; Alan D.B. Clarke, Senior Clinical Psychologist, at the Manor Hospital, Epsom, and Neil O'Connor, from the Medical Research Council's Unit for Research in Occupational Adaptation, at the Maudsley Hospital. In an earlier generation, the Burdon Trust had been funded by a eugenist sympathiser for eugenic research on the mentally defective, and administered by R.J.A. Berry, also a eugenist.[163] The Maudsley Hospital, too, had been an institution that could be counted upon: its connections with the Kraepelin clinic in Munich had been maintained from the days of Henry Maudsley up to those of Sir Aubrey Lewis. The memorandum, which represented the views of a post-war generation, made its position on the eugenist point of view absolutely explicit:

> At the time of the passing of the first Mental Deficiency Act [sc., 1913], a much simpler view of human genetics was taken by the experts than is now considered warranted by available evidence and modern research techniques. Studies of relevant documents of that period (*Hansard, The Eugenics Review*, 1909–1911, *The Poor Law Commission Report*, etc.) indicates that the fear of national degeneracy assumed great importance in the minds of the experts giving evidence: e.g. 'National degeneracy is no myth but a very serious reality ... the chief evil we have to prevent is undoubtedly that of propagation' (Tredgold). 'Cases are not wanting to show that pauperism is hereditary' (Sir E. Brabrook). This point of view naturally led to the segregation of many of those considered to be potential biological dangers to the community. The practice of custodial care, as opposed to remedial treatment, thus developed. Although the possibility of a decline in national intelligence is still a matter of controversy, Penrose (*Biology of Mental Defect*, 1949) states that, '... the great majority of defectives of all grades are born to parents who cannot be classed as defectives themselves. ... There is no precise genetics of social inefficiency, so the idea that it can be prevented on the basis of genetical theory is essentially invalid' (op. cit., p. 234).[164]

The influence of Penrose on professional expert opinion thus combined with the break-up of the once unitary functions of the Poor Law, to weaken both these aspects of the eugenic problematic.

251

Penrose, indeed, was the Society's most persistent critic in the years after the Second World War. He never let slip an opportunity for pointing out the flaws in every aspect of the eugenists' arguments. He often showed a slide of one of Lidbetter's pedigrees as an example of naïve confusion, and he pointed out that, in spite of the high fertility of the class with the lowest height and the lowest measured intelligence, it now appeared that intelligence had not gone down, and heights had been steadily increasing ever since measurements had been being made.[165] The Wood Committee had agreed in 1929 that the true criterion of mental defect was social incompetence, but incompetence varied from society to society. In towns it was closely linked to success in school, whereas in the country that had much less importance. Penrose calculated that the age incidence of mental defect coincided precisely with the age incidence of schooling: epidemiologically, the greatest risk was in the 11-to-14 age group, with infants and adults being much less susceptible to this disease. An epidemiologist, he said, would have to conclude that its chief cause was probably exposure to education. In the changed climate of post-war thinking on mental defect, his remarks were cited as an indication of the social determination of mental defect, and its effect on the number of cases ascertained in a community.[166]

Penrose thought that it was quite likely that intelligence was in genetic equilibrium, in the sense explored by Fisher and

Table 5.1 Penrose's model of a population in genetical equilibrium, in which the numbers of the class with a high IQ are replenished from the class below

Mating	Frequency (%)	No. of offspring	Types of offspring		
			AA	Aa	aa
AA × AA	90	1.89	17	–	–
Aa × Aa	10	4.0	1	2	1
aa × aa	0	0.0	–	–	–
Total offspring			18	2	1

AA: normal, with IQ 108
Aa: defective, with IQ 66, and high fertility: they represent the 'submerged 10%' or social problem group
aa: very defective, with IQ 24, do not reproduce

Average IQ for the population is 100

Source: L.S. Penrose, 'Genetical influences on the intelligence level of the population' (1950), n. 146

Haldane: the eugenists had failed to take into account that the lowest intelligence levels were almost completely infertile. It was an idea that he often made use of in talks to audiences of non-geneticists. He worked out a model of a population in which there was differential fertility and assortative mating for intelligence, which would nevertheless be in genetic equilibrium.

According to the model, this population is in genetical equilibrium. The defectives' matings not only keep up their own numbers, but contribute to replenishing the numbers in the AA class, while their aa offspring do not reproduce and die out. If the numbers of the superior group were reduced, lowering the average IQ, the numbers would rise again in each succeeding generation, replenished from below, until they were again in equilibrium. Penrose concluded that the part of the population that is most fertile, but least well-adapted to scholastic training, was important both in maintaining the numbers of the whole population, and giving it genetical stability for IQ.[167] His model and his argument are a parody of the eugenists' prognoses for the future of the race, that ended with the decline of the population into imbecility due to the luxuriant fecundity of the pauper class.

As Penrose said, during his tenure of the Galton Chair, at the Department of Eugenics, Biometry and Genetics, nobody taught eugenics, and the Galton Professor of Eugenics was not a eugenist.[168] By 1954, he had changed the name of the house journal, the *Annals of Eugenics*, to *Annals of Human Genetics*. In 1963, he managed to have the title of his chair changed too, to the Galton Professorship of Human Genetics.[169]

It is interesting to compare the picture of Penrose's work that I have presented in this chapter with his own account of the history of human genetics, written in 1966. His history begins with Wilhelm Weinberg and G.H. Hardy, moves to R.A. Fisher's reconciliation of correlation and Mendelism of 1918, and then to the criticism of Fisher's belittlement of environmental influence by Haldane and Hogben, which, he says, 'enlivened the picture'. The 'fine opportunities for the application of mathematical and statistical methods' offered by human genetics were realised by Fritz Lenz and Gunnar Dahlberg with their models of consanguinity, and by Felix Bernstein's work on the triple allele hypothesis and on linkage. The linkage lead was followed up by R.A. Fisher and his blood-grouping unit at the

Galton Laboratory during the 1930s. Another feature of the work of the thirties was the gradual acceptance of the necessity for defining not only the presence or absence of a given trait in a family, but also its frequency in the general population. This was a perception that had originated in the programme of Rüdin's group in Munich, though Penrose does not name them specifically. He ends his account with a denunciation of the 'cult of eugenics':

> My reason for taking this stand is that eugenics was based upon *arbitrary valuations of individuals and social groups*, [my emphasis] supported by unjustified and premature assumptions about the nature of hereditary influences.[170]

A knowledge of genetics will benefit the human race eventually, he says, but the social and biological values of hereditary differences are continually altering as the environment changes, and it is not possible to be sure that a given gene will be bad in all circumstances.

In this account of the history of human genetics, Penrose lists the techniques of investigation that he himself had used, emphasising particularly the *Vererbungsmathematik*, the mathematical models, and the empirical data-collection methods, both of them originating in the German eugenics movement. Weinberg and Lenz, and the Munich empiricists, and R.A. Fisher in Britain, were all committed to eugenics. In his rejection of eugenics, Penrose appears to separate the methods from the broader questions that they were designed to answer, and from the interests of the thinkers who developed them. But Hogben and Haldane, and especially Penrose himself, the enemies of the movement, were no less involved in it than its supporters. The questions they answered were those which had been proposed by the eugenists, and so were the new and powerful methods they used. Although all three of the *contras* felt that ordering the genes on the chromosome was the proper study of mankind, the questions that their studies were to answer were the same ones that were being asked by their opposite numbers on the other side of the fence. Neither were they opposed to the idea that genetics in itself might be used to upgrade the human race, as Penrose's statement and the 'Geneticists' manifesto' of September 1939 show. The *Colchester Survey*, as well as Penrose's post-war preoccupation with trouncing the eugenists, demonstrates the pervasiveness of the eugenist problematic even where the writer was plainly hostile to the aims and the traditional methods of eugenics. The attackers from the left found weaknesses in the scientific method used by the British eugenists, and they upgraded them by demonstrating the use of the methods introduced by eugenists in Germany. The British methods were not very sophisticated, but they could be improved. The attackers were far more deeply offended by the eugenists' conflation of social class and social worth, and, in the case of Penrose, by the conflation of mental defect and the social problem group. The changes in method that the *contras* advocated were designed to eliminate class as a unit-character from human genetics.

The disintegration of the eugenist problematic that followed the Second World War must be ascribed not only to the changes in genetics, but also to the social changes that were associated with the reconstruction of the welfare system and the final disappearance of the Poor Law. The timing is significant: the Society had survived the attacks by the geneticists of the left which took place in the early thirties. It had survived the war, and the disgrace of the German movement. It emerged in 1945 ready to re-start its projects on the social problem group, or the problem families, as the group had come to be called as it became less and less certain that it was in fact a group. It could not, however, survive the break-up of the Poor Law and the new *mentalité* of the egalitarian welfare state. The loss of the old clarity of the class dimension, in public opinion, if not in any other way, meant the end of the British eugenics movement.

In 1968, Charles Blacker was forced to admit that the there was no longer any reason for the continuation of the *Eugenics Review*. With the sixtieth volume, containing reprints of some of the best of its old articles, some essays on the history of the Society, and a very useful index, the *Review* came to an end. Its mandate had been mainly to promote the interests of the movement by propaganda. Blacker could see that its time had now passed.[171] In the new *Journal of Biosocial Science* that succeeded the *Eugenics Review*, the Society withdrew on to the safer ground of a quantitative bio-demography, in which the informed observer might discern shadows of its former concerns with differential fertility, social problems and intelligence, now often set in the Third World.

EPILOGUE AND
CONCLUSION

Up to this point, this book has been dealing with an era in the history of human genetics in Britain that appeared to wind down with the weakening of the peculiar problematic that had held it together. It analyses the eugenics movement in terms of a single unifying theme: the focus of the movement upon the concept of a hereditary pauper class.

From the early seventies, it has been clear to historians that the membership of the Eugenics Society was highly homogeneous from the point of view of class. There have been several attempts since then to divide the membership into finer categories. It was a logical extension of this thinking, or perhaps an idea derived from Michel Foucault's *Archéologie du Savoir*, to expand the examination synchronically, and to look at the Society as a member of a broad archaeological stratum containing a tangle of interlocking and overlapping groups of middle-class activists, some medical, some sociological, some educational and some political, whose statements of purpose all reveal a common focus upon the urban poor.[1] It was this relationship, established by the Victorian social reform movements long before the founding of the Eugenics Education Society, that defined the nature of the eugenic problematic in Britain. The key concept of the movement was the inheritance of social worth in terms of social class. The Society's direct forerunners in the Charity Organisation Society had discussed a residuum, a class of destitutes which was beyond the help of charity, and which must be left to the Poor Law. The Eugenics Education Society itself, very soon after its founding, began its research project on the pauper families of East London, which was to continue to the end of its active life. The residuum evolved into the pauper class, which evolved into the social problem group, which in turn became the problem families. The project was brought to an end only by the flattening out of the old forms of class consciousness, and by the disappearance of the pauper class as an administrative category after the end of the war.

Class, then, as well as hereditarianism, was an essential part of the eugenist problematic. A problematic has been defined simply as a choice of problems, but perhaps it should be more strongly stated: certain concepts are rendered all-important, and others more or less invisible. The all-important problem of the British eugenists was the inheritance of pauperism. The specific pathology of pauperism was feeble-mindedness, which provided the biological basis for its inheritance.

The attacks on eugenics that came from the left during the thirties were essentially attacks on this problematic. It was this that had set the programme of work on human inheritance in Britain up to this time, so it was not easy for the geneticists of the left to disentangle from the existing field those elements of human genetics that were worth preserving. They were them-selves affected by it: there were already ongoing lines of thought, such as that on mental defect, to which they contributed. Only one methodology seemed to be perfectly safe. If a character were found to be genetically linked to a blood group, it *must* be truly biological, and free of class-bias. The non-scientific intru-sion of class values could be controlled for mathematically: blood grouping was the perfect value-free science, and the mapping of genes along a chromosome was the first duty of human geneticists.

The attack from the left was, broadly speaking, successful. The *Annals of Eugenics* became the *Annals of Human Genetics* in 1955, and the *Eugenics Review* came to an end in 1968. The Society continued to pursue a social biology in the journals that it started in place of the old *Review*, but the articles published addressed a group that was more interested in fertility patterns in the Third World than in persuading the legislature to deal with a pauper class at home. By 1989, the Society had given up its efforts to educate the public. It changed its name and moved out of town, leaving the field to human genetics. The problem of mapping the human chromosomes, the value-free science which J.B.S. Haldane had called the proper study of mankind, was left, the legacy of the struggles of the thirties.

The disintegration of the eugenic problematic after the end of the war was mainly a product of changed social attitudes. Post-war reconstruction was dominated by the idea that a time of triumphant social justice was now here, and that the expected continuous economic growth would deal with the remaining problems of inequality. A depressed class defined administratively or biologically seemed no longer to be possible. It has now become all too clear that class distinctions, in life chances, morbidities and mortalities, have not been equalised by the Welfare State. At the time, however, class distinction appeared to be levelled already, or was soon to be so. It was a feeling that Winston Churchill, speaking of the *Beveridge Report* of 1942, had called 'dangerous optimism'.

The change in social structure and social attitudes was felt generally by the political left and the right. Sociologists, trying to apply theory to existing conditions, were among the most sensitive indicators of the change. The rise of a post-war conservative sociology predicated on the 'end of ideology', as in the work of Daniel Bell and Edward Shils, to mention only two of a large group of writers, was a product of this new feeling. The loss of confidence in a class analysis affected the Marxist as much as the conservative or eugenist. Norman Birnbaum, writing in the late sixties on the 'crisis in Marxist sociology', put the problem in terms that, like all good abstractions, are useful in more than one situation:

A doctrinal or theoretic crisis in a system of thought occurs when either of two sets of abstract conditions obtains. In one case, the possibilities of internal development exhaust themselves. ... In the other case, the realities apprehended by the system in its original form change, so much so that the categories are inapplicable to the new conditions.[2]

It is Birnbaum's second case that seems to apply here: the old categories appeared to be inapplicable to the new conditions. The eugenic problematic had grown out of the union of a middle-class activism focused upon the pauper class, with a biological view of human failings. In the egalitarian world of welfare and economic growth, the pauper class had disappeared. A class analysis no longer carried weight, and with the loss of the class dimension, the eugenic problematic could no longer survive in its original form.

But what about Birnbaum's first case? Have the possibilities of internal development of the eugenics movement exhausted themselves? The most recent answer now seems to be that they have not. Instead, they have been renewed by the new methods of research upon the human genome.

It is easy to interpret eugenics as a precursor of human genetics, which had to disappear when human genetics became a mature science. The terror of forced sterilisation has now given way to genetic counselling sought by patients for themselves. However, the developments of the 1980s in human genetics have raised anew some of the old fears about eugenics.

The chromosome mapping programme of the sixties and seventies continued along the lines chalked out before the war. There were a large number of linkage studies using blood groups and other inherited marker systems. Many of the workers in this field were blood-group serologists, whose bible was a beautifully written book by the married team of Robert Race and Ruth Sanger, entitled *Blood Groups in Man*.[3] Race and Sanger themselves and the serologists around them at the Lister Institute in London, such as Sylvia Lawler and Marie Cutbush, searched for new blood-group markers, investigated possible linkages and provided an expert reference service to the community of interested parties.[4] One of these was J.H. Renwick, working at the London School of Hygiene and Tropical Medicine, who claimed a 99 per cent chance that the gene determining *Myotonia dystrophica* was linked to the *Secretor* locus, which determined the presence or absence of blood-group substances in the saliva.[5] Victor McKusick, the leading American human geneticist, working at Johns Hopkins Hospital in Baltimore, Maryland, wrote optimistically in 1977 that there were now more than fifty usefully polymorphic traits that could serve as markers for linkage.[6]

In spite of McKusick's enthusiastic assessment of progress and of future possibilities, others were not so positive about the prospects of mapping the chromosomes by existing methods. Serologists in the Netherlands had collected 198 blood samples from three extended families showing the inheritance of Huntington's disease. They used twenty-seven markers, including seven blood group systems, ten plasma proteins, nine red cell enzymes and the human lymphocyte antigen (HLA) groups, and analysed the results using two different computer programmes.

No evidence of a linkage was found, either in their own material, or in a second batch of thirteen more kindreds sent to them by Renwick from London. The Dutch workers concluded that no more than about 15 per cent of the human genome had been excluded as a site for the Huntington's gene, which left a depressingly large percentage untouched. There was little to be expected, they felt, from more random linkage studies of families with Huntington's.[7] Other projects, including a particularly large one in the United States, in spite of thousands of man-hours of effort, found next to nothing. The author of this book worked on one such project in 1961; many years later, it reported the expected negative results. It was a depressing experience.

It could be said that, using the methods based on serology and mathematics, the blood-groupers had done all they could. Linkage had seemed very promising, and huge numbers of blood samples had been collected and family data analysed all over the world. Both the serology and the mathematics were highly skilled and time-consuming, and very few useful results had appeared so far.

In the last years of the decade, however, linkage mapping was transformed by a new, more concrete methodology, the technique of examining the chromosomal DNA sequence itself for markers, without waiting to find out what it was that the sequence controlled. The DNA was divided up using enzymes that attacked it wherever they found a specific sequence of base-pairs; in many cases the fragments produced differed in the two members of a homologous chromosome pair — that is, they represented genetic polymorphisms. The fragments, called restriction-fragment length polymorphisms or RFLP, were separated electrophoretically, and then identified using a strand of DNA whose sequence was known, which bound to the fragment whose sequence was complementary to its own. The known strand was radioactively labelled, and could be identified. Where there was a polymorphism, the radioactivity appeared at different spots in different individuals. This neat technique was known as the Southern blot, after its inventor, Edward M. Southern of Edinburgh University. Among its first results was the mapping to the X-chromosome, by two different groups of English workers, of the gene for muscular dystrophy, which the serologists had already picked out fairly successfully.[8]

The next achievement, which followed in 1983, was the localisation to chromosome 4 of a marker very close to the gene for Huntington's chorea. This was the result of work by a group that included Nancy Wexler, and used blood samples from an extended kindred of over 7,000 members, with many cases of Huntington's among them, living near Lake Maracaibo in Venezuela.[9]

Several different laboratories as well as private firms in the United States and in Europe now began to collect libraries of cloned DNA probes. Other physical mapping methods helped to localise a gene and its marker on the larger-scale map. This could be expected to lead, with time and sufficient funding, to a full, high-resolution map of the complete genome. A report to the US Office of Technology Assessment advised mapping the genome one chromosome at a time, dividing and subdividing the fragments until the level of restriction enzyme mapping and lining up of fragments in their original order was reached.[10]

First predictions, made in 1980 by American workers, suggested that a random scatter of about 150 markers would be enough to provide fixed points for a linkage map of all human genes.[11] But those located were not evenly spaced, and later estimates by the group working at the Howard Hughes Medical Institute of the University of Utah revised this 150 to 'thousands'. By 1987, 475 of them had been reported. By 1988, genetic markers for ten single-gene diseases had been picked out, including muscular dystrophy, cystic fibrosis, Huntington's chorea, sickle cell anaemia, haemophilia, beta-thalassaemia, Alzheimer's disease and phenylketonuria. In most of them, the gene had been cloned, and the abnormal protein identified.[12]

The genetics community regarded these developments with tremendous excitement. As Victor McKusick wrote in 1988,

> The general enthusiasm that greeted these reports was entirely justified. All of these conditions shared in common the characteristic that at the time the mapping was achieved, there was no clue as to the nature of the fundamental biochemical defect, and therefore it was impossible to devise a specific diagnostic test for carrier detection, pre-clinical diagnosis or prenatal diagnosis and impossible to develop any methods of treatment that would serve to correct or counteract the ill effects of that biochemical

defect. A leading and immediate effect of the mapping of
the disorders ... is that it permits the elucidation of the
fundamental fault and the devising of specific diagnostic
methods.[13]

Not only could genetic defects be firmly predicted, but the
possibility now arose, at least in the future, for correction of the
defects.

Projects on a large scale, and with international cooperation,
began to be set up. In Europe, the European Molecular Biology
Laboratory in Heidelberg arranged to share its DNA sequence
data with GenBank, one of the private American companies.
The Paris *Centre d'Étude du Polymorphisme Humaine* (CEPH) was
founded in 1983 by Jean Dausset, well known for his work
on human lymphocyte polymorphisms, with funding from an
anonymous donor and from his own Nobel Prize. The CEPH
panel of family material was partly contributed by a research
unit of the Howard Hughes Institute in Utah. Jean-Marc
Lalouel, a mathematical geneticist at Utah, designed computer
programmes that would analyse linkages and also sketch mapping possibilities. CEPH organised a programme of open
international cooperation, based on its panel of forty families.
Any investigator who already had a set of DNA probes might
use the centre's DNA samples and its computer programmes,
and, in return, agreed to make the results of testing with its
DNA probes available to the centre. Significantly, the investigators
did not have to make the probes themselves available. Some of
them were likely to be patented.[14]

Governments were also interested. By 1987, the US National
Institute of Health was already providing $110 million for a
range of different projects involving mapping and sequencing.
In 1988, the NIH received $17.3 million in new funds specially
for the genome project, and in 1989, the Presidential Budget
request increased that to $28 million. This funding enabled it to
set up the NIH Office of Human Genome Research, with the
mandate of coordinating existing genome research within the
NIH, planning new initiatives and, in particular, promoting
technological developments.[15] Like the NIH, the US National
Research Council's Committee on Mapping and Sequencing the
Human Genome saw the acquisition of a complete map as being
so important that it justified a specially organised effort outside

the normal course of biological research. It recommended that, 'in view of the importance and magnitude of the task, a rapid scale-up to $200 million of additional funding per year' would be appropriate, and that this should be new funding, not money diverted from the current federal research budget for bio-medical sciences.[16]

In Britain, mapping and sequencing projects were funded through the Medical Research Council, in 1985–86 to a total of £4.2 million, centred on the Molecular Genetics Unit at Cambridge. There was no suggestion of setting up a special project or a special unit for the purpose of mapping alone, although the Council had the power to do that, and had done it in the past for other areas of research.[17] But it did support the plan of an individual, the geneticist Sydney Brenner, to map the human genome with funds from a prize he had received, as long as the work cost his Medical Research Council Unit nothing.[18] The Council excluded collaboration with private firms by stipulating that all information and all clones were to remain in the public domain. In spite of this imbalance in funding, according to figures collected by the US Office of Technology Assessment on numbers of publications in the international genetics journals, Britain ranked second (a distant second, however) to the United States in the number of articles on human gene mapping.

In Japan, the Science and Technology Agency of the government set aside a Special Coordination Fund of $3.8 million beginning in 1981 for the development of automated robotic technology in the area of DNA sequencing studies. A prototype machine made by Seiko appeared, but had not (by 1988) been very widely accepted. In spite of that, the news of the Japanese interest in sequencing instrumentation aroused American fears that the sales of American machines would suffer.[19]

Outside the genetics community, however, and outside those political circles concerned, like the US Congress, with inter-national rivalry disguised as international cooperation, the mapping project was not regarded nearly so favourably. Problems that had been invisible while the linkage studies had been having little success suddenly became real problems now that people could imagine a world in which the contents of one's genome might be made public. Many of those currently worrying about ethical issues looked back to the eugenics movement as their example of a dangerous and inhumane human genetics. American ethicists, such as Dorothy Nelkin, Professor of Sociology at New York University, and Laurence Tancredi, a psychiatrist-lawyer, director of the University of Texas Health Law Centre, linked the impulse to multiply tests, medical, educational and judicial, with the biological reductionism that had legitimised the American eugenics movement. The eugenists had used biological science to justify large-scale sterilisation, the exclusion of immigrants and the loss of access to education. Nelkin and Tancredi noted that post-war understanding of the effects of the eugenics movement in Germany had toned down the popularity of biological explanations as a guide to social policy for a time, but that the sixties had seen a revival, at least among scientists. There had been some reaction against this, but the genetic discoveries of the eighties seemed, they thought, to have shifted the balance in the nature-versus-nurture controversy decisively to the side of nature. The 'new eugenics', they admitted, has tried to avoid the cruder biologism of race and class. It appears instead to be focusing upon individuals and their fate as predicted by their genes.[20]

There are, it is true, many advantages to such knowledge for the individual. However, troubling fears, as expressed in articles in the daily press and in magazines directed to the general reader, have tended to focus on the problem of the use of genetic information in a market-oriented society by insurance companies and employers. It may not be to people's advantage to know that they carry an oncogene which renders them susceptible to toxic chemicals, even though the knowledge should allow them to take steps to avoid contact with that type of chemical. If the information comes out as part of an examination for insurance, an insurance company may refuse to accept them: there are already several categories of medical uninsurables, a tragic fate in the United States, where there is no state responsibility for medicine. An employer may decide to screen applicants for the gene, and not employ them, rather than cleaning up the environment of the factory. Nelkin and Tancredi cite a trade-union leader as predicting that the 1980s would be 'the decade of genetic struggles in the workplace'.[21] Perhaps he spoke too soon: the decade in question may turn out to be the nineties.

The daily press has also taken up the problem. An article on genetic screening in the Toronto daily *Globe and Mail* is headed 'Genetic screening: employees under a microscope'.[22] The *New York Times* cites Nelkin and Tancredi at length and repeats their warnings about the recovery of eugenic patterns of thought.[23] A *Time* magazine cover says, 'The drive to map human genes could revolutionize medicine, but it also raises troubling ethical questions.' Inside, the article again compares current thinking with the thinking of the eugenists in America and in Nazi Germany.[24] American *Vogue* interviewed Nancy Wexler, one of the team that located the Huntington's gene, who told them that the suicide rate for diagnosed Huntington's patients was seven times the national average. She had noticed, she said, an emotional upheaval, 'survivor's syndrome', even in those who are given the good news that they do not carry the gene.[25] Each of these sources, in rehearsing the dangers of the new genetics, makes some reference to the eugenics movements of the recent past.

In Europe, closer still to a dangerous eugenics movement, and well aware of its history, fears were even more overt. As *Science* reported, the genome project was given a rough ride there.[26] In 1988, the Commission of the European Communities produced a proposal to adopt a research programme entitled *Predictive Medicine: Human Genome Analysis*.[27] It was referred to the Committee on Energy, Research and Technology of the European Parliament for comment. The *rapporteur* entrusted with it was Benedikt Härlin, a member of the left-wing group called *Arc en Ciel*, a party which includes members of the German Greens, among other ecologically minded European parties.[28] The proposal itself had been a fairly positive document. Its title, *Predictive Medicine*, indicated its generally sympathetic tenor. But Härlin's treatment of it was anything but sympathetic, and demonstrated in the clearest possible way the equation of the genome projects with eugenics. His first objection was to the title: *Predictive Medicine* was to be cut, leaving only *Human Genome Analysis*. Throughout the report, Härlin excised sections that presented the goals of the programme as 'improvements', and inserted cautionary remarks on its dangers. To a section dealing with 'Research on the improvement of advanced genetic technologies', Härlin added a list of additional desiderata:

Amendment No 18

New paragraph to be added ... :
Evaluation of the risk of using genetic engineering and processes in analysing the human genome, definition of conditions and development of procedures to ensure absolute protection for individual genetic data, ... to assess the medical, social, economic, political and moral implications of the use of knowledge obtained from human genome research, development of programmes for public information on the possibilities offered by, and the dangers of, human genome research, study of the history of and current trends in eugenics.[29]

Härlin insisted on the importance of including the study of the history of eugenics, and of listing desirable measures of preventing misuse of the scientific knowledge, in the proposal that was to be debated by the European Parliament. Härlin warns that this technologically 'clean' type of eugenics differs from traditional eugenics only in form but not in its basic goal. Every attempt, he wrote, to use genetic knowledge for the benefit of mankind is inseparable from decisions concerning health and social policy which in one form or another are eugenic in nature. And, he pointed out, the US study *Mapping our Genes* had been very limited in its criticism of the eugenics of the past. According to the Americans, it was only the means, not the goals, of that movement that were at fault: today's technologies would allow us to achieve eugenic objectives by technical, rather than social, control.[30]

In the debate that followed upon the amendments that Härlin's committee had proposed, he himself again made the point that

> history teaches us to be extremely cautious and extremely distrustful of our own ability to exercise democratic and social control, especially within an international framework. ... Even before the first findings of this research are available, there is danger of our declining into a kind of bio-deterministic conception of the world, of our subscribing to the mistaken belief that everything is already predetermined in our genes. This would run counter to the very substance of our present concept of freedom and equality.[31]

The members of the European Parliament took Härlin's fears very seriously indeed: the reference to eugenics clearly touched them. The Vice-President of the Commission, however, disclaimed any connection of the programme with those of the past:

> here I have to be very firm in saying what this programme isn't. It is not – and it would be horrible to think it was, and I refuse to believe that anyone inside or outside this Chamber could think it to be – a programme for some eugenic purpose, or for the so-called selection of the human species. We do not mean to evoke spectres of the past; our roots are in today's society, which fortunately is immunised to the highest degree against risks of this kind, and if it were not sufficiently so immunised, we should strive to immunise it further.[32]

The disintegration of the eugenic problematic that occurred in the years following the Second World War was more a product of the changed social attitudes that came to Britain with the post-war welfare state than a product of the attacks made on it by the geneticists of the left. One way or another, however, human genetics was left in posession of a field that now coincided almost exactly with the programme the geneticists had advocated. The old class-centred problematic has almost disappeared, as the *contras* had hoped. Ironically, the American statement that we could now achieve eugenic goals by technical, rather than social, control, which was cited with polemic intent by Härlin, mirrored almost exactly the polemic statements of the thirties of men like Lancelot Hogben. Hogben had compared the safely value-free technology of linkage studies with the Eugenics Society's crude attempt at displaying the inheritance of human failings in its pauper pedigrees. But it is the alternative programme which has become the new eugenics, and which in its turn is raising ethical problems.

The virus has mutated, and we are not as well immunised as we thought. The emergence of what many now see as a new eugenics points up for us even more clearly the exquisitely close relationship between human genetics and eugenics that was evident in the struggles of the thirties. The critics of eugenics did not manage to give us a human genetics that would create no victims. That seemed to be true only so long as the attempts to map the human chromosome were safely confined to the abstract, mathematical and generally unsuccessful. With more powerful methods, more concrete results began to come, and they no longer appeared to be as harmless as before. The projects that seemed in the thirties to represent a truly value-free science, by contrast with the cruder social biases of the eugenists, have come in the nineties to stand for the possibility of a new eugenics.

NOTES

INTRODUCTION

1 R. Johnson, 'Three problematics: elements of a theory of working-class culture', in J. Clarke, C. Critcher and R. Johnson, eds, *Working-Class Culture: Studies in History and Theory* (New York, NY: St Martin's, 1980), 201; cited by Philip Abrams, 'History, sociology, historical sociology', *Past & Present* 87 (1980): 3–16 (9, n. 21).

2 Daniel Kevles, *In the Name of Eugenics: Genetics and the Uses of Human Heredity* (New York, NY: Knopf, 1985), 57–84.

3 Pauline M.H. Mazumdar, 'Two models for human genetics: blood grouping and psychiatry in Germany between the wars' (in preparation).

1 THE EUGENICS EDUCATION SOCIETY

1 On Sybil Gotto see n. 73, below.

2 This account is taken from [Lady Chambers] 'Notes on the early days of the Eugenics Education Society', written at C.P. Blacker's suggestion and dated 17 January 1950. Georgina Chambers was on the Council of the Society from 1908, Hon. Secretary of the Educational Committee, and from 1920 to 1926 Joint Hon. Secretary of the Society along with R.A. Fisher. In 1930 she was elected a Vice-President. She was married to Sir Theodore Chambers, also a member of the Society.

3 Cited by Chambers, 'Notes', 1950, n. 2, from Sir Francis Galton, 'Eugenics, its definition, scope and aims', *Sociological Papers* 1 (1904): 43–99.

4 Chambers, 'Notes', 1950, n. 2.

5 Eugenics Education Society, *Annual Report* (1908–09).

6 Lyndsay A. Farrall, 'The origin and growth of the British eugenics movement', dissertation, University of Indiana, 1970, Ann Arbor, MI, University Microfilms, 1970.

7 Farrall, 'British eugenics movement' (1970), n. 6, pp. 213–30; Frank Parkin, *Middle Class Radicalism: The Social Bases of the British Campaign for Nuclear Disarmament* (Manchester: University Press, 1968); Harold

Silver, *English Education and the Radicals, 1780–1850* (London: Routledge, 1971).

8 Donald MacKenzie, 'Eugenics in Britain', *Social Studies of Science* 6 (1976): 499–532, esp. p.501; MacKenzie, 'Sociobiologies in competition: the biometrician–Mendelian debate', in Charles Webster, ed., *Biology, Medicine and Society, 1840–1940* (Cambridge: University Press, 1981), 243–88.

9 MacKenzie, 'Eugenics in Britain', (1976), n. 8, p. 511.

10 G.R. Searle, 'Eugenics and class', in Webster, *Biology, Medicine and Society* (1981), n. 8, pp. 217–42, esp. p. 235.

11 Lawrence Ritt, 'The Victorian conscience in action: the National Association for the Promotion of Social Science, 1857–1886,' dissertation, Columbia University, 1959 (Ann Arbor, University Microfilms, 1959).

12 Margaret Fison, *Handbook of the National Association for the Promotion of Social Science* (London: Longmans, 1859), 71–2, 206–18. A history of the Social Science Association appears as Chapter III, pp. 67–116.

13 Silver, *English Education* (1971), n. 7; see especially Chapter III, 'Middle class radicals and education'.

14 Pauline M.H. Mazumdar, 'Anatomical physiology and the reform of medical education, 1825–1835', *Bull. Hist. Med.*, 1983, vol. 57, pp. 230–46.

15 Fison, *Handbook*, 1859, n. 16, pp. 11–12.

16 M.W. Flinn, ed. and intro., *Report on the Sanitary Condition of the Labouring Population of Great Britain by Edwin Chadwick*, 1842 (Edinburgh: University Press, 1965), pp. 1–75.

17 E.P. Thompson, *The Making of the English Working Class* (New York, NY: Vintage, 1963), 267–8; see n. 120 on the link between the New Poor Law and the views of T.R. Malthus.

18 For an account of the education movement of the nineteenth century, including the schools for the 'respectable' working class as well as for the subclass, see J. Lawson and H. Silver, *A Social History of Education in England* (London: Methuen, 1973), 267–313, includes bibliography. At the time of the formation of the Association, government support for Ragged and other special schools had come first in 1854 under the Juvenile Offenders Act, and from 1857 onwards by a share in the grants from the Committee of the Council on Education. Mary Carpenter had campaigned for this support.

19 James Estlin Carpenter, *The Life and Work of Mary Carpenter* (London: Macmillan, 1881). No more recent work on Mary Carpenter seems to add much to this account by her nephew. Mary Carpenter, *Reformatory Schools for the Children of the Perishing and Dangerous Classes and for Juvenile Offenders* (1851) (Montclair, NJ: Patterson Reprint, 1970). On the 'ragged and dangerous classes' see Gertrude Himmelfarb, *The Idea of Poverty: England in the Early Industrial Age* (New York, NY: Vintage, 1985), 371–400.

20 Fison, *Handbook* (1859), n. 16, pp. 88 and 107.

21 Mary Carpenter, 'Juvenile delinquency in its relation to the educational movement', in A. Hill, ed., *Essays on Educational Subjects Read at the Educational Conference of June 1857, with a Short Account of the Objects and Proceedings of the Meeting* (London: Longmans, 1857), 320–33.

22 W.M. Williams, cited in Fison, *Handbook* (1859), n. 16, pp. 21–2.

23 Editorial, 'Article I. Meliora', *Meliora, a Quarterly Review of Social Science in its Ethical, Economical and Ameliorative Aspects*, 1 (1858): 1–16, esp. p. 8.

24 Warnings against the loose use of this concept come from F.M.L. Thompson, 'Social control in Victorian Britain', *Econ. Hist. Rev.* 34 (1981): 189–208; Gareth Stedman Jones, 'Class expression vs. social control? A critique of recent trends in the history of leisure', in his *Languages of Class: Studies in English Working Class History, 1832–1982* (Cambridge, University Press, 1983), 76–89.

25 *Meliora*, 1858, n. 25, p. 10; Peter McCandless, 'Curses of civilization: insanity and drunkenness in Victorian Britain', *Brit. J. Addiction*, 79 (1984): 49–58.

26 Alexander Peddie, MD, 'Dipsomania, a proper subject for legal decision', *Trans. Nat. Assoc. for Promotion of Soc. Sci.* (1860): 538–46.

27 The standard work on the nineteenth-century temperance movement is Brian Harrison's centenary history, *Drink and the Victorians: the Temperance Question in England, 1815–1872* (London: Faber, 1971). The year 1872 is that of the first British Licencing Act; see also R.M. MacLeod, 'The edge of hope: social policy and chronic alcoholism, 1870–1900', *J. Hist. Med.* 22 (1967): 215–45.

28 Gareth Stedman Jones, *Outcast London: a Study in the Relationship between Classes in Victorian Society* (1971) (Harmondsworth, Middlesex: Penguin, 1976), 239–314; Asa Briggs and Anne Macartney, *Toynbee Hall: the First Hundred Years* (London: Routledge, 1985); C.L. Mowat, *The Charity Organisation Society, 1869–1913, Its Ideas and Work* (London: Methuen, 1961).

29 Jones, *Outcast London* (1971), n. 11, pp.129–51.

30 Idem, pp. 291–5, 301, 305.

31 Beatrice Webb, *My Apprenticeship* (London: Longman, 1926), 179; for a short discussion of interlocking membership of these societies, see Pauline M.H. Mazumdar, 'The eugenists and the residuum: the problem of the urban poor', *Bull. Hist. Med.* 54 (1980): 204–15.

32 Mowat, *The Charity Organisation Society* (1961), n. 28, p. 83.

33 Bernard Bosanquet, *Aspects of the Social Problem, by Various Writers* (London: Macmillan, 1895), v.

34 Helen Dendy, 'The industrial residuum', in Bosanquet, *Social Problem* (1895), n. 34, pp. 82–102, p. 83.

35 Idem, p. 91.

36 Charles Booth, 'Notes on social influences and conclusion', in *Life and Labour of the People in London*, 17 v (London: Macmillan, 1902–3), v. 17, p. 9; also referred to by Webb, *My Apprenticeship* (1926), n. 31, pp. 216–56.

37 E.J. Hobsbawm, 'Trends in the British Labour Movement', in

Labouring Men: Studies in the History of Labour (London: Weidenfeld, 1st. ed., 1968), 316–46.

38 E.J. Hobsbawm, 'The labour aristocracy in XIXth century Britain', in his *Labouring Men* (1968), n. 37, pp. 272–315; and 'Trends in the British Labour movement since 1850', in his *Labouring Men* (1968), pp. 316–43, (p. 321).

39 E.J. Hobsbawm, *Labour's Turning Point, 1880–1900* (1948) (Hassocks, Sussex: Harvester, 2nd ed., 1974) 3.

40 H. and V. Joshi, *Surplus Labour and the City. A Study of Bombay* (Delhi: Oxford University Press, 1976).

41 Dipak Mazumdar, 'The Urban Informal Sector', *World Development*, Oxford, 5 (1976): 655–80; Mazumdar, 'Labour supply in early industrialisation: the case of the Bombay textile industry', *Econ. Hist. Rev.* 26 (1973): 477–96.

42 Richard Sandbrook and J. Arn, *The Labouring Poor and Urban Class Formation*, No. 12 in Monograph Series, Centre for Developing-Area Studies (Montreal: McGill University Press, 1977).

43 C.S. Loch's influence on the Royal Commission is discussed by Mowat, *The Charity Organisation Society*, (1961), n. 28, pp. 159–66.

44 Great Britain, Royal Commission on the Poor Laws and Relief of Distress, v. 1 being Parts I to VI of the Majority Report. Cd. 4499 of Session 1909 (London: HMSO, 1909), *Majority Report*, p. 286, para. 529.

45 B. Webb, *Our Partnership* B. Drake and M.I. Cole, eds (London: Longman, 1948), p. 403.

46 *Majority Report* (1909), n. 44, p. 293, para. 556.

47 Webb, *Our Partnership* (1948), n. 45, p. 341.

48 Webb, *Our Partnership* (1948), n. 45, p. 195, calls the Charity Organisation Society 'my friend the enemy'; for her discussion of the National Minimum campaign, see pp. 422–91, 481.

49 [B.Webb], *Break up the Poor Law and Abolish the Workhouse: Being Part I of the Minority Report of the Poor Law Commission* (London: Fabian Society, 1909). The Minority Report was signed by Beatrice Webb, George Lansbury, Francis Chandler and Henry Russell Wakefield, Dean of Norwich. Webb, Lansbury and Chandler were 'representatives of labour'. Wakefield, who later became Bishop of Birmingham, was a convert to their cause. [B. Webb, *Our Partnership* (1948), n. 45.]

50 Eugenics Education Society, a good summary of its foundation in 1907 is given in F. Shenk and A.S. Parkes, 'The activities of the Eugenics Society', *Eugen. Rev.* 60 (1968): 142–61; also see Lady Chambers, 'Notes' (1950), n. 2.

51 C.S. Loch, 'Eugenics and the Poor Law: the Majority Report', *Eugen. Rev.* 2 (1910–11): 229–32; Sidney Webb, 'Eugenics and the Poor Law: the Minority Report', *Eugen. Rev.* 2 (1910–11): 233–7, and reprinted in *Eugen. Rev.* 60 (1968): 71–5.

52 [Montague Crackanthorpe], Presidential Address of 5 May 1910 in Eugenics Education Society, *Second Annual Report*, (1909–10), 1–16, especially pp. 10–16.

53 August Henri Forel, 'Alcohol und Keimzellen (Blastophthorische Entartung)', *Münch. Med. Wschr.* 58 (1911): 2596–601.

54 National Association for the Care and Protection of the Feeble-Minded, founded 1896, and closely connected to the Charity Organisation Society's campaign for government action on the problem. See Kathleen Jones, *Mental Health and Social Policy, 1845–1959* (London: Routledge, 1972), 43–60, 186–7, 196.

55 [Mrs Walter Slater], *The Problem of the Feeble-minded: an Abstract of the Report of the Royal Commission on the Care and Control of the Feeble-Minded* with an introduction by the Rt. Hon. Sir Francis Galton, FRS, the Rev. W.R. Inge, DD, Professor Pigou and Miss Mary Dendy (London: King, 1909); from Great Britain, Royal Commission on the Care and Control of the Feebleminded, *Minutes of Evidence and Reports*, Cmd 4515–4221, 4202, (London: HMSO, 1908), *(Bath-Radnor Report).*

56 Arthur C. Pigou, 'The economic aspect of the problem', in [Slater], *Problem of the Feebleminded* (1909), n. 55, pp. 97–101, 99.

57 Eugenics Education Society, Council Minute Book, Oct. 1909–Dec. 1912, p. 26. Meeting of Council 6 July 1919, and see Jones, *Mental Health* (1972), n. 54, for an account of this campaign; the textbook is A.F. Tredgold, *Mental Deficiency (Amentia)* (New York, NY: Wood, 1912).

58 Council Minute Book, 1909–12, n. 57, p. 53; meeting of Executive Committee, 1 March 1911.

59 Council Minute Book, 1909–12, n. 57, p. 66; report of A.F. Tredgold to the Council, 1 June 1911.

60 Eugenics Education Society, *Fifth Annual Report* (1912–13), 22.

61 Eugenics Education Society, *Sixth Annual Report* (1913–14), 5–6.

62 This account of the Moral Education League is mainly from G.A.S. [i.e., G.A. Spiller] 'The growth of an idea', *Moral Ed. League Q.* 35 (1914): 2–4.

63 M.E. Sadler, 'The International Congress on Moral Education', *Int. J. Ethics* 7 (1909): 158–73.

64 'List of authorities and other bodies represented at the Congress', *Record of Proceedings, 1st International Moral Education Congress, University of London, 25–29 September, 1908* (London: Nutt, 1908), 11–13.

65 J.H. Muirhead, 'The central problem of the International Congress on Moral Education', *Hibbert J.*, 6 (1909): 346–51.

66 [Editorial], *Moral Ed. Q.* 35 (1914): 1.

67 E.J. Hobsbawm, 'The Fabians Reconsidered', in *Labouring Men* (1968), n. 37, pp. 250–71. He points to the 'large bloc of emancipated and presumable middle class women' and 'independent women, often earning their livelihood as writers, or even typists' who made up a large part of the Fabian Society; for the eugenists, see Farrall, *Origin and Growth* (1970), n. 6, p. 223.

68 J.S. MacKenzie, 'Moral education and social progress', *Moral Ed. Q.* 29 (1912): 1–3.

69 'Biology and moral education', report of talk, 'Eugenics', by

J.W. Slaughter, *Proc. 1st Intl. Moral Education Cong.*, n. 64, p. 67.

70 'The close of the Moral Education Congress', *Manchester Guardian*, 30 Sept. 1908.

71 E. Sayer, reported in *Daily Mail*, 30 Sept. 1908. According to Farrall, 'British Eugenics Movement', (1970), n. 6, p. 233, Ettie Sayer was a strong supporter of the women's suffrage movement, and a member of the National Society for the Welfare of the Feeble-minded. By this time she was also a member of the Eugenics Education Society.

72 The London Positivist Society maintained the Church of Humanity at 19 Chapel Street, Lamb's Conduit, WC1, until 1932, when their lease came to an end. They then offered the set of busts of the 52 Scientific Saints of Comte's Positivist Calendar to University College, London, 'to be attached to the Galton Bequest in perpetuity'. The College authorities saw no interest beyond quaintness in them, and turned down the offer. UCL Coll. Records, 33 (Eugenics), 22 Nov. 1932; on Galton's naturalistic religion, see C.P. Blacker, *Eugenics: Galton and After* (London: Duckworth, 1972), 96–7.

73 Sybil Gotto was born in 1887, daughter of Admiral Sir Cecil Burney, married Lt Corry Gotto, RN, who died soon after. Hers was the original inspiration for the foundation of the Eugenics Society, and she worked for it as Honorary Secretary until 1920. In 1917 she married Lt Commander Cecil Neville Rolfe, RN, and thereafter used the name of Mrs Neville Rolfe. In 1914, she was instrumental in forming the National Council for Combating Venereal Disease, later the British Social Hygiene Council, whose Honorary Secretary she was until her retirement in 1944. She organised a number of joint activities by the two societies. She was awarded the Order of the British Empire for her war work. See Appeal from British Social Hygiene Council to C.P. Blacker, Secretary, Eugenics Society, 14 Feb. 1944, Eugen. Soc. Papers, C294; Schenk and Parkes, 'Eugenics Society' (1968), n. 50; Obituary notices, *Eugen. Rev.* 47 (1955–56): 149(n), 249(n).

74 Chambers, 'Notes', (1950), n. 2; Schenk and Parkes, 'Eugenics Society' (1968), n. 50.

75 Farrall, 'British eugenics movement' (1970), n. 6, pp. 206–7, citing Galton's 'Eugenics: its definition, scope and aims' (1904), n. 3; and his 'Eugenics', *Sociological Papers* 2 (1905): 1–54. These papers were reprinted by the Eugenics Education Society in F. Galton, *Essays in Eugenics* (London: Eugenics Education Society, 1909).

76 Farrall, 'British eugenics movement' (1970), n. 6, p. 207, lists A.C. Haddon, F.W. Mott, A.C. Crawley, Havelock Ellis, Professor Poulton, Archdall Reid, C.W. Saleeby and Dr Alice Vickery.

77 Farrall, 'British eugenics movement' (1970), n. 6, cites G. Archdall Reid, 'The biological foundation of sociology', *Sociological Papers* 3 (1906): 3–52; J. Arthur Thomson, 'The sociological appeal to biology', *Sociological Papers* 3 (1906): 157–96.

78 Unlike the other interested 'sociologists' who were doctors or

biologists, the American James W. Slaughter was a lawyer who had studied under the American educationalist Stanley Hall, author of *Adolescence*, 2 v (New York, NY: Appleton, 1904); *Youth* (New York, NY: Appleton, 1907), and *The Physical and Mental Life of Schoolchildren* (London: Longman, 1913). The Moral Educationalists frequently cited the first two. Slaughter himself wrote on *The Adolescent* (London, Allen, 1912). He later returned to the United States and became a judge.

79 Sybil Neville Rolfe [Mrs Gotto] to C.P. Blacker, 11 November 1945: Eugen. Soc. Papers, C294.

80 [Sybil Gotto] 'Scheme of Organisation', n.d., Eugen. Soc. Papers, B1.

81 Eugenics Education Society, Committee Meeting, 23 July [1907 ?] Eugen. Soc. Papers, B1.

82 Eugenics Education Society, Council Minute Book, Nov. 1907–June 1909, meeting of Provisional Council, 25 Nov. 1907, James Slaughter in the chair. It is possible that Marion Hunter was the woman doctor who was later to object to Slaughter's presentation at the Moral Education Congress, above, n. 71.

83 Robert Jones, 'Mental integrity and how to attain it', Monthly meeting for June 1908. Eugen. Ed. Soc., *First Annual Report* (1907–08), 17; Dr Stanton Coit, 'Moral education', a drawing-room lecture, March 1908. Eugenics Education Society, *First Annual Report* (1907–08), 17.

84 'Origin and work of the Society, 1907–8', Eugen. Ed. Soc., *First Annual Report* (1907–8), 16–18.

85 Eugenics Education Society, First Minute Book, Nov. 1907–June 1909. Council Meeting, 3 June 1908, p. 47.

86 Letter on behalf of Education Committee, to Headmistresses of Girls' Schools, 12 Dec. 1912, Eugen. Soc. Papers B7.

87 First Minute Book, 1907–09, n. 85, p. 47.

88 Society for the Study of Inebriety: a brief summary of its history from its foundation in 1884 is given in 'The Foundation of the Society for the Study of Inebriety', *Brit. J. Inebriety*, 1 (1903): i–iv; Virginia Berridge, Editorial, *Brit. J. Addiction*, 79 (1984): 1–6.

89 Membership lists for the Society for the Study of Inebriety, see *Brit. J. Inebriety*, 1 (1903): v–xv, and for the Eugenics Education Society, see its *First Annual Report*, pp. 26–32.

90 G. Archdall Reid, 'The biological foundations of sociobiology', *Sociological Papers* 3 (1906): 3–52.

91 Berridge, Editorial (1984), n. 88.

92 William P. Bynum, 'Alcohol and degeneration in twentieth century European medicine and psychiatry', *Brit. J. Addiction* 79 (1984): 59–70; G. Archdall Reid, *Alcoholism, a Study in Heredity* (London: Unwin, 1901), 272–87.

93 Frederick W. Mott, 'Heredity and Insanity', *Lancet*, i (1911): 1251–9.

94 Benedict-Augustin Morel, *Traité des Dégénérescences Physiques, Intellectuelles et Morales de l'Espèce Humaine*, (Paris: Ballière, 1857); Morel,

Traité des Maladies Mentales (Paris: Masson, 1860), 515ff.; on Morel and degeneration, see Eric T. Carlson, 'Medicine and degeneration: theory and praxis', in J. Edward Chamberlin and Sander L. Gilman, eds, *Degeneration: the Dark Side of Progress*, (New York, NY: Columbia University Press, 1985), 121–44.

95 G. Archdall Reid, 'Human evolution and alcohol', *Brit. J. Inebriety* 1 (1903–04): 186–201.

96 Frederick W.Mott, 'Alcohol and insanity', *Brit. J. Inebriety* 9 (1911–12): 5–27; Mott was an active supporter of the Eugenics Society until his death in 1926. For biography and bibliography, see W.D. Haliburton, 'Some personal reminiscences', and C. von Monachow, 'Sir Frederick Mott, CBE: his life and work', in J.R. Lord, ed., *Contributions to Psychiatry, Neurology and Sociology, dedicated to the late Sir Frederick Mott, K.B.E.* (London: Lewis, 1929).

97 E.C. Taylor, 'The pauper inebriate: a note on the aetiology of poverty', *Brit. J. Inebriety* 2 (1904–5): 112–16.

98 Farrall, 'British eugenics movement', (1970), n. 6.

99 Eugenics Education Society, *Record and Programme 1908–1914* Section III, Legislative and Administrative Reform.

100 Majority Report, 1909, n. 44, v. 1, Part V, pp. 355–6, esp. p. 356.

101 Eugenics Education Society, Council Minute Book, Oct. 1909–Dec. 1912, pp. 76–7.

102 Eugenics Education Society, *Fifth Annual Report*, (1911–12), 22–3.

103 Royal Commission on Venereal Disease, *Report* Cmd 7474, 7475, 8189, 8190 (London: HMSO, 1916), Chair: Lord Sydenham *(Sydenham Report)*; on economic effects of venereal disease, paras. 100–7. Summary of Recommendations, General Conclusions, paras. 230–9.

104 Lord Sydenham, George Sydenham Clarke, 'The work of the National Council', *First Annual Report of the National Council for Combating Venereal Disease*, June 1916, 12–17.

105 Eugenics Education Society, *First Annual Report*, (1908–09), 2–7.

106 Eugenics Education Society, *Eighth Annual Report*, 1915–16, p. 4.

107 *Sydenham Report* (1916), n. 103, para. 177, and Conclusions, para. 230, no. 18.

108 British Social Hygiene Council Inc., *Foundations of Social Hygiene* (London: British Social Hygiene Council Inc., 1926). Contributions to this collection of statements on social hygiene include (Sir) Cyril Burt, Professor Winifred Cullis, Professor Julian Huxley, Professor B. Malinowski, Sir Arthur Newsholme, T. Percy Nunn and Professor Arthur Thomson.

109 Greta Jones, *Social Hygiene in Twentieth Century Britain* (London: Croom Helm, 1986), 'A dynasty of experts', pp. 43–65.

110 Angus McLaren, *Birth Control in Nineteenth Century England* (New York, NY: Holmes & Meier, 1978), 141–56.

111 Farrall, 'British eugenics movement' (1970), n. 6, pp. 10–53, citing Charles Darwin, *Origin of Species* (1859), and his *Descent of Man and Selection in Relation to Sex* (1871); Thomas Huxley, *Evidence as to Man's Place in Nature* (1863), and the work of Herbert Spencer,

A.R. Wallace and a number of others. See also J.W. Burrow, *Evolution and Society: a Study in Victorian Social Theory* (Cambridge: University Press, 1966).

112 D.E.C. Eversley, *Social Theories of Fertility and the Malthusian Debate* (Oxford: Clarendon, 1959), 38.

113 Eversley, *Malthusian Debate* (1959), n. 113, p. 53 cites R.R. Kuczynski, 'British demographer's opinions on fertility, 1660–1760', in L. Hogben, ed., *Political Arithmetic* (London: Macmillan, 1938).

114 For biographical material on Malthus and the debate on his views among contemporaries, see Patricia James, *Population Malthus, His Life and Times* (London: Routledge, 1979), esp. pp. 116–59; 369–406. See also J.A. Banks and D.V. Glass, 'A list of books and articles on the population question, published in Britain in the period 1793–1880', in David V. Glass, *Introduction to Malthus* (London: Watts, 1953), 79–112.

115 Thomas Robert Malthus, *An Essay on the Principle of Population, or, a View of its Past and Present Effects on Human Happiness, with an Inquiry into our Prospects Respecting Future Removal or Mitigation of the Evils which it Occasions*, 1798, London, 2nd ed. 1803. This enlarged edition contains the references to the 'prudential check' as an alternative to the 'misery check', pp. 483–93. For an overview of Malthus's theory written towards the end of his life, see Malthus, *Summary of the Principle of Population*, (London: Murray, 1830), reprinted in Glass, *Malthus* (1953), n. 115, pp. 115–81.

116 David V. Glass, 'Malthus and the limitation of population growth', in his *Malthus* (1953), n. 115, pp. 38–47; J. Knodel, 'Law, marriage and illegitimacy in nineteenth century Germany', *Population Studies*, March 1967, pp. 279–94; for an account of the literature of cameralism, see George Rosen, 'Cameralism and the concept of medical police', *Bull. Hist. Med.* 27 (1952): 21–42, reprinted in his *From Medical Police to Social Medicine: Essays on the History of Health Care* (New York, NY: Science History 1974), pp. 120–41.

117 J.J. Spengler, 'French population theory since 1800 I', *J. Econ.* 44 (1926): 577–611, 743–66, cited by William Coleman, *Death is a Social Disease: Public Health and Political Economy in Early Industrial France* (Madison, WI, University Press, 1982), 80–5.

118 Support for this view is still widespread among demographers, see David M. Heer, 'Economic development and the fertility transition', in D.V. Glass and R. Revelle, eds, *Population and Social Change* (London: Arnold, 1972), 99–113. Heer discusses the various factors that might be involved in the decision to have children.

119 H.L. Beales, 'The historical context of the *Essay on Population*', in Glass, *Malthus* (1953), n. 115, pp. 1–24.

120 See Ronald L. Meek, ed., *Marx and Engels on Malthus: Selections from the Writings of Marx and Engels dealing with the Theories of Thomas Robert Malthus* (New York, NY: International, 1954). Engels's words are from *The Condition of the Working Class in England* (1845), translated W.O. Henderson and W.H. Chaloner (Stanford, CA:

Stanford University Press, 1968), 320–31, and cited in Meek, p. 69, with no page reference and a different translation.

121 James, *Population Malthus* (1979), n. 115, pp. 136–9.

122 On the New Poor Law and the opposition to it see Derek Fraser, *The Evolution of the British Welfare State: a History of Social Policy since the Industrial Revolution* (London: Macmillan, 1973), 34–51. Fraser also gives a bibliography of useful articles on the Old and New Poor Laws, 283–4.

123 Thomas Robert Malthus, *A Letter to Samuel Whitbread, Esq., MP on his Proposed Bill for the Amendment of the Poor Laws* (London: Hatchard's, 1807), reprinted in Glass, *Malthus* (1953), n. 115, pp.183–285; James, *Population Malthus* (1979), n. 115, pp. 136–9.

124 *Chadwick Report* (1842), n. 18, pp. 254–61; M.J. Cullen, *The Statistical Movement in Early Victorian Britain: the Foundations of Empirical Social Research* (Hassocks, Sussex: Harvester, 1975), 53–64, esp. p. 59.

125 Great Britain, Commissioners for Inquiring into the State of Large Towns and Populous Districts, *First Report* (London: HMSO, 1844); *Second Report* (London: HMSO, 1845).

126 Cullen, *Statistical Movement* (1975), n. 125, p. 62.

127 For the special importance of race in American eugenics, see Kenneth Ludmerer, *Genetics and American Society: a Historical Appraisal* (Baltimore, MD: Hopkins, 1972), 87–90, 95–131, and see Charles Rosenberg, ed., *The History of Hereditarian Thought*, a 32-volume reprint series (New York, NY: Garland, 1984). Rosenberg's collection traces the roots of eugenics exclusively to hereditarianism. He emphasises the importance of such influentials as de Gobineau, whose book on the moral and intellectual diversity of races of 1853 was reprinted in the United States with a commentary pointing out how it applied to the American racial situation, particularly slavery: Count Joseph Arthur de Gobineau, *The Moral and Intellectual Diversity of Races, with particular Reference to their Respective Influence in the Civil and Political History of Mankind ... (1853) from the French ... with an Analytical Introduction and Copious Historical Notes by H.Hotz. to which is Added an Appendix containing a Summary of the Latest Scientific Facts bearing upon the Question of the Unity or Plurality of Species*, Philadelphia, 1865, rpt. (New York, NY: Garland, 1984). For the influence of de Gobineau on European and especially German thought, see Daniel Gasman, *The Scientific Origins of National Socialism: Social Darwinism in Ernst Haeckel and the German Monist League* (New York, NY: Elsevier, 1971), xii–xxiii; and see also Gerhard Baader, 'Zur Ideologie des Sozial-Darwinismus', in *Medizin und Nationalsozialismus: tabuisierte Vergangenheit-ungebrochene Tradition*, G. Baader and U. Schultz, eds, (Berlin: Verlag Gesundheit, 2nd ed., 1983), 39–54.

128 Karl Pearson, *Francis Galton, 1882–1922: a Centenary Appreciation* (London: Cambridge University Press, 1922), 5–6. The word 'eugenics' was invented by Galton and first used in his *Inquiries into Human Nature* (1883) (London: The Eugenics Society, 1951), 17;

he says in a note that it is a neater word than 'viriculture'. See also Pearson, *Life, Letters and Labours of Francis Galton*, 3 v in 4 (Cambridge: University Press, 1914–30); v. 3a covers eugenics; Francis Galton, *Memories of my Life* (London: Methuen, 1908); Blacker, *Eugenics* (1952), n. 75.

129 Ruth Schwartz Cowan, Introduction to Francis Galton, *English Men of Science, their Nature and Nurture*, 1874 (London: Cass, 1970), viii; Cowan, 'Sir Francis Galton and the study of heredity in the nineteenth century', dissertation, Johns Hopkins University, 1969.

130 Francis Galton, 'Hereditary talent and character', *Macmillan's Mag.* 12 (1865): 157–66, 318–27.

131 Francis Galton, *Hereditary Genius: an Enquiry into its Laws and Consequences* (London: Macmillan, 1869).

132 Francis Galton, 'Presidential Address', *Transactions of the International Congress of Hygiene and Demography*, Section of Demography, Tuesday, 11 Aug. 1891 (London: 1892), 7–12.

133 Karl Pearson, 'On the inheritance of the mental and moral characters in man and its comparison with the inheritance of physical characters', Huxley Lecture for 1903, *J. Anthropol. Inst. Brit. Ireland* 33 (1903): 179–237.

134 Sir William Taylor, KCB, Director-General of Army Medical Service, 'Memorandum', in Great Britain, Interdepartmental Committee on Physical Deterioration, *Report* Cmd 2175, 2210, 2186 (London: HMSO, 1904), v. 1, pp. 95–7, Appendix 1 *(Fitzroy Report)*.

135 *Fitzroy Report* (1904), n. 135, v. 1, p. 39.

136 Great Britain, Poor Law Commissioners, *Report to Her Majesty's Principal Secretary of State for the Home Department from the Poor Law Commissioners, on an Inquiry into the Sanitary Condition of the Labouring Population of Great Britain* with Appendices (London: HMSO, 1842) *(Chadwick Report)*; for a historical introduction to the *Chadwick Report*, see Flinn (1965), n. 16 above.

137 *Fitzroy Report* (1904), n. 135, v. 1, p. 6.

138 C.S. Loch, 'Some recent investigations as to the number of "poor" in the community', in *Fitzroy Report* (1904), n. 135, v. 1, pp. 104–11, Appendix III, p. 107.

139 *Fitzroy Report* (1904), n. 135, v. 1, p. 39.

140 David Heron, *On the Relation of Fertility in Man to Social Status and on the Changes in this Relation that have Taken Place during the Last Fifty Years*, No. 1 in series, Drapers Company Research Memoirs, Studies in National Degeneration (London: Dulau, 1906).

141 Idem, p. 22.

142 Eugenics Education Society, *First Annual Report*, (1907–08), List of members.

143 Minute Book, Nov. 1907–June 1909, n. 85, AGM, 9 March 1909, p. 73.

144 Karl Pearson, cited in indirect speech in Minute Book, Nov. 1907–June 1909, n. 85, Council Meeting, 12 Feb. 1908, p. 19.

145 Francis Galton, cited in indirect speech from a letter, in Minute

Book, Nov. 1907–June 1909, n. 85, Council Meeting, 12 Feb. 1908, p. 19.
146 Minute Book, Council Meeting, 8 July 1908, p. 49.
147 Idem, p. 50.
148 Ethel M. Elderton, A. Barrington, H.G. Jones, E.M. de G. Lamotte, Harold J. Laski and Karl Pearson, *On the Correlation of Fertility with Social Value. A Cooperative Study*, series, Eugenics Laboratory Memoirs XVIII (London: Dulau, 1913).
149 Idem, p. 45.
150 Sir Shirley Murphy, in *Fitzroy Report* (1904), n. 140, v. 3, pp. 50–5, Appendix XIII. The reference given by Elderton *et al.* (1913), n. 148, is to Murphy's paper, 'Sanitary science and preventive medicine: Presidential Address to the Congress of the Royal Sanitary Institute, 'Some points in the decline of birth and death rates', *J. Roy. Sanitary Inst.* 33 (1912): 345–9.
151 Webb, 'Eugenics and the Poor Law' (1910), n. 51, p. 71.
152 Hobsbawm, 'The Fabians reconsidered', in *Labouring Men* (1968), n. 37, pp. 150–271. Hobsbawm cites the Webbs, p. 258, and G.B. Shaw, p. 269, as giving this *nouvelle couche sociale* the responsibility for guiding the working class to its betterment.
153 S. and B. Webb, *The Decay of Capitalist Civilisation* (London: Fabian Society, 1923). The Webbs' respect and loyalty towards this class is plain:

> this *nouvelle couche sociale*, comprising now the vast majority of the active brain-workers in each country – honest, diligent and highly qualified for their work … which has reduced to absurdity the claim of the capitalist that only by the stimulus of profit-making … could efficient service to the community in this industrial realm be obtained. (pp. 124–5)

A similar assessment is to be found in A.M. Carr-Saunders and P.A. Wilson, *The Professions* (Oxford: University Press, 1933).
154 Ansley K. Coale, 'The decline of fertility in Europe from the French Revolution to World War II', in S.J. Behrman, L. Corsa, and R. Freedman, eds, *Fertility and Family Planning: a World View*, (Ann Arbor, University of Michigan Press, 1970), 3–24.
155 John Hajnal, 'European marriage patterns in perspective', in D.V. Glass and D.E.C. Eversley, eds, *Population in History* (London: Arnold, 1964), 101–43.
156 David V. Glass, *The Struggle for Population* (Oxford: Clarendon, 1936); Glass, *Population: Policies and Movements in Europe* (1940), reprinted with new Introduction (London: Cass, 1967); pp. 145ff., France; pp. 219ff., Italy; pp. 269ff., Germany.
157 D.V. Glass, 'Changes in fertility in England and Wales, 1851–1931', in Hogben, *Political Arithmetic* (1938), n. 114, pp. 6–7.
158 Idem, pp. 35, 13.
159 [――――] 'The dwindling family; a case for enquiry', 19 Sept. 1936. Leader accompanied by two articles from a Special Correspondent: 'A menace to the future: I Britain and Europe', 28 Sept.

1936, and 'II Planning for population: Germany and Italy', 29 Sept. 1936. These articles were based on Glass, *Struggle for Population* (1936), n. 156, and A.M. Carr-Saunders, *World Population* (Oxford: Clarendon, 1936).

160 *The Declining Birth Rate: Its Causes and Effects. Being the Report and the Chief Evidence Taken by the National Birth Rate Commission, instituted with Official Recognition by the National Council of Public Morals, for the Promotion of Race Regeneration – Spiritual, Moral and Physical*, (London: Chapman, 1916).

161 [———] 'The Commission of Inquiry into the national birth rate', *The Times*, 13 Oct. 1913.

162 *Declining Birth Rate*, n. 160, pp. 3–7, citing E.M. Elderton, *Report on the English Birth Rate Part I* (London: Dulau, 1914).

163 Leonard Darwin, *Quality not Quantity* (London: Eugenics Education Society, n.d.), 22. Reprinted from *Eugen. Rev.* 8 (1916–17): 297–321.

164 Eugenics Education Society, *Eighth Annual Report*, (1915–16), 4.

165 Darwin, *Quality not Quantity* (1916), n. 163, p. 14.

166 Eugenics Education Society, *Tenth Annual Report* (1917–18), 10–13.

167 Leonard Darwin, 'Memorandum on the evidence proposed to be given before the Royal Commission on Income Tax', *Eugen. Rev.* 11 (1919–20): 213–18.

168 President of the Eugenics Society [Major Leonard Darwin], Letter to the Chancellor of the Exchequer. Pamphlet d. Jan. 1927, and published in *Eugen. Rev.* 19 (1927–28): 96–7.

169 See *Outline of a Practical Eugenic Policy* approved by the Council of the Eugenics Education Society . . ., London, Eugenics Education Society, n.d., but before 1926, and 'The aims and objects of the Eugenics Society', Eugenics Society, *Annual Report* (1936–37), p. 5.

170 R.A. Fisher, 'Family allowances and the contemporary economic situation', *Eugen. Rev.* 24 (1932): and reprinted in idem, 60 (1968): 109–17. The eugenists generally conflated the unemployed with the 'Social Problem Group'.

Unemployment was of course a major concern of all political parties during the inter-war period: D. Frazer, *Evolution of the British Welfare State* (London: Macmillan, 1973), 172–83, 'The central problem of unemployment'.

171 Michael Freeden, 'Eugenics and progressive thought: a study in ideological affinity', *Historical J.* 22 (1979): 645–71, esp. pp. 661–8.

172 'Sir William Beveridge as Chairman put the eugenics aspect with clearness, moderation and most convincing seriousness', account of a meeting at the British Institute of Philosophical Studies, *Eugen. Rev.* 19 (1927–28): 98.

173 Freeden, 'Eugenics and progressive thought', (1979), n. 171, pp. 633–4. Freeden describes a Malthusian controversy in the twenties between Keynes and Beveridge; the anti-Malthusian position was later taken by Clifford Sharp, editor of the left-wing weekly *New Statesman*. Sharp too wished to encourage those 'who ought to be encouraged to bear children'.

174 F.J. Allaun, 'Eugenics and capitalism', Letter to the Editor, *Eugen. Rev.* 24 (1932–33): 345, cited by Lawrence S. Waterman, 'The Eugenics movement in Britain in the nineteen thirties', dissertation, University of Sussex, 1975, p. 12.

175 Raymond E. Fancher, *The Intelligence Men: Makers of the IQ Controversy* (New York, NY: Norton, 1985), 87–93.

176 Charles Spearman, 'General intelligence objectively determined and measured', *Am. J. Psychol.* 15 (1904): 201–93.

177 Bernard J. Norton, 'Charles Spearman and the general factor in intelligence: genesis and interpretation in the light of socio-personal considerations', *J. Hist. Behav. Sci.* 15 (1979): 142–54.

178 See Stephen Jay Gould, *The Mismeasure of Man* (New York, NY: Norton, 1981), 239–72, for an explanation of Spearman's original calculations of *g* and the statistical methods that were evolved from it.

179 Charles Spearman, 'The heredity of abilities', *Eugen. Rev.* 6 (1914–15): 219–37.

180 Gould, *Mismeasure* (1981), n. 178, pp. 265–9, citing Charles Spearman, *The Abilities of Man* (New York, NY: Macmillan, 1927), 407–8.

181 For biographical material on Burt, see L.S. Hearnshaw, *Cyril Burt, Psychologist* (London: Hodder, 1979).

182 Sir Cyril Burt, *Mental and Scholastic Tests: Report by the Education Officer ...* (London County Council, 1921).

183 Cyril Burt, 'The inheritance of mental characters', *Eugen. Rev.* 4 (1912–13): 168–200.

184 Burt's data on the heritability of IQ were based on studies of monozygotic twins reared apart. His results were criticised first by Leon J. Kamin, *The Science and Politics of IQ* (1974) (Harmondsworth, Middlesex, Penguin, 1977), 52–71. Kamin calculated that the results showed a consistent bias towards the hereditarian viewpoint. In 1976 Oliver Gillie, medical correspondent of the *Sunday Times*, made public the doubts that had already collected around Burt's post-second World War articles in his 'Crucial data was faked by eminent psychologist', *Sunday Times*, 24 Oct. 1976. For a detailed and sympathetic account of 'the Burt case', see Hearnshaw, *Cyril Burt* (1979), n. 181, pp. 227ff., 'Posthumous controversies'.

185 For a discussion of IQ testing and British education, see Gillian Sutherland, 'Measuring intelligence: English Local Education Authorities and mental testing, 1919–1939', in Charles Webster, ed., *Biology, Medicine and Society 1840–1940* (Cambridge: University Press, 1981), 315–35.

186 R.B. Cattell, 'Is national intelligence declining?' *Eugen. Rev.* 28 (1936): 181–203.

187 British Population Society 'aims, members, rules', *Bulletin of the Intl. Union for the Scientific Investigation of Population Problems* 1 (1930): 23–5.

188 F.A.E. Crew and E. Moore, 'Outline of problems to be investigated

by Commission II, on differential fertility, fecundity and sterility', *Bull. Intl. Union* 1 (1930): 17–22.

189 Eugenics Education Society, *Annual Report* (1936–37), 8.

190 Idem.

191 Idem.

192 Carr-Saunders, Introduction to Glass, *Struggle for Population* (1936), n. 156, p. x.

193 Benito Mussolini, Speech on Ascension Day, 26 May 1937, cited by Glass, *Struggle for Population* (1936), n. 156, p. 34.

194 Idem, 26–7.

195 David V. Glass, 'The Berlin Population Congress and recent population movements in Germany', *Eugen. Rev.* 27 (1935–36): 207–12.

196 Eugenics Education Society, *Annual Report* (1936–37), 12.

197 Eugenics Education Society, *Annual Report* (1936–37), 13.

198 [———] 'The practice of eugenics', Eugenics Education Society, *Annual Report* (1937–38), 5.

199 D. Caradog Jones, 'Eugenics and the decline in population', essay review of Glass, *Struggle for Population* (1936), n. 156, and Carr-Saunders, *World Population* (1936), n. 159, *Eugen. Rev.* 28 (1936–37): 213–15.

200 Trygve Tholfsen, ed., *Sir James Kay-Shuttleworth on Popular Education* (New York, NY: Teacher's College Press, 1974), Introduction, pp. 2ff.

2 THE AGE OF PEDIGREES

1 Karl Pearson, Preface to Julia Bell, *Treasury of Human Inheritance*, name and subject index to vol. 1, no. 16 in series Eugenics Laboratory Memoirs (London: Dulau, 1912), iii–iv.

2 William B. Provine, *The Origins of Theoretical Population Genetics* (Chicago, IL, Chicago University Press, 1971), 25–56; Lyndsay Farrall, 'The role of controversy and conflict in science – a case study: the English biometric school and Mendel's laws', *Social Stud. Sci.* 5 (1975): 269–301.

3 For an account of the Eugenics and Biometrical Laboratories at University College under Galton and Pearson, see Lyndsay A. Farrall, 'The origins and growth of the British eugenics movement, 1865–1925', dissertation, Indiana University, 1970 (Ann Arbor, MI, University Microfilms, 1970), 102–26; Bernard J. Norton, 'Karl Pearson and statistics: the social origin of scientific innovation', *Soc. Stud. Sci.* 8 (1978): 3–34.

4 Bernard Norton, 'Biology and philosophy: the methodological foundation of biometry', *J. Hist. Biol.* 6 (1975): 85–93; Norton, 'The biometric defense of Darwinism', idem, 14 (1983): 283–316.

5 William Bateson, *Mendel's Principles of Heredity* (Cambridge: University Press, 1909), 54; 76–80.

6 R.A. Fisher, 'The correlation between relatives on the supposition of Mendelian inheritance', *Trans. Roy. Soc.* (Edinburgh) 52 (1918):

399–433; republished as no. 41 in series, Eugenics Laboratory Memoirs, edited and introduced by P.A. Moran and C.A.B. Smith (Cambridge: University Press, 1966).

7 [Montague Crackanthorpe], Presidential Address, 5 May 1910, Eugenics Education Society, *Second Annual Report* (1909–10), 1–16, p. 5.

8. 'Origins and work of the Society', Eugenics Education Society, *First Annual Report* (1907–08), 16–18, 17.

9. Eugenics Education Society, *Fifth Annual Report* (1912–13), 21.

10 Clifford Dobell is best known to historians of biology for his *Anthony van Leeuwenhoek and his Little Animals* (London: Ball, 1932). He also wrote many papers on medical protozoology.

11 Clifford Dobell and F.W. O'Connor, *Intestinal Protozoa of Man* (London: Ball, 1921).

12 Eugenics Education Society, *Sixth Annual Report* (1913–14), 13–15.

13 Reginald C. Punnett, *Mendelism* (London, Macmillan, 1905, 1907, 1911); references are to edition of 1911, p. 27.

14 Punnett, *Mendelism* (1911), n. 13, vi.

15 Andrew Mearns (pseudonym), *The Bitter Cry of Outcast London* (London: Congregational Union, 1883); see Gareth Stedman Jones, *Outcast London: a Study in the Relationship between Classes in Victorian Society* (Harmondsworth: Middlesex, Penguin, 1976), 222–5.

16 Charles Booth, 'The inhabitants of Tower Hamlets (School Board Division), their conditions and occupations', *J. Royal. Stats. Soc.* 50 (1887): 326–401; p. 374, table 330 and p. 335; Booth divides the Tower Hamlets population into eight classes; the 'indoor paupers' are not included, but the 'ins-and-outs' come mainly from class 2. The classes are: 1. Lowest: loafers, semi-criminals, street sellers, homeless outcasts (1.5%). 2. Casual earners: 'shiftless hand-to-mouth, pleasure-loving and always poor' (11%). 3. Irregular labourers, poorer artisans – Booth recommends these as the 'most proper field for charitable assistance' (7.5%). 4. Small but regular earners: home industries, small shops. 'No class deserves greater sympathy than this one: its members live hard lives very patiently' (15%). 5. Regular and standard earners (45%). 6. Higher class labour: foremen. 7. Lower middle class: small employers, clerks, lower professional. 8. Upper middle class: 'the servant-keeping class'.

17 Charles Booth, *The Aged Poor in England and Wales: Condition* (London: Macmillan, 1894), 56–103; on his method, p. 56; on the rural unions, p. 59 ff.; on the London unions, pp. 96–8; concern about the aged poor was linked to the Royal Commission on the Aged Poor, appointed to Consider whether any Alterations in the System of Poor Law Relief are Desirable in the Case of Persons whose Destitution is Occasioned by Incapacity for Work resulting form Old Age, or whether Assistance could otherwise by Afforded in these Cases, *Report and Minutes of Evidence* (London: HMSO, 1895).

18 C.S. Loch, 'Mr Charles Booth on the aged poor', *Econ. J.* 4 (1894):

468–87; Booth's answer appears in Charles Booth, 'Poor Law statistics', *Econ. J.*, 6 (1896): 70–4

19 The technique was developed by Francis Galton during the late 1870s and 1880s; see Donald A. MacKenzie, *Statistics in Britain, 1865–1930: the Social Construction of Scientific Knowledge* (Edinburgh: University Press, 1981); on Yule's work see Helen M. Walker, *Studies in the History of Statistical Method* (Baltimore, MD: Williams, 1929), 111, 137–8.

20 George Udny Yule, 'Note on the teaching of the theory of statistics at University College', *J. Royal. Stats. Soc.* 60 (1897): 456–8; Udny Yule and L.N.C. Filon wrote the obituary notice for Pearson in *Obituary Notices of the Fellows of the Royal Society* (London) 2 (1936): 73–110.

21 George Udny Yule, 'On the correlation of total pauperism with the proportion of out-relief, I. All ages, II. Males over 65', *Econ. J.* 5 (1895): 603–11; idem 5 (1896): 613–23, esp. p. 614.

22 George Udny Yule, 'On the theory of correlation', *J. Roy. Stats. Soc.* 60 (1897): 812–54.

23 George Udny Yule, 'Notes on the history of pauperism in England and Wales from 1850, treated by the method of frequency curves, with a note on the method', *J. Roy. Stat. Soc.* 59 (1896): 318–49; Yule, 'Investigation into the causes of changes in pauperism in England, chiefly during the last two intercensal decades', idem, 62 (1899): 249–86.

24 George Udny Yule, *Introduction to the Theory of Statistics* (London: Griffin, 1st ed., 1911), Preface. Chapter 10 is on 'Practical applications and methods'. New editions appeared until 1932, with additions at the end but no changes.

25 George Udny Yule, 'Statistical methods in relation to eugenics: syllabus of the course given in the autumn of 1913 at the offices of the Society', Eugenics Education Society, *Sixth Annual Report* (1913–14).

26 Major Greenwood, the statistician who gave the course the following year, however, did become a member; see M. Greenwood, 'Instruction in statistical methods as applied to problems in eugenics', Syllabus of a course given in summer 1914 at the Lister Institute. Eugenics Education Society, *Sixth Annual Report* (1913–14), p. 15. One of his lectures was entitled 'Mendelian proportions and their testing'.

27 W.T. Calman, 'Ernest William MacBride', *Obituary Notices of Fellows of the Royal Society* (London), 3 (1940): 747–59.

28 Ernest W. MacBride, *Zoology: the Study of Animal Life*, in series, The People's Books (London: Jack, 1913), 98.

29 Ernest W. MacBride, *An Introduction to the Study of Heredity* (London: Williams, 1924), 240ff.

30 Leon Poliakov, *The Aryan Myth: a History of Racism and Nationalist Ideas in Europe* (New York, NY: Basic Books, 1974). The connection between settled farming and the Nordic race was to be of central importance under Nazism.

31 Kammerer's experiments showing the inheritance of acquired characteristics were violently attacked by William Bateson; attacks which seem to have led to Kammerer's suicide; Arthur Koestler, *The Case of the Midwife Toad* (London: Hutchinson, 1971).

32 MacBride, *Study of Heredity* (1924), n. 29, p. 105.

33 Idem, p. 243.

34 Ernest W. MacBride, 'Biological memory: a new theory of life', *Scientia* (Bologna) 38 (1925): 153–64.

35 The effectiveness of the eugenists in the United States in creating so-called eugenic, i.e., racist, immigration laws has been pointed out by Kenneth Ludmerer, *Genetics and American Society* (Baltimore, MD: Johns Hopkins University, 1972), 95–113.

36 Peter J. Bowler, 'E.W. MacBride's Lamarckian eugenics and its implications for the social construction of scientific knowledge', *Ann. Sci.* 41 (1984): 245–60.

37 Eugenics Education Society, policy pamphlet, 1922–23, Eugen. Soc. Papers, C108.

38 MacBride to Sir Bernard Mallet, letter d. 30 Nov. 1930, Eugen. Soc. Papers, C223/1; 'E.W. MacBride, resignation from the Society', *Eugen. Rev.*, 23–4 (1931–32): 4. According to the Society, he resigned over a matter of office routine only, but Kathleen Hodson reveals that there had been an acrimonious row over the editorial policy of the *Eugenics Review*. Kathleen Hodson, 'The *Eugenics Review* 1909–1968', *Eugen. Rev.* 60 (1968): 162–75.

39 MacBride, *Study of Heredity* (1924), n. 29, 158–62.

40 Idem, 117–29.

41 Eugenics Education Society, Council Minute Book, Oct. 1909 – Dec. 1912, p. 4, Council Meeting of 3 Nov. 1909.

42 Karl Pearson, 'The law of ancestral heredity', *Biometrika* 2 (1909): 211–36; Pearson, 'Letter to the Editor', *Brit. Med. J.* ii (1908): 1720; idem, i (1909): 184, 372, 568, 694; and see P. Froggatt and N.C. Nevin, 'Galton's law of ancestral heredity: its influence on the early development of human genetics', *Hist. Sci.* 21 (1971): 1–27; Froggatt and Nevin, 'The "law of ancestral heredity" and the Mendelian–ancestrian controversy in England, 1899–1906', *J. Med. Genet.* 8 (1971): 1–36.

43 Three pamphlets attacking Charles Davenport were issued in the series 'Questions of the Day and of the Fray', under the aegis of the Department of Applied Statistics, University College, London. They were:

VII. David Heron, *Mendelism and the Problem of Mental Defect: a Criticism of Recent American Work* (London: Dulau, 1913).

VIII. Karl Pearson and G.A. Jaederholm, *Mendelism and the Problem of Mental Defect II. On the Continuity of Mental Defect* (London: Dulau, 1914).

IX. Karl Pearson, *Mendelism and the Problem of Mental Defect III. On the Graded Character of Mental Defect and on the Need for Standardising Judgements as to the Grade of Social Inefficiency that shall Involve Segregation* (London: Dulau, 1914).

44 Pearson, *Mendelism and Mental Defect II* (1914), n. 43, p. 33.
45 Pearson, *Mendelism and Mental Defect III* (1914), n. 43.
46 Charles Rosenberg, *No Other Gods: Science and American Social Thought* (Baltimore, MD: Johns Hopkins Press, 1976), 89–97.
47 Garland E. Allen, 'The Eugenics Record Office at Cold Spring Harbor, 1910–1940: an essay in institutional history', *Osiris* 2 (1986): 225–64; Barbara Kimmelman, 'The American Breeders Association: genetics and eugenics in an agricultural context, 1903–1913', *Social Studies of Science* 13 (1983): 163–204.
48 'Ardent Mendelian', 'The present position of the Mendelians and the Biometricians', in Methods and Results, *Mendel J.* 1 (1909): 159–63, esp p. 160.
49 Bernard J. Norton and E.S. Pearson, 'A note on the background to and refereeing of, R.A. Fisher's 1918 paper, "On the correlation between relatives on the supposition of Menelian inheritance",' *Notes and Records of Roy. Soc.* (London), 31 (1976): 151–62.
50 Eugenics Education Society, *Third Annual Report* (1910–11), 18.
51 Report of the Committee appointed to consider the Eugenic Aspect of Poor Law Reform, 'Section I. The eugenic principle in Poor Law administration', *Eugen. Rev.* 2 (1910–11): 167–77, esp. p. 173 (*Poor Law Committee Report*).
52 E.J. Lidbetter, 'Eugenics and the prevention of destitution: a paper read at the Conference on Prevention of Destitution', *Eugen. Rev.* 3 (1911–12): 170–3.
53 E.J. Lidbetter, *Heredity and the Social Problem Group* (London: Arnold, 1933), v. 1, p. 12; no more appeared.
54 *Poor Law Committee Report*, (1910), n. 51, 174, 177.
55 Idem, 175.
56 Biographical information from Leonard Darwin, Introduction to Lidbetter, *Social Problem Group* (1933), n. 54, 5–6; and from Obituary, 'E.J. Lidbetter (1878–1962)', *Eugen. Rev.* 54 (1962–63): 191.
57 Eugenics Education Society, *Fifth Annual Report* (1912–13), 24–6.
58 Lidbetter spoke on 4 Oct. 1912 to Liverpool University; 1 Nov. 1912 to St Matthews Literary and Debate Society; 7 July 1913 to Croydon Women's Liberal Association; 24 Sept. 1913 to National Relieving Officers' Association; Eugenics Education Society, *Sixth Annual Report* (1913–14), 20.
59 Eugenics Education Society, *Sixth Annual Report* (1913–14), 13.
60 Eugenics Education Society, *Fifth Annual Report* (1912–13), 18.
61 For a list of the officers of the Society, see Faith Schenck and A.S. Parkes, 'The activities of the Eugenics Society', *Eugen. Rev.* 60 (1968): 142–61, esp. p. 159.
62 Council meeting of 1 June 1911. Eugenics Education Society, Council Minute Book, Nov. 1909 to Dec. 1912, p. 65.
63 Eugenics Education Society, Council Minute Book, Nov. 1909 to Dec. 1912.
64 Alexander M. Carr-Saunders, Major Greenwood, Eric J. Lidbetter

and Alfred F. Tredgold, 'The standardisation of pedigrees: a recommendation', *Eugen. Rev.* 4 (1912–13): 383–90.

65 Eugenics Education Society, Council Minute Book, Nov. 1909 to Dec. 1912, pp. 68, 70.

66 Eric J. Lidbetter, 'Nature and nurture: a study in conditions', *Eugen. Rev.* 4 (1912–13): 54–73.

67 Eugenics Education Society, *Fifth Annual Report* (1912–13), 18.

68 Charles P. Blacker, *Eugenics: Galton and After* (London: Duckworth, 1952). The phrases are Galton's, as cited by Blacker.

69 Francis Galton and Edgar Schuster, *Noteworthy Families (Modern Science): an Index to Kinships in Near Degrees between Persons whose Achievements are Honourable and have been Publicly Recorded*, v. 1 in series, Publications of the Eugenics Record Office of the University of London (London: Murray, 1906).

70 Edgar Schuster and Ethel M. Elderton, *The Inheritance of Ability. Being a Statistical Examination of the Oxford Class Lists from the Year 1800 Onwards, and of the School lists of Harrow and Charterhouse*, No. 1 in series, Eugenics Laboratory Memoirs (London: Dulau, 1907); Schuster, *The Promise of Youth and the Performance of Manhood. Being a Statistical Examination into the Relation existing between Success in the Examinations for the B.A. Degree at Oxford and Subsequent Success in Professional Life. (The Professions considered are the Bar and the Church)*, No. 3 in series, Eugenics Laboratory Memoirs (London: Dulau, 1907).

71 Schenk and Parkes, 'The Eugenics Society' (1968), n. 61; Alexander M. Carr-Saunders, *World Population* (Oxford, University Press, 1936).

72 Alfred F. Tredgold, *Mental Deficiency (Amentia)* (London: Ballière, 1st ed., 1908), 36–7.

73 Tredgold, *Mental Deficiency* (1908), n. 72, 7.

74 Idem.

75 Eugenics Education Society, *Fourth Annual Report*, (1911–12), 27, 28.

76 Francis Galton, *Hereditary Genius: an Inquiry into its Laws and Consequences* (London: Macmillan, 1869).

77 Kimmelman, 'American Breeders' Association' (1983), n. 47, 163–204.

78 Charles B. Davenport, *Heredity in Relation to Eugenics* (New York, NY: Holt, 1911), 25, 66. Chapter 2. 'The methods of eugenics' is an explanation of Mendelism, and Chapter 3, 'The inheritance of family traits', includes a collection of 150 pedigrees.

79 H.H. Goddard, 'The heredity of feeblemindedness', *Bulletin of the Eugenics Record Office* 1 (1911): 1–14.

80 Harry H. Laughlin, *Eugenical Sterilisation in the United States* (Chicago, IL: Municipal Court, 1922). Laughlin's sterilisation campaign is discussed by Ludmerer, *Genetics* (1972), n. 35, 90–5.

81 Karl Pearson, Julia Bell and others, *A Treasury of Human Inheritance: Pedigrees of Physical, Psychical and Pathological Characters in Man*, Nos

VI, IX, XII, XV, XVII in series Eugenics Laboratory Memoirs (London: Dulau, 1912), v. I, parts I–VIII, and Index volume.
82 Pearson, Preface to Bell (1912), n. 81.
83 *Poor Law Committee Report* (1910), n. 51, 181–2.
84 Idem, 194.
85 Idem, 187.
86 Idem, 190.
87 Leonard Darwin, introduction to Lidbetter, *Social Problem Group* (1933), n. 53.
88 *Problems in Eugenics: Papers Commuinicated to the First International Eugenics Congress,* University of London, 24–30 July 1912; *Catalogue of the Exhibition* (London: Knight, 1912), 75.
89 Booth, 'Inhabitants of Tower Hamlets' (1887), n. 16.
90 *Catalogue of the Exhibition* (1912), n. 88, 52–3.
91 Idem, 75.
92 Frederick W. Mott, 'Heredity and eugenics in relation to insanity', *Problems in Eugenics* (1912), n. 88, 400–28; the published version of the essay contains two Lidbetter pedigrees (see Fig. 2.10) but Mott's slides for the lecture are listed on the back of a box among the Eugenics Society's Papers, and include only one, a different one. All but one of the slides themselves are missing: Eugen. Soc. Papers, G 38.
93 Kimmelman, 'American Breeders' Association' (1983), n. 47.
94 Max von Gruber and Ernst Rüdin, eds, *Fortpflanzung Vererbung Rassenhygiene Illustrierte Führer durch die Gruppe Rassenhygiene der Internationalen Hygiene-Ausstellung 1911 in Dresden* (Munich: Lehmann, 1911).
95 *Catalogue of the Exhibition* (1912), n. 88, 17.
96 Idem, 1–2.
97 'Worst family in the world: interesting and curious exhibition: pedigrees of the great', *Pall Mall Gazette* (29 July 1912), report of exhibition.
98 *Catalogue of the Exhibition* (1912), n. 88, 3, 26.
99 Karl Pearson, *A First Study of the Statistics of Pulmonary Tuberculosis (Inheritance),* No. 2 in series, Studies in National Deterioration, Drapers' Company Research Memoirs (London: Dulau, 1910); Pearson's answer to his critics appeared in his *On the Handicapping of the First-born,* No. 10 in Eugenics Lecture series, Galton Laboratory Publications (London: Dulau, 1914).
100 Friedrich Martius, 'Die Vererbbarkeit des konstitutionellen Factors bei Tuberculose', *Berl. klin. Wschr.* 38 (1901): 1125–30.

3 IDEOLOGY AND METHOD

1 F. Yates and K. Mather, 'Ronald Alymer Fisher', in *Biographical Memoirs of Fellows of Roy. Soc.* (London) 9 (1963): 91–120; Karl Pearson, 'Contributions on the mathematical theory of evolution', *Phil. Trans. Roy. Soc.* (London) A 185 (1894): 70–110; Pearson, 'Mathematical contributions to the theory of evolution.

On the law of ancestral heredity', *Proc. Roy. Soc.* (London) 62 (1898): 386–412.

2 The 'Cambridge University Eugenics Society's Minute Book' runs from May 1911 to May 1913. It was restarted in 1920 with F.L. Engledon as Honorary Secretary (letter from Engledon to C.S. Stock, 1 March 1920, stuck in back of book) and ceased again 1922–23. See Eugenics Education Society, *Fifteenth Annual Report* (1922–23), 6.

3 Eugenics Education Society, *Sixth Annual Report* (1913–14), 36–51, gives details of societies in the provinces and elsewhere.

4 Cambridge Minute Book, n. 2, printed announcement of Inge's lecture and Society's inauguration.

5 *Cambridge Daily News*, 23 May 1911, copied into Cambridge Minute Book, n. 2.

6 Cambridge Minute Book, n. 2; announcement, n. 4, lists Society's officers.

7 William R. Inge, 'Some moral aspects of eugenics', *Eugen. Rev.* 1 (1909–10): 26–36.

8 C.S. Stock, 'Eugenics: introductory paper read in Mr R.A. Fisher's rooms ... October 29, 1911', reading script stuck into Cambridge Minute Book, n. 2.

9 R.A. Fisher, 'Heredity: paper given in Mr C.E. Shelley's rooms ... 10 November 1911', reading script stuck into Cambridge Minute Book, n. 2. This paper was not published by Fisher himself, but was brought out recently, n. 10.

10 Bernard Norton and Egon S. Pearson, 'A note on the background to and refereeing of, R.A. Fisher's 1918 paper, "On the correlation between relatives on the supposition of mendelian inheritance"', *Notes & Records Roy. Soc.* (London) 31 (1976): 151–62. The authors print Fisher's paper (1911), n. 9, and point out that he is already attempting to unite Mendelism and biometry at this time.

11 C.S. Stock, 'The principles of eugenics', *Cambridge Mag.*, 18 May 1912.

12 R.C. Punnett, 'Genetics and eugenics', a paper read at the second public meeting of the Cambridge University Eugenics Society, 5 Dec. 1911, Cambridge Minute Book, n. 2.

13 C.S. Stock, 'Secretary's Report for the end of his year of office, 1911–1912', in Cambridge Minute Book, n. 2, report of Committee Meeting, 10 March 1912.

14 L. Doncaster, 'Sex limited inheritance', paper read to Cambridge University Eugenics Society, 14 Feb. 1912; report in Cambridge Minute Book, n. 2.

15 F. Kidd, 'Natural selection and Mendelism', paper read at the fourth undergraduate meeting of the Cambridge University Eugenics Society, 13 Feb. 1912 in the author's rooms at K Staircase, 2nd Court, St Johns College. Cambridge Minute Book, n. 2; announced by C.S. Stock as a preliminary to Doncaster's lecture, 1912, n. 14.

16 R.C. Punnett, 'Genetics and eugenics', report in *Cambridge Daily News*, 6 Dec. 1911.

17 R.K. Webb, *Harriet Martineau, a Radical Victorian* (London; Heinemann, 1960).

18 E.P. Thompson, *William Morris: Romantic to Revolutionary* (London: Merlin, 2nd ed., 1977) 139.

19 Leonard Darwin, 'First steps towards eugenic reform', lecture delivered at Cambridge University, 8 Feb. 1912, under the auspices of the Cambridge University Eugenics Society, *Eugen. Rev.* 4 (1912–13): 26–38.

20 Darwin, 'First steps' (1912–13), n. 19, report in *Cambridge Daily News*, 12 Feb. 1912.

21 Stock, 'Secretary's Report' 1912, n. 13.

22 Idem.

23 Cambridge Minute Book, n. 2, announcement lists members of the university who had promised support.

24 Cambridge Minute Book, n. 2, printed prospectus for October term 1912.

25 Kenneth M. Ludmerer, *Genetics and American Society* (Baltimore, MD: Hopkins, 1972), 156. 'From its beginning, the Eugenics Education Society largely consisted of a collection of social snobs very conscious of being "well-born", who expressed silly views on heredity. To most observers they appeared foolish and haughty, but few onlookers thought of them as pernicious.' Ludmerer's view seems to be a reflection of his conversations with Lancelot Hogben, who attacked the eugenists in the thirties for their class prejudice and snobbery.

26 Karl Mannheim, *Ideologie und Utopie*, in Series, Schriften zur Philosophie und Soziologie, K. Mannheim, ed. (Bonn: Lohen, 1929), 123. 'Jene nicht eindeutig festgelegt, relativ klassenlose Schicht ins (in Alfred Weber's Terminologie gesprochen) die *sozial freischwebende Intelligens*. . . .'

27 R.A. Fisher, 'Some hopes of a eugenist', *Eugen. Rev.* 5 (1913–14): 309–15. Read at the Second Annual Meeting of the Cambridge University Eugenics Society, 12 Oct. 1913.

28 Idem.

29 Joan Fisher Box, *R.A. Fisher: the Life of a Scientist* (New York, NY: Wiley, 1978), 8.

30 Maximilian Mügge, 'Eugenics and the superman: a racial science and a racial religion', *Eugen. Rev.* 1 (1909–10): 184–93. Mügge was also the author of *Friedrich Nietzsche, his Life and Work* (London: Unwin, 1909), a copy of which was in the Society's library.

31 On Ellis's Nietzschean writings, see D.S. Thatcher, *Nietzsche in England 1890–1914: the Growth of a Reputation* (Toronto: University Press, 1970), 93–120, 114.

32 The Society's collection includes the first English translations, *The Case of Wagner* translated by Thomas Common, introduced by Alexander Tille (London: Henry, 1896), and *Thus Spake Zarathustra*, translated by Alexander Tille (London: Henry, 1896), edition of 1908; 'beyond-man' is Tille's version of *Übermensch*.

33 This is Tille's interpretation, e.g., in introduction to *Wagner*, 1896, n. 32.

34 The reinterpretation seems to have begun with Karl Jaspers' *Nietzsche: an Introduction to the Understanding of his Philosophical Activity*, 1935, translated by C.F. Wallraff and F.J. Schmitz (Flagstaff, AR: University of Arizona Press, 1965); Jaspers associated Nietzsche with existentialism, in order, as he wrote in the 'Preface to the second and third edition', 'to marshall against the National Socialists the world of thought of the man whom they had proclaimed as their own philosopher', and to show that the 'phraseological materials' used by the Nazis were aberrations in the writings of a man on the verge of insanity.

35 Georges Chatterton-Hill, *The Philosophy of Nietzsche: an Exposition and an Appreciation* (London: Ousely, 1912),: 188.

36 Idem, 192.

37 J.A. Lindsay, Review of G. Chatterton-Hill, *The Philosophy of Nietzsche*, in *Eugen. Rev.* 5 (1913–14): 72.

38 Details of Fisher's life are from Box, *Fisher* (1978), n. 29; Joan Box very kindly allowed me to see a draft of her manuscript. I must also thank her for a long and very enjoyable discussion we had in May 1977 on Fisher and the eugenics movement.

39 R.A. Fisher and C.S. Stock, 'Cuenot on preadaptation', *Eugen. Rev.* 7 (1915–16): 184–92.

40 R.A. Fisher, Report on progress of the bibliography of eugenics over the past year, Executive Council Meeting, 18 April 1916. Eugenics Education Society, Council Minute Book, 1912.

41 Box, *Fisher* (1978), n. 29, p. 38.

42 R.A. Fisher, 'The evolution of sexual preference', *Eugen. Rev.* 7 (1915–16): 184–92.

43 Box, *Fisher* (1978), n. 29, p. 43.

44 Fisher, 'Some hopes' (1913–14), n. 27, p. 313.

45 R.A. Fisher, 'Positive eugenics', *Eugen. Rev.* 9 (1917–18): 206–12.

46 George Udny Yule, 'Mendel's laws and their probable relations to intraracial heredity', *New Phytologist* 1 (1902): 226–7.

47 Karl Pearson, 'On a generalised theory of alternative inheritance with special reference to Mendel's laws', *Phil. Trans. Roy. Soc.* (London) 203 (1904): 53–86.

48 George Udny Yule, 'On the theory of inheritance of quantitative compound characters on the basis of Mendel's laws – a preliminary note', *Report of the Third International Conference on Genetics* (London: Spottiswoode, 1907), 140–2.

49 R.A. Fisher, 'The biometrical study of heredity', two lectures delivered at the London School of Economics on 6 and 11 June 1924, *Eugen. Rev.* 16 (1924–25): 189–210.

50 Fisher, 'Biometrical study' (1924), n. 49, p. 204.

51 P.A. Moran and C.A.B. Smith, *Commentary on R.A. Fisher's Paper on The Correlation between Relatives on the Supposition of Mendelian Inheritance*, No. 41 in series, Eugenics Laboratory Memoirs (Cambridge: University Press, 1966), 50. This reprint of Fisher's 1918 paper is accompanied by an interlined commentary. References hereafter are to this edition.

52 Moran and Smith, *Commentary* (1966), n. 51, p. 49.
53 William B. Provine, *The Origins of Theoretical Population Genetics*, in series, Chicago History of Science and Medicine, A.G. Debus, ed. (Chicago, IL: University Press, 1971), 144.
54 Rothamsted Experimental Station, *Guide to the Experimental Farms* (Harpenden, Hertfordshire: Lawes Agricultural Trust, 1962). Sir E. John Russell, *Plant Nutrition and Crop Production* (Berkeley, CA: University of California Press, 1926), 1–26.
55 $Ca_2H_2(PO_4)_2$ was known to be converted to $CaH_4(PO_4)_2$ or 'superphosphate'; see S. Hare Collins, *Chemical Fertilizers and Parasiticides* (London: Ballière, 1920), 119–46; 175–8.
56 Sir E. John Russell, *History of Agricultural Science in Great Britain* (London: Allen, 1966), 88–109; 143–75.
57 Sir John Bennett Lawes and Sir J. Henry Gilbert, 'On agricultural chemistry', *J. Roy. Agric. Soc.* 8 (1847): 226–60; Lawes and Gilbert, 'On agricultural chemistry, especially in relation to the mineral theory of Baron Liebig', *J. Roy. Agric. Soc.* 12 (1851): 1–40; they refer to Justus Liebig, *Principles of Agricultural Chemistry with Special Reference to the late Researches made in England* (1855).
58 Sir A. Daniel Hall, *The Book of the Rothamsted Experiments* (London: Murray, 1905); Hall, *Fertilizers and Manures* (London: Murray, 1909); 2nd ed., 1913; 3rd ed., 1920.
59 Sir E. John Russell, *The Land Called Me: an Autobiography* (London: Allen, 1956).
60 Sir E. John Russell, *Soil Conditions and Plant Growth* (London: Longmans, 4th ed., 1921), vii [1st ed., 1912].
61 Box, *Fisher* (1978), n. 29, pp. 93–112.
62 Fisher's lectures to the London School of Economics of 1924 were still maintaining this position in respect of human heights.
63 R.A. Fisher, 'Studies in crop variation, I. An examination of the yield of dressed grain from Broadbalk', *J. Agric. Sci.* 11 (1921): 107–35, esp. p. 109.
64 Rothamsted Experimental Station, *Guide to the Classical Field Experiments* (Harpenden, Hertfordshire: Lawes Agricultural Trust, 1984), 16–17.
65 D.G. Dalrymple, *Development and Spread of High Yielding Varieties of Wheat and Rice in the Less Developed Nations*, No. 95 in series, Foreign Agriculture Reports (Washington DC, Dept. of Agriculture, 6th ed., 1978).
66 Kenneth A. Dahlberg, *Beyond the Green Revolution: the Ecology and Politics of Global Agricultural Development* (New York, NY: Plenum, 1979), 'Resumé of the development of new seeds', 48–90.
67 Fisher's innovations are discussed by Box, *Fisher* (1978), n. 29, pp. 100–12.
68 Idem, pp. 158–61.
69 Idem, p. 158, citing R.A. Fisher, 'Statistical Methods in Genetics', Bateson Lecture 1951, *Heredity* 6 (1952): 1–12.
70 Fisher, 'Correlation between relatives' (1918/1966), n. 51, p. 12.
71 R.A. Fisher and W.A. Mackenzie, 'Studies in crop variation, II. The

manurial response of different potato varieties', *J. Agric. Sci.* 13 (1923): 311–20.

72 Ian Hacking, 'Telepathy: origins of randomisation in experimental design', *Isis* 79 (1988): 427–51.

73 T. Eden and R.A. Fisher, 'Studies in crop variation, IV. Experiments on the response of the potato to potash and nitrogen', *J. Agric. Sci.* 19 (1929): 201–13.

74 F. Yates, 'Sir Ronald Fisher and the design of experiments', *Biometrics* 20 (1964): 307–21; R.A. Fisher, 'The arrangement of field experiments', *J. Min. Ag.* 33 (1926): 503–13. Fisher's own explanation of his new techniques is in R.A. Fisher, *The Design of Experiments* (Edinburgh, Oliver, 1935), 48–67, 'An agricultural experiment in randomized blocks'; pp. 68–90, 'The Latin square'; pp. 91–8, 'The factorial design in experimentation'. For a recent treatment of this important technigue see H.H. Harman, *Modern Factor Analysis* (Chicago, IL: University Press, 3rd ed., 1976).

75 Rothamsted, *Experimental Farms* (1962), n. 54, p. 27; Sir John Russell, 'Field experiments: how they are made and what they are', *J. Min. Ag.* 32 (1926): 989–1001.

76 The Board of Control was set up under the Mental Deficiency Act of 1913 to oversee certification, detention and care of lunatic and feeble-minded paupers. For its history and functions see the account in *Report of the Royal Commission on Lunacy and Mental Disorder*, Cmd 2700 (London: HMSO, 1926), pp. 9–14 (*Macmillan Report*).

77 Hodson to Burt, letter d. 12 April 1923, Eugen. Soc. Papers, C52; Cora Hodson was the General Secretary from 1920 to 1931; she was succeeded by Charles Blacker; Faith Schenk and A.S. Parkes, 'Activities of the Eugenics Society', *Eugen. Rev.* 60 (1968): 142–61.

78 Protocol of Research, Eugen. Soc. Papers, C52.

79 Hodson to Burt, letter d. 16 April 1923, Eugen. Soc. Papers, C52.

80 Burt to Hodson, letter d. 13 April 1923, Eugen. Soc. Papers, C52.

81 Eugen. Ed. Soc., Research Committee Minute Book, 1923–25, Meeting of 12 May 1923.

82 Burt enthusiastically describes this Committee as having as its members 'almost every psychologist and educationalist of note in the country ... and one or two members of the staff of the Board of Education. I feel quite sure that they would willingly place themselves at the disposal of you or Mr Lidbetter. ...' Burt to Hodson, letter d. 14 April 1923. Eugen. Soc. Papers, C52.

83 Hodson to Burt, letter d. 10 Sept. 1923, Eugen. Soc. Papers, C52.

84 Hodson to Burt, letter d. 29 Aug. 1923, Eugen. Soc. Papers, C52.

85 Research Minute Book, 1923–25, Meeting of 6 Oct. 1923.

86 Hodson to Burt, letter d. 2 Feb. 1925, Eugen. Soc. Papers, C52.

87 Hodson to Burt, letter d. 25 May 1925, Eugen. Soc. Papers, C52.

88 Hodson to Rathbone, letter d. 3 April 1925, Eugen. Soc. Papers, C210.

89 Eleanor Rathbone, *The Disinherited Family*, introduction by S. Fleming (London: Falling Wall Press, 1986).

90 Hodson to J. Sandeman Allen, letter d. 3 June 1925, Eugen. Soc. Papers, C210.
91 Hodson to Elton Mayo, letter d. 27 June 1927, Eugen. Soc. Papers, C210.
92 'Enquiry into Causes and Continuance of Destitution (Poor Law)', Circular letter to firms, with covering letter d. 4 Feb. 1927, Eugen. Soc. Papers, J22.
93 Research Minute Book, 1923–25, Meeting of 6 Oct. 1923.
94 Research Minute Book, 1923–25, typewritten memorandum attached at end of book.
95 R.A. Fisher, 'The elimination of mental defect', Eugen. Rev, 16 (1924–25): 114–16.
96 R.C. Punnett, 'Eliminating feeblemindedness', J. Heredity 8 (1917): 464–5.
97 Fisher, 'Elimination of mental defect' (1925), n. 95, p. 115.
98 Research Minute Book, 1923–25, typed document, unsigned, stuck into back of book. It appears to be Lidbetter's reply to Fisher, n. 93.
99 Research Minute Book, 1923–25, typed document, unsigned, in same typewriting as n. 98. It appears to be Lidbetter's reply to Fisher's questions after he had seen them in written form, n. 94.
100 E.W. MacBride, 'Do we inherit our habits?' Radio Times, 12 Oct. 1923.
101 Fisher, 'Elimination of mental defect' (1925) n. 95.
102 Research Minute Book, 1923–25, Meeting of 6 Oct. 1923.
103 Research Minute Book, 1923–25, Meeting of 3 March 1925.
104 Research Minute Book, 1923–25, Meeting of 3 March 1925, typescript stuck into record, same typing as that assumed to be by Lidbetter (n. 98, n. 99).
105 G. Udny Yule, 'On the method of measuring association between two attributes', (1912), reprinted in Alan Stewart and Maurice G. Kendall, Statistical Papers of George Udny Yule (London: Griffith, 1971), 107–70.
106 G. Udny Yule, 'On the association of attributes in statistics' (1900), in Stewart and Kendall (1971), n. 105, pp. 7–69. Yule explains the technique of association at length in his Introduction to the Theory of Statistics (London, Griffin, 1st ed., 1911); 7th ed., 1924; 10th ed, 1932. Subsequent editions to 14th ed., 1950, were carried out by M.G. Kendall. My references are to the 7th ed., 1924, chapters III and IV.
107 L.H.D. Buxton to Hodson, letter d. 1 March 1925; Research Minute Book, 1923–25. Pearson is referring to the method first proposed in his On the Theory of Contingency and its Relation to Association and Normal Correlation, Drapers' Company Research Memoirs, Biometric Series T (London: Dulau, 1904); Karl Pearson, 'On a new method of determining correlation when one variable is given by alternative and the other by multiple categories', Biometrika 7 (1910): 248–57; this paper gives a method for the relationship between a quantitative character and another that is

present or absent, and would presumably be the method he had in mind.

108 See Yule, *Introduction* (1911/1924), n. 106, Chapter V.

109 The controversy over the two methods and its social roots in eugenics are discussed by D.A. Mackenzie, *Statistics in Britain 1865–1930, the Social Construction of Scientific Knowledge* (Edinburgh: University Press, 1981), Chapter 7, 'The politics of the contingency table', pp. 153–82.

110 Yule, *Introduction* (1911/1924), n. 106, pp. 31, 34.

111 Hodson to Burt, letter d. 16 May 1925, Eugen. Soc. Papers, C53.

112 Hodson to Martin, letter d. 21 Oct. 1925, Eugen. Soc. Papers, C53.

113 D. Ward Cutler was Secretary of the Society along with Lady Chambers from 1927 to 1934; see Schenk and Parkes (1968), n. 77. He was the author of a book on the mechanism of evolution, *Evolution, Heredity and Variation* (London: Christopher, 1925), in which he opposed MacBride's position on the inheritance of acquired characters. He discusses multifactorial inheritance of stature, but says that 'a complete Mendelian analysis has not yet been made for this character', p. 132. He does not seem to be aware of Fisher's work, or perhaps ascribes less significance to it than is now the case.

114 Research Minute Book, 1923–25, Meeting of 25 Nov. 1925.

115 Research Minute Book, 1923–25, Meeting of 8 Dec. 1925.

116 Burt to Hodson, letter d. 10 Aug. 1925, Eugen. Soc. Papers, C52.

117 Hodson to Burt, letter d. 14 Dec. 1925, Eugen. Soc. Papers, C52.

118 Hodson to L. Darwin, letter d. 14 Dec. 1925, Eugen. Soc. Papers, C52.

119 Research Minute Book, 1923–25, Meeting of 16 Dec. 1925.

120 Research Minute Book, 1925–31, Meeting of 23 Dec. 1925. This meeting begins a new book. The last minutes in the old book, 1923–25, are very crossed out and altered. Fisher had asked for several amendments relating to the things he had said; a fresh copy was to be prepared and a space was left, but it was never done. The rest of the book is blank.

121 Research Minute Book, 1925–31, Meeting of 5 March 1926. Report to the Henderson Trust, submitted by Dr Carter [*sic*; should probably be Dr Cutler].

122 Cutler, *Evolution* (1925), n. 112, p. 114.

123 Research Minute Book, 1925–31, Meeting of 30 June 1926.

124 Research Minute Book, 1925–31, Meeting of 27 Oct. 1926.

125 'Research into Pauperism', annotated 'sent to Prof. Huxley 5.7.1928', Eugen. Soc. Papers, D162.

126 Secretary, P. B[oyd], to Martin, 30 March 1926, Eugen. Soc. Papers, C53.

127 Research Minute Book, 1925–31, Meeting of 27 Oct. 1926.

128 [———] 'Population studies in Edinburgh', *Eugen. Rev.*, 18 (1926–27): 227–30.

129 Research Minute Book, 1923–25, Meeting of 6 Oct. 1923, also in n. 85, n. 93, n. 102.

130 Leonard Darwin, 'The aims and methods of eugenics societies', *Eugenics and the Family: Scientific Papers Presented at the Second International Eugenics Congress, New York, 1922* (Baltimore, MD: Williams, 1923), 5–19, esp. p. 6.

131 Ernest J. Lidbetter, 'Nature and nurture: a study in conditions', *Eugen. Rev.* 4 (1912–13): 54–73.

132 Ernest J. Lidbetter, 'Eugenics Society population research, Draft Report', n.d., 1929?, Eugen. Soc. Papers, D162.

133 'Research into the social qualities of a sample of our population', n.d., Eugen. Soc. Papers, C210.

134 R.A. Fisher, *Statistical Methods for Research Workers* (London: Oliver, 1925), 138.

135 Ernest J. Lidbetter, *Heredity and the Social Problem Group*, introduced by Leonard Darwin (London: Arnold, 1933), v.1; no others appeared.

136 Ernest J. Lidbetter, 'Eugenics Society population research, Draft Report', n.d., 1929?, Eugen. Soc. Papers, D162.

137 See, for example, the explanations in the famous German textbook, 'Baur-Fischer-Lenz', Fritz Lenz, 'Die krankhaften Erbanlagen', in Erwin Baur, Eugen Fischer and Fritz Lenz, *Grundriss der menschlichen Erblichkeitsforschung*, 2 v, (Munich: Lehmann, 1921), v. 1, p. 244, Weinberg's *Geschwister-Probanden-Methode*; p. 246, cousin marriage. This text was not translated into English until the 3rd edition of 1927. By then it contained a detailed exposition of the now highly-developed *Vererbungsmathematik* or mathematical Mendelism by Lenz; for example, pp. 422–3, 432–3, Weinberg's *Geschwister-Probanden-Methode*, its problems and the means of correcting for them; p. 435, cousin marriage and the method for comparing its frequency in general population and in tainted stocks. The translation, by Eden and Cedar Paul, did not appear until 1931.

138 Otto Diem, exhibit C16, showing 'Distribution of particular taints in every hundred of tainted members among the nearest relations (parents, grandparents, uncles, aunts, brothers and sisters)'. First International Congress of Eugenics, *Catalogue of the Exhibition*, London, Knight, 1912, pp. 5–6, Chapter II, n. 99; Diem, 'Die psycho-neurotische erbliche Belastung der Geistesgesunden und Geisteskranken: eine statistische-kritische Untersuchung auf Grund eigener Beobachtungen', *Arch. f. Rassen- u. Gesellsch. biol.* 2 (1905): 215–52, 336–68.

139 Lidbetter, *Social Problem Group* (1933), n. 135.

140 Crewe to Blacker, letter d. 6 May 1930, Eugen. Soc. Papers, C79.

141 Fisher to Bramwell, letter d. 6 Jan. 1934, Eugen. Soc. Papers, C108.

142 D.J. Kevles, 'Genetics in the United States and Britain, 1890–1930: a review with speculations', *Isis* 71 (1980): 441–55.

143 Maria Günther, *Die Institutionalizerung der Rassenhygiene an den deutschen Hochschulen vor 1933*, Inaugural Dissertation zur

Erlangung der Würde des Doktors der Medizin der Johann Gutenberg Universität, Mainz, 1982.

144 Davenport to Secretary of the Society, letter d. 26 March 1926, informing her that eugenics would be presented at the Fifth International Genetics Congress; Eugen. Soc. Papers, D80.

145 See correspondence between Charles P. Blacker and Ernst Rüdin, Eugen. Soc. Papers, C300, C301; further discussion Chapter V.

4 THE ATTACK FROM THE LEFT

1 Frederick W. Mott, 'Heredity and insanity', last of a series of six lectures on heredity delivered at the Royal Institution, *Lancet* i (1911): 1251–9; see Chapter 1, n. 93.

2 Alfred Grotjahn and J. Kaup, eds, *Handwörterbuch der sozialen Hygiene*, 2 v (Leipzig: Vogel, 1912).

3 Myron Kantorovitz, 'Alfred Grotjahn as a eugenist', *Eugen. News* 25 (1940): 15–19.

4 A. Grotjahn, *Erlebtes und Erstrebtes: Erinnerung eines sozialistischen Ärztes* (Berlin: Herbig, 1932), 246.

5 A. Grotjahn, 'Der Unterricht der Studierenden und der Ärzte', in A. Gottstein, A. Schlossman and L. Telecky, eds, *Handbuch der sozialen Hygiene und Gesundheitsfürsorge*, 8 v (Berlin: Springer, 1925), v. 1, 391–400.

6 M. von Gruber, 'Hygienische Aufgaben der Gegenwart', in R. Eucken and M. von Gruber, *Ethische und hygienische Aufgaben der Gegenwart, Vorträge gehalten den 8 januar 1916 in der neuen Aula der Berliner Universität* (Berlin: Massigkeits-Verlag der Deutschen Vereins gegen den Missbrauch geistiger Getränke, 1916), 21–47.

7 Loren Graham, 'Science and values: the eugenics movement in Germany and Russia in the 1920s', *Am. Hist. Rev.* 82 (1977): 1133–64, and in his *Between Science and Values* (New York, NY: Columbia University Press, 1981), 217–56.

8 Graham, *Between Science and Values* (1981), n. 7, 228.

9 Max Levien, 'Stimmen aus dem deutschen Urwald (Zwei neue Apostel des Rassenhasses)', *Unter dem Banner des Marxismus* 2 (1928): 150–95; cited in Graham, *Between Science and Values* (1981), n. 7, 230.

10 Pauline M.H. Mazumdar, 'Two models for human genetics: blood grouping and psychiatry in Germany between the wars', in preparation.

11 Pauline M.H. Mazumdar, 'Blood and soil: the serology of the Aryan racial state', *Bull. Hist. Med.* 64 (1990): 187–219.

12 Lancelot Hogben, *The Nature of Living Matter* (London: Kegan Paul, 1930), 207–8.

13 Hogben, *Living Matter* (1930) n. 12, 213–14. The phrase 'a national minimum of parenthood' refers to Beatrice Webb, *The Case for the National Minimum* (London: National Committee for the Prevention of Destitution, 1913).

14 Obituary notice, 'Lancelot Hogben', *The Times* (23 Aug. 1975), 14;

Gary Werskey, *The Visible College* (London: Lane, 1978), 60–7; Lancelot Hogben, 'An unauthorised autobiography of Lancelot Hogben', edited by Adrian and Anne Hogben, Chapter I; my grateful thanks to them for allowing me to cite this unpublished manuscript.

15 Lancelot Hogben, *Science for the Citizen: a Self-Educator based on the Social Background of Scientific Discovery*, second of the Primers for the Age of Plenty (London: Allen, 1938), 1054–7.

16 Werskey, *Visible College* (1978), n. 13, 101–15.

17 Lancelot Hogben, 'Modern heredity and social science', *Socialist Rev.* 16 (1919): 147–56, cited in Werskey, *Visible College* (1978), n. 15, 105. Hogben's essays appear in almost every one of the isssues of the *Socialist Review* at this time.

18 Lancelot Hogben, 'Origins of the Society', in M. Sleigh and J. Sutcliffe, *The Society for Experimental Biology: Origins and History* (Cambridge: Company of Biologists, 1974), 6–12.

19 J.A. Frazer Roberts, 'Reginald Ruggles-Gates, 1882–1962', *Biographical Memoirs of Fellows of Roy. Soc.* (London) 10 (1964): 83–106.

20 Crew to Hodson, letter d. 12 Aug. 1919, Eugen. Soc. Papers, C79.

21 Crew to Blacker, letter d. 6 May 1930, Eugen. Soc. Papers, C79.

22 Lancelot T. Hogben, *The Pigmentary Effector System*, No. 1 in series, Biological Monographs and Manuals, edited by F.A.E. Crew and D. Ward Cutler (Edinburgh: Oliver, 1924).

23 Frank A.E. Crew, *Animal Genetics: the Science of Animal Breeding* (Edinburgh: Oliver, 1925); other volumes in the series included Ward Cutler's *Soil Protozoa* and R.A. Fisher's *Statistics for Biological Research Workers* (1924).

24 Lancelot T. Hogben, *Comparative Physiology*, in series, Textbooks of Animal Biology, edited by Julian S. Huxley (London: Sidgwick, 1926).

25 E. Babak *et al.*, *Handbuch der vergleichende Physiologie* 4 v in 9 (Jena: Fischer, 1910–14).

26 See, for example, Lancelot Hogben, 'The pigmentary effector system, IV. A further contribution to the role of pituitary secretion in amphibian colour response,' *Brit. J. Exper. Biol.* 1 (1923): 249–70.

27 Hogben, 'Origins of the Society', (1974), n. 18, 8.

28 Hogben, *Comparative Physiology* (1926), n. 24, 183; 186.

29 The term 'factorial analysis' was used in several different senses. It was introduced by R.A. Fisher for the methods used in the analysis of factors affecting crop yields, as elaborated and explained by F. Yates, *Design and Analysis of Factorial Experiments* (London: Commonwealth Bureau of Soil Science, 1937), Technical Communication No. 35. Fisher himself chose the name, he stated, because the method was derived from the Mendelian 'factors' by way of his famous reconciliation of biometry and Mendelism. Fisher's method is based on partial correlation. It is used in this sense by the psychologists, such as Spearman; see, for example, Godfrey H. Thomson, *The Factorial Analysis of Human Ability* (London: University Press, 1939). Hogben, however, uses the phrase 'factorial analysis'

to mean the type of Mendelian mathematics used by Weinberg and Bernstein to calculate gene frequencies according to the binomial expansion. In order to distinguish these two uses – an important distinction for my argument – and to emphasise the German origin of the method, I have kept to the German term *Vererbungsmathematik* for this kind of analysis.

30 L.T. Hogben, *Principles of Animal Biology* (London: Christophers, 1930), x.

31 L.T. Hogben, *Principles of Evolutionary Biology* (Cape Town: Juta, 1927), 105.

32 L. Hogben, 'Contemporary philosophy in Soviet Russia', *Psyche* 12 (1931): 2–18, 4.

33 Hogben, *Evolutionary Biology* (1927), n. 31, 107.

34 William H. Beveridge, 'Origin of social biology in the School of Economics', London School of Economics, Archives, File no. 213 E (1925), dated 16 July 1935.

35 Beveridge, 'Origin of social biology' (1925), n. 34, 1, and in a letter to Beardsley Ruml, Director of the Laura Spelman Rockefeller Memorial dated 16 July 1925. On Beveridge and the sociobiology chair, see José Harris, *William Beveridge: a Biography* (Oxford: Clarendon, 1977), 286–90.

36 Editorial note, *Eugen. Rev.* 19 (1927–28): 98.

37 Hogben, *Evolutionary Biology* (1927), n. 31, 100.

38 L. Hogben, 'Memorandum concerning the scope and development of a science of Social Biology, together with a programme of research and a statement of its financial requirements', in LSE Archives, File no. 312 A (n.d., but this is the first item in the file; the next is dated 18 March 1931).

39 Hogben, *Evolutionary Biology* (1927), n. 30, 100.

40 Hogben, *Living Matter* (1930), n. 12, 193. The poem is Campbell's 'The flaming terrapin'. It is also quoted in *Evolutionary Biology* (1927), n. 30, 94.

41 Hogben, *Living Matter* (1930), n. 12, 199–200.

42 Blacker to Lidbetter, letter d. 27 June 1931, Eugen. Soc. Papers, C209.

43 E.J. Lidbetter, 'Eugenics Society population research Draft Report', n.d., Eugen. Soc. Papers, D167. For a discussion of the new provisions, see B.B. Gilbert, *British Social Policy 1914–1939* (London: Batsford, 1970), 213–19, and Charles Webster, 'Health welfare and unemployment during the depression', *Past and Present* 109 (1985): 204–30.

44 Hogben to Beveridge, letter d. 7 July 1931, LSE Archives, File no. 312 A 1931.

45 Hogben, 'Memorandum on social biology', (1931), n. 38, 4.

46 This meeting has been discussed by P.G. Werskey, in his introduction to N.I. Bukharin *et al.*, *Science at the Cross-roads: Papers Presented to the International Congress of the History of Science and Technology held in London from June 29th to July 3rd, 1931 by the delegates of the USSR* (London: Cass, 1971), and also by C. Holmes, 'Bukharin in

England', *Soviet Studies* (July 1972): 86–90, and by J.G. Crowther, *Fifty Years of Science* (London: Barrie, 1970), 76–80.

47 Hogben, 'Contemporary philosophy in Soviet Russia' (1931), n. 32, 4.

48 Idem, 11.

49 Idem, 12–13.

50 Idem, 13.

51 David Joravsky, 'Soviet views on the history of science', *Isis* 46 (1955): 3–13, suggests that the famous paper by Boris Hessen read at this meeting was the product of an ex-idealist brought into line by Stalin. In that case, Bukharin's paper with its emphasis on the determining effect of practice must be seen as belonging to the same style of thought. See also Loren Graham, 'The socio-political roots of Boris Hessen: Soviet Marxism and the History of Science', *Soc. Stud. Science* 15 (1985): 705–22.

52 N.I. Bukharin, 'Theory and practice from the standpoint of dialectic materialism', *Science at the Crossroads* (1931), n. 46, 1–23.

53 Hogben, 'Contemporary philosophy in Soviet Russia', (1931), n. 32.

54 B.M. Zavadovskii, 'The "physical" and "biological" in the process of organic evolution', *Science at the Crossroads* (1931), n. 46, 1–12 [each paper separately paginated], p. 7; see Joravsky, 'Soviet views on the history of science' (1955), n. 51, 4. Zavadovskii was also one of those classed as an idealist by Stalin. Here, after Stalin's condemnation of this school, Zavadovskii was attacking bourgeois scientists in the style which now had official approval – the class-determinateness of scientific theories being equated with Stalin's primacy of the influence of ownership of the means of production.

55 Hogben, 'Contemporary philosophy in Soviet Russia' (1931), n. 32, 14.

56 Joseph Needham, 'Integrative levels: a revaluation of the idea of progress', first given as a Herbert Spencer Lecture, Oxford, 1937, later appeared in Needham, *Time, the Refreshing River: Essays and Addresses* (London: Allen, 1943), and in Needham, *Moulds of Understanding: a Pattern of Natural Philosophy*, edited by Gary Werskey (London: Unwin, 1976), 131–69 (p. 166, n. 39; p. 138).

57 Lancelot Hogben, *Genetic Principles in Medicine and Social Science* (London: Williams, 1931), 169.

58 Lancelot Hogben, 'The genetic analysis of family traits: I. Single gene substitution; II. Double gene substitution, with especial reference to hereditary dwarfism; III. Mating involving one parent exhibiting a trait determined by a single recessive gene substitution with special reference to sex-linked conditions', *J. Genet.* 25 (1931): 97–112; 211–40; 293–314.

59 Torsten Sjögren, 'Die juvenile amaurotische Idiotie: klinische und erblichkeitsmedizinische Untersuchungen', *Hereditas* (Lund) 14 (1931): 197–425.

60 Fritz Lenz, 'Methoden der menschliche Erblichkeits-forschung', in E. Gotschlich, ed., *Handbuch der hygienischen Untersuchungsmethoden*, 3 v (Jena: Fischer, 1926–29), for an exposition of the method of

Mendelian mathematics, v. 3, 697–701; for Lenz's critique of Weinberg's methods of correcting for the sampling bias in human families, pp. 700–1, 'Mangel der Geschwister-methode und Ersatz'; for Felix Bernstein's critique of Weinberg's methods, see below, n. 61.

61 Felix Bernstein, 'Über die Ermittlung und Prüfung von Genhypothesen aus Vererbungsbeobachtungen am Menschen und über die Unzulässigkeit der Weinbergschen Geschwister-methode als Korrektur der Auslesewirkung', *Arch.f.Rassen- u. Gesellsch.biol.* 22 (1929): 241–4. This controversy was over the corrections proposed by Weinberg for dealing with the sampling bias in human families: see above, n. 60.

62 Wilhelm Weinberg, 'Mathematischen Grundlagen der Probandenmethode', *Z.f.indukt.Abstammungs- u.Vererbungs-lehre* 48 (1927): 179–228; Sjögren's bibliography contains many more of these men's papers, but these were the ones cited by Hogben.

63 Hans Luxenburger, 'Wilhelm Weinberg', *Allgem.Z.f. Psychiatrie u.ihre Grenzgebiet* 108 (1938): 378–81.

64 Wilhelm Weinberg, 'Über die Nachweis der Vererbung beim Menschen', *Jb. d. vaterl. Naturkunde in Württemberg* 64 (1908): 368–82. G.H. Hardy, 'Mendelian proportions in a mixed population', *Science* 28 (1908): 49.

65 Fritz Lenz, 'Die Bedeutung der statistisch ermittelten Belastung mit Blutverwandschaft der Eltern', *Münch. med. Wschr.* 66 ii (1919): 1340–2, cited by Hogben, *Genetic Principles*, (1931), n. 57, 49.

66 This controversy is discussed by Pauline M.H. Mazumdar, 'Two models for human genetics', (n. 10).

67 Felix Bernstein, 'Ergebnisse einer biostatistischen zusammenfassenden Betrachtung über die erblichen Blutstrukturen des Menschen', *Klin. Wschr.* 3 (1924): 1495–7; Bernstein, 'Zusammenfassenden Betrachtungen über die erblichen Blutstrukturen des Menschen', *Z.f. indukt. Abstammungs- u.Vererbungslehre* 37 (1925): 237–70; see Mazumdar, 'Two models for human genetics' (n. 10).

68 Felix Bernstein, 'Über mendelistische Anthropologie', *Verhandlungen des V Internationalen Kongresses f. Vererbungswissenschaft*, Berlin, 1927 (Leipzig: Bornträger, 1928), 431–8.

69 Hogben, *Genetic Principles* (1931), n. 57, 64.

70 Felix Bernstein, 'Zur Grundlegung der Chromosomentheorie der Vererbung beim Menschen, mit besonderer Berücksichtigung der Blutgruppen', *Z.f. indukt. Abstammungs- u. Vererbungslehre* 57 (1931): 113–38.

71 The number of human chromosomes was not found to be 46 until 1956: Joe-Hin Tjio and Albert Levan, 'Chromosome number in man', *Hereditas* (Lund) 42 (1956): 1–6.

72 Hogben, *Genetic Principles* (1931), n. 57, 42.

73 Idem, 69.

74 Idem, 214.

75 Hogben to Beveridge, letter d. Oct. 1931. LSE Archives, File no. 312B 1931.

76 Anon., Review of Hogben, *Genetic Principles* (1931), n. 57, *The*

Medical Officer 47 (6 Feb. 1932): 59; *Lancet* i (14 May 1932): 1049; *Brit. Med. J.* i (13 Feb. 1932): 293–4; J.B.S. Haldane, 'A programme for human genetics', a review of Hogben, *Genetic Principles* (1931), n. 57, *Nature* 129 (5 March 1932): 345–6; Anon., Review of Hogben, *Genetic Principles* (1931), n. 57, *The Times* (1 July 1932), 8d; *Times Lit. Suppl.* (7 July 1932), 492; Anon., 'Social biology', *New Statesman and Nation* (n.s.) 2 (26 Dec. 1931): 816–17; Solly Zuckerman, 'Human genetics', *Spectator* 148 (13 Feb. 1932): 221.

77 Anon, 'Social biology' (1931), n. 76, 816.

78 Carr-Saunders to Blacker, letter d. 17 Feb. 1932, Eugen. Soc. Papers C56.

79 Blacker to Carr-Saunders, letter d. 23 Feb. 1932, Eugen. Soc. Papers C56.

80 Hogben, *Genetic Principles* (1931), n. 57, 213.

81 Idem, 210.

82 Lancelot Hogben, *Nature and Nurture: being the William Withering Memorial Lectures on the Method of Clinical Genetics, Delivered at the Faculty of Medicine of the University of Birmingham, 1933* (London: Williams, 1933), 9–33: 91–121.

83 A contemporary account of these experiments is given in E.V. McCollum, Elsa Orent-Keiles and H.G. Day, *The Newer Knowledge of Nutrition* (New York: Macmillan, 4th ed., 1929), 15–30.

84 Lancelot Hogben, 'The limits of applicability of correlation technique in human genetics', *J. Genet.* 27 (1933): 379–406; the relationship between class and height was re-investigated by Mary N. Karn, beginning in 1934; see for example her 'Comparison of the mean physique in the schools of the three suburban boroughs, and of the variance of physique within the schools', *Ann. Eugen.* 7 (1936): 226–39. She states, 'It is assumed these differences are due to a great extent to differences in nutrition and until this factor is diminished or removed it is not possible to say what are the genetic differences of social or occupational groups.'

85 J.L. Gray and Pearl Moshinsky, 'Ability and opportunity in English education', *Social Rev.* 27 (1935): 113–62.

86 A.S. Russell, 'Ability and educational opportunity', *The Listener* (2 Oct. 1935), 554.

87 For example, he gave the 'William Withering Memorial Lectures' to the University of Birmingham for 1933 on 'The method of medical genetics', later published as *Nature and Nurture* (1933), n. 82. It is dedicated to J.B.S. Haldane.

88 Hogben to Beveridge, letter d. 9 June 1931, telling him that the Medical Research Council had agreed to set up a Committee to organise research in human genetics, LSE Archives, File no. 312 A (1931). The MRC Committee on Human Genetics was set up in 1932. Its members were J.B.S. Haldane, Chairman; Julia Bell; E.A. Cockayne; R.A. Fisher; L. Hogben; L.S. Penrose and J.A. Fraser Roberts. The Secretary was J.A. Thomson (later Sir Arthur Landsborough Thomson). Reports on the work of the Committee are to be found in Great Britain, Medical Research Council, *Reports*.

89 L.T. Hogben, R.L. Worrall and I. Zieve, 'The genetic basis of alcaptonuria', *Proc. Roy. Soc.*(Edinburgh) 52 (1932): 264–95.

90 David Slome, 'The genetic basis of amaurotic family idiocy', *J. Genet.* 25 (1931): 363–78. L. Hogben, 'Factorial analysis of small families', *J. Genet.* 26 (1932): 75–9.

91 L.T. Hogben and R. Pollack, 'A contribution to the relation of the gene loci involved in the iso-agglutinin reaction, taste blindness and major brachydactyly of man', *J. Genet.* 31 (1935): 353–61. The expense accounts are in the files in the LSE Archives. The trips were funded by the Medical Research Council's Committee. Fisher later claimed that using a more efficient scoring system, he could show that one of Hogben's twelve families did strongly favour linkage: Hogben had found it but missed it. See R.A. Fisher, 'Heterogeneity of linkage data for Friedreich's ataxia and the spontaneous antigens', *Ann. Eugen.* 7 (1936–37): 17–21.

92 I. Zieve, A.S. Wiener and J.H. Fries, 'On the linkage relations of the genes of allergic disease and the genes determining blood groups, MN groups and eye colour in man', *Ann. Eugen.* 7 (1936): 163–78; A.S. Wiener, I. Zieve, and J.H. Fries, 'The inheritance of allergic disease', *Ann. Eugen.* 7 (1936): 141–62. As in the case of Friedreich's families, D.J. Finney, a statistician from Rothamsted Experimental Station, analysed these papers again a few years later and suggested that there might be a linkage in the data: see D.J. Finney, 'The detection of linkage', *Ann. Eugen.* 10 (1940): 171–214.

93 There is a very large number bio/ergo-graphical memoirs on J.B.S. Haldane. One of the most interesting and useful is the *New York Times* (1 Dec. 1964), 1 and 45. Others include: N.W. Pirie, 'John Burdon Sanderson Haldane' *Biographical Memoirs of Fellows of Roy. Soc.* (London) 12 (1966): 212–49; C.A.B. Smith, 'Professor J.B.S. Haldane', *Ass. Scientific Workers J.* 2 (1965): 3–4; [L.S. Penrose], *Brit. Med. J.* ii (1964): 1536; L.S. Penrose, 'Presidential Address: the Influence of the English Tradition in Human Genetics', *Proc. III Intl. Congr. Human Genetics*, Chicago, 5–10 Sept. 1966 (Baltimore, MD: Johns Hopkins, 1967), 13–25; R. Wurmser, 'Haldane as I knew him', in K.R. Dronamraju, ed., *Haldane and Modern Biology* (Baltimore, MD: Johns Hopkins, 1968), 313–17. Historians who have discussed his Marxism and eugenics include: P. Gary Wersky, *The Visible College* (1978), n. 15; Diane Paul, 'Eugenics and the left', *J. Hist. Ideas* 45 (1984): 567–90; R.W. Clark, 'Haldane, John Burdon Sanderson', in C.C. Gillespie, ed., *Dictionary of Scientific Biography* (New York: Charles Scribner's Sons, 1972).

94 Naomi Mitchison, 'Beginnings', in Dronamraju, *Haldane and Modern Biology* (1968), n. 88, 299–305.

95 Eugenics Education Society, *Sixth Annual Report* (1913–14), 51.

96 J.B.S. Haldane, 'What I think about', in Haldane, *The Inequality of Man and Other Essays* (London: Chatto, 1932), 225–30, 229.

97 Haldane, 'The inequality of man', in *Inequality of Man* (1932), n. 96, 12–26, 16.

98 Charlotte Franken Haldane, (Mrs J.B.S.), *Truth will Out* (London: Vanguard, 1951).

99 Erwin Baur, Eugen Fischer and Fritz Lenz, *Human Heredity*, translated by Eden and Cedar Paul from *Grundriss der menschliche Erblichkeitsforschung* (3rd ed.,1927) (London: Allen, 1931).

100 Eden and Cedar Paul, *Population and Birth Control: a Symposium* (New York, NY: Critic and Guide, 1917), 121–46; cited by Diane Paul, 'Eugenics and the left', *J. Hist. Ideas* 45 (1984): 567–90.

101 Haldane, 'My philosophy of life', a talk broadcast in Nov. 1929, *Inequality of Man* (1932), n. 96, 211–24, 220.

102 On this dialogue see the work of William B. Provine, 'The role of mathematical models in the evolutionary synthesis of the 1930s and 1940s', *Stud. Hist. Biol.* 2 (1978): 167–92; Provine, *The Origins of Theoretical Population Genetics* (Chicago, IL: University Press, 1971).

103 J.B.S. Haldane, *The Causes of Evolution* (1932) (Ithaca, NY: Cornell University Press, 1966), 98–9; 179–82; 184.

104 Ernst Mayr, 'Where are we?' *Cold Spring Harbor Symposia on Quantitative Biology* 24 (1959): 1–14; and Mayr, 'Prologue: Some thoughts on the history of the evolutionary synthesis', in Ernst Mayr and William B. Provine, *The Evolutionary Synthesis: Perspectives on the Unification of Biology* (Cambridge, MA: Harvard University Press, 1980), 1–48. Haldane's reply to this pejoration is in J.B.S. Haldane, 'A defense of bean-bag genetics', *Persp. Biol. & Med.* 7 (1964): 343–59.

105 J.B.S. Haldane and A.E. Gairdner, 'A case of balanced lethal factors in *Antirrhinum majus*', *J. Genet.* 21 (1929): 315–25; J.B.S. Haldane and D. DeWinton, 'The genetics of *Primula sinensis*, II. Segregation and interaction of factors in the diploid', *J. Genet.* 27 (1933): 1–44; Haldane's course of lectures were published as J.B.S. Haldane, *Enzymes* (London: Longmans, 1930). He also wrote a number of papers on the statistics of enzyme action.

106 J.B.S. Haldane, *The Chemistry of the Individual* (Oxford: University Press, 1936), 17.

107 Haldane, *Chemistry of the Individual* (1936), n. 103, 6.

108 J.B.S. Haldane, *Human Biology and Politics*, Tenth Annual Norman Lockyer Lecture to the British Science Guild (London: British Science Guild, 1935). See Chapter V for the 'social problem group', a phrase introduced by the *Wood Report* of 1929.

109 J.B.S. Haldane, *Heredity and Politics* (New York, NY: Norton, 1938), 136–7.

110 Hogben, *Living Matter* (1930), n. 12, 207–8.

111 J.B.S. Haldane, 'A method for investigating recessive characters in man', *J. Genet.* 25 (1932): 251–5; for Haldane's account of this chain of thought, see Haldane, *New Paths in Human Genetics* (London: Allen, 1941), 158–9.

112 J.B.S. Haldane, 'A provisional map of a human chromosome', *Nature* 137 (1936): 398–400; Haldane, 'A search for incomplete sex-linkage in man', *Ann. Eugen.* 7 (1936): 28–57.

113 Haldane, *Heredity and Politics* (1938), n. 109, 91.
114 Idem, 95.
115 Reviews of Haldane, *New Paths in Human Genetics* (London: Allen, 1941), n. 108: C.H. Waddington, 'The expansion of genetics', *New Statesman and Nation* 23, n.s. (1942): 246; *Times Lit Suppl.* (27 Jan. 1942), 28.
116 Great Britain, Interdepartmental Committee on Physical Deterioration, *Report* (London: HMSO, 1904), Cmd 2175, 2210, 2186 (*Fitzroy Report*).
117 Sir George Newman, *The Building of a Nation's Health* (London: Macmillan, 1939), 322–59.
118 Leslie J. Harris, 'The discovery of vitamins', in J. Needham, ed., *The Chemistry of Life: Lectures on the History of Biochemistry* (Cambridge: University Press, 1971), 156–70; C. Petty, 'The MRC's interwar dietary surveys', *Soc. Social Hist. Med. Bull.* (London) 37 (1985): 76–8.
119 Newman, *Nation's Health* (1939), n. 117, 337–8, 357; see also, Sir John Boyd Orr, *As I Recall* (New York, NY: Doubleday, 1967), 114–22.
120 Great Britain, Medical Research Council, *Vitamins: a Survey of Present Knowledge* (1932), No. 167 in series, Special Reports; see also Special Reports, Nos. 187, 213, 218 for contemporary views of nutrition and dietetics.
121 Sir John Boyd Orr, *Food Health and Income: Report on a Survey of Adequacy of Diet in Relation to Income* (London: Macmillan, 1936), 38.
122 John R. Marrack, 'A national food policy', *Labour Monthly* 20 (1938): 502–7; F. LeGros Clark, 'Food prices and poverty', *Labour Monthly* 20 (1938): 231–6.
123 *Final Report of the League of Nations on the Relation of Nutrition to Health, Agriculture and Economic Policy* (Geneva, 1938) (*Astar Report*), cited in Newman, *Nation's Health* (1939), n. 114, 358; Boyd Orr, *As I Recall* (1967), n. 119, 118–20.
124 Mary N. Karn, 'Comparison of mean physique' (1936), n. 84.
125 Haldane, *Heredity and Politics* (1938), n. 109, 93.
126 I owe the clarification of this point to discussion with Gordon McOuat, and to his unpublished essay, 'Was Haldane a eugenist?' (in preparation), in which he discusses the evidence brought forward by Diane Paul, 'Eugenics and the left' (1984), n. 100.
127 Haldane, *Heredity and Politics* (1938), n. 109, 135; see also, J. Needham, 'The nature of biological order' (1936) in Needham, *Order and Life* (Cambridge, MA: MIT Press, 1968), 6–48, 45.
128 Paul, 'Eugenics amd the left' (1984), n. 100.
129 Lancelot Hogben, *Mathematics for the Million: a Popular Self-Educator*, No. 1 in series, Primers for an Age of Plenty (London: Allen, 1st imp. Sept. 1936; 2nd imp. Oct. 1936; 4th ed., 1967); Lancelot Hogben, *Science for the Citizen*, No. 2 in series, Primers for an Age of Plenty (London: Allen, 1938). Two further books were planned as Primers: F. Bodmer, *The Loom of Language: a Guide to*

Foreign Languages for the Home Student (London: Allen, 1943), and H. Hamilton, *History of the Homeland* (London: Allen, 1947).

130 J.G. Crowther, *British Scientists of the Nineteenth Century* (London: Kegan Paul, 1935), see ix, for Crowther's acknowledgement of Hessen; Hogben cited Crowther's treatment of Joule and the quantification of work; J. Desmond Bernal, *The Social Function of Science* (London: Macmillan, 1939).

131 Boris Hessen, 'The social and economic roots of Newton's *Principia*', in Wersky, ed., *Science at the Crossroads* (1931/1971), n. 46.

132 Lancelot Hogben, 'Our social heritage', *Science and Society* 1 (1936): 137–51.

133 Lancelot Hogben, 'Marxism and the middle class', an address to the Midlands Conference of the Workers' Education Association, March 1939, in Hogben, *Lancelot Hogben's Dangerous Thoughts* (London: Allen, 1939), 194–208, 199.

134 Lancelot Hogben, 'The creed of a scientific humanist', in *Hogben's Dangerous Thoughts* (1939), n. 133, 13–24, 17.

135 Lancelot Hogben, *Author in Transit* (New York, NY: Norton, 1940), 270–7.

136 Hogben, *Author in Transit* (1940), n. 135, 270.

137 T.H. Huxley, 'Autobiography' (1889), in Gavin de Beer, ed. *Charles Darwin, Thomas Henry Huxley: Autobiographies* (London: Oxford University Press, 1974), 109. Part of this passage is cited by P. Gary Werskey, 'Haldane and Huxley: the first appraisals', *J. Hist. Biol.* 4 (1971): 171–83.

138 J.B.S. Haldane, 'Science and ethics', a Conway Memorial Lecture, delivered on 18 April 1928, published separately and also reprinted in J.B.S. Haldane, *Science and Human Life* (New York, NY: Harper, 1933), 98–119.

139 J.B.S. Haldane, 'Science in western civilization', a lecture to the Fabian Society, 25 Oct. 1928 in *Science and Human Life* (1933), n. 138, 120–41, 126–7.

5 HUMAN GENETICS AND THE EUGENICS PROBLEMATIC

1 See the geneticists' manifesto, 'Social biology and population improvement', *Nature* (16 Sept. 1939), 521–2, signed by, among others, F.A.E. Crew, J.B.S. Haldane, L.T. Hogben, and J.S. Huxley. L.S. Penrose did not sign.

2 Great Britain, Parliamentary Papers, *Report of the Mental Deficiency Committee* being a Joint Committee of the Board of Education and the Board of Control (*Wood Report*) (London: HMSO, 1929).

3 See Chapter 1, nn. 55–60.

4 On the Board of Control (sc., of Pauper Lunatics) and its history, see Great Britain, Parliamentary Papers, *Report of the Royal Commission on Lunacy and Mental Disorder* presented to Parliament ... (London: HMSO, 1926) Cmd 2700 (*Macmillan Report*), Section 1,

No. 9, Historical Note; Section 2, No. 12, Outline of Present System; see also *Percy Report* (1957) n. 149, 109–200. The Lunacy Commission was set up in 1845 to supervise public and private care of lunatics; it was separate from the Poor Law Board. In 1871, the Local Government Board took over the functions of the Poor Law Board, and assumed responsibility for public health, but not for lunatics. In 1919, the Local Government Board was replaced by the Ministry of Health, which took over some of the administration of the Lunacy and Mental Deficiency Acts. Pauper lunatics, however, remained under the Board of Control, which succeeded the Lunacy Commission in 1913.

5 *Wood Report* (1929), n. 2, Section 4, 136–7.

6 See Chapter 2, n. 72, Fig. 2.4.

7 The Central Association for Mental Welfare 'came out officially' against sterilisation in 1923: see *Mental Welfare* (previously *Studies in Mental Inefficiency*) 3 (1923). It maintained this position until 1934: see *Ann. Rep. CAMW* (1934–35), 21. The social problem group and the sterilisation campaign are discussed by Greta Jones, *Social Hygiene in Twentieth Century Britain* (London: Croom Helm, 1986), 88–112.

8 Great Britain, Parliamentary Papers, Ministry of Health: *Report of the Departmental Committee on the Casual Poor* Cmd 3640 (London: HMSO, 1930) (*Phelps Report*) 71.

9 British Medical Association, 'Report of Mental Deficiency Committee', *Brit. Med. J.* i (1932) Supplement, 25 June, 322–44.

10 F. Douglas Turner, 'Mental deficiency: the Presidential Address at the 92nd Annual Meeting of the Royal Medico-Psychological Association, Colchester, July 1933', *J. Mental Sci.* 79 (1933): 563–77.

11 Lord Brackenbury, 'Sterilisation of the unfit', *Brit. Med. J.* i (1933): Supplement, 11 Feb., 42–3.

12 K.B. Aikman, C.P. Blacker, R.A. Gibbons, Lord Horder of Ashford, and J.A. Ryle, 'Sterilisation of mental defectives', Letter to the Editor, *Brit. Med. J.* i (1933): 483; the signatories were all members of the Society's Committee for Legalising Eugenic Sterilisation, set up in 1930; they were also all physicians.

13 Charles P. Blacker, 'Voluntary sterilisation: the last sixty years. Introduction and summary', *Eugen. Rev.* 53 (1961–62): 145–7; Blacker, 'Voluntary sterilisation: the last sixty years', idem, 54 (1962): 9–23; Blacker, 'Voluntary sterilisation: transitions throughout the world', idem, 54 (1962–63): 143–62. These papers were reprinted by the Society under the title *Voluntary Sterilisation*, with an Appendix by the Legal Correspondent of the *Brit. Med. J.* and was reprinted from *Brit. Med. J.* ii (1960), Nov. 19; also Editorial, 'The sterilisation proposals; a history of their development', *Eugen. Rev.* 22 (1930): 239–47.

14 The Committee for Legalizing Sterilization, *Eugenic Sterilization* (London: Eugenics Society, 1930).

15 Ernst Rüdin, 'Einige Wege und Ziele der Familienforschung, mit Rücksicht auf die Psychiatrie', *Z. f. die ges. Neurol. u. Psychiatrie* 7

(1911): 487–585; Rüdin, *Studien über Vererbung und Entstehung geistiger Störungen, I. Zur Vererbung und Neuentstehung der* Dementia praecox, No. 12 in series, Monographien aus dem Gesamtgebiete der Neurologie und Psychiatrie (Berlin: Springer, 1916).

16 Gregory Zilboorg with George W. Henry, *A History of Medical Psychology* (New York, NY: Norton, 1941) 450–9; Emil Kraepelin, *Dementia praecox and Paraphrenia*, translated by R. Mary Barclay and edited by G.M. Robertson, from his *Clinical Psychiatry*, 3 v, 8th German ed. (1916) (Edinburgh: Livingstone, 1919).

17 Walther Spielmeyer, 'Die Eröffnung des Neubaues der Deutschen Forschungsanstalt für Psychiatrie (Kaiser Wilhelm Institut) in München', *Z.f. die ges. Neurol. u. Psychiatrie* 113 (1928): 117–84.

18 Ernst Rüdin, 'Praktische Ergebnisse der psychiatrischen Erblichkeitsforschung', *Arch. f. Rassen-u. Gesellsch. biol.* 24 (1930): 228–37; Rüdin, 'Empirische Erbprognose', idem, 27 (1933): 271–83; see also Pauline M.H. Mazumdar, 'Two models for human genetics: blood grouping and psychiatry in Germany between the wars' (in preparation).

19 The Committee for Legalizing Sterilization, *The Elimination of Mental Defect* by R.A. Fisher (London: Eugenics Society, n.d.). Reprint with update of R.A. Fisher, 'The elimination of mental defect', *Eugen. Rev.* 16 (1924–25): 114–16. The work by Goddard referred to by Fisher and in *Eugenic Sterilization* (1930), n. 14, is H.H. Goddard, *Feeble-Mindedness* (New York, NY: Macmillan, 1914), 440–1.

20 Hodson to Rüdin, letter d. 24 July 1930, Eugen. Soc. Papers, C300. The American work may have been 'largely discounted in this country' because of the attack on it by Karl Pearson and his group in 1914; see Chapter 2, n. 45.

21 Ernst Rüdin, 'Psychiatrische Indikation zur Sterilisierung', *Das kommende Geschlecht* 5 (1929): 1–19; the Society had this paper translated and published as a pamphlet. Eugen. Soc. Papers, C300.

22 Great Britain, Board of Control, Committee on Sterilisation, *Report* (*Brock Report*) Cmd 4485 (London: HMSO, 1934), 21 paragraph 7; 23–6 paragraph 38ff.

23 Blacker to Rüdin, letter d. 11 Nov. 1932, Eugen. Soc. Papers C301. A copy of the Society's brief is in Eugen. Soc. Papers A108.

24 Rüdin to Blacker, letter d. 18 Nov. 1932, Eugen. Soc. Papers C301.

25 Rüdin, 'Empirische Erbprognose' (1933), n. 18.

26 Blacker to Rüdin, letter d. 6 Feb. 1933, Eugen. Soc. Papers C301.

27 *Brock Report* (1934), n. 22, 122–5, 'Law for the Prevention of Hereditary Disease in Posterity, 14 July 1933'. The provisions are listed in full in the *Report*; Section XII provides for involuntary sterilisation. The law came into force on 1 Jan. 1934.

28 On the significance of this legislation under Nazism, see Ernst Rüdin, ed., *Erblehre und Rassenhygiene im volkischen Staat* (Munich: Lehmann, 1934); Kurt Nowak, *'Euthanasie' und Sterilisierung im 'Dritten Reich': die Konfrontation der evangelischen und katholischen Kirche mit dem 'Gesetz zur Verhütungerbkranken Nachwuchses'*, und

der Euthanasie'-Aktion (Göttingen: Vandenhoek, 1984); Götz Aly, ed., *Totgeschwiegen 1933–1945: Die Geschichte der Karl-Bonhoeffer-Nervenklinik,* Arbeitsgruppe zur Erforschung der Geschichte der Karl-Bonhoeffer-Nervenklinik (Berlin: Hentrich, 1988).

29 Rüdin, 'Psychiatrische Indikation' (1929), n. 21.
30 Blacker to Fisher, letter d. 9 Nov. 1932, Eugen. Soc. Papers, C107.
31 Ernst Rüdin, 'Veröffentlichungen aus der genealogischen Abteilung', typed bibliography of 153 items plus Nos. 154–73 from outside the *Genealogische Abteilung*; Eugen. Soc. Papers, C301.
32 Blacker to Carl Brugger, letter d. 25 April 1933, regarding his 'Genealogischen Untersuchungen an Schwachsinnigen' *Z.f.d. gesamte Neurol. u. Psychiatrie* 130 (1930): 66–103. Similar letter to Werner Pleger, 24 April 1933, regarding his 'Erblichkeitsuntersuchungen an schwachsinnigen Kindern', *Z.f.d. ges. Neurol. u. Psychiatrie* 135 (1931): 225–52. Eugen. Soc. Papers, C301.
33 Charles P. Blacker, 'Memorandum regarding foreign investigations into mental deficiency', *Brock Report* (1934), n. 22, Appendix IX, 131–4.
34 R.A. Fisher, 'Report of an enquiry into children of mental defectives', *Brock Report* (1934), n. 22, Chapter 3, 60–74.
35 Correspondence between Fisher and Blacker shows Fisher looking for British work similar to Rüdin's: Blacker to Fisher, letter d. 9 Nov. 1932; 'I take it you approve of my writing to Popenoe and to Rüdin. I am inclined to think that the Bristol authority to whom you refer is Professor Berry. To my knowledge he has not instituted researches comparable to those of Rüdin', Eugen. Soc. Papers C107.
36 Charles P. Blacker, 'Voluntary sterilisation: the last sixty years' (1962), n. 13.
37 Blacker to Brock, letter d. 25 May 1936, Eugen. Soc. Papers D50.
38 Idem.
39 George Gibson, 'Sterilisation of the unfit', *Report of Proceedings at the 66th Annual Trades Union Congress ... Sept. 3–7, 1934* (London: Cooperative Printing Society, 1934), 399–400; Jones, *Social Hygiene* (1986), n. 7; Jones uses Gibson's remark as a chapter-head, but does not appear to discuss its implications directly.
40 T. O'Brien, *Trades Union Congress* (1934), n. 39, 400.
41 Fisher to Blacker, letter d. 20 April 1951, Eugen. Soc. Papers, C108.
42 Joint Committee on Voluntary Sterilisation, Lecturer's Reports, 1935–39, Eugen. Soc. Papers, D245.
43 Letitia Fairfield, *The Case against Sterilisation* (London: Catholic Truth Society, 2nd ed., 1935); see also her *Catholics and the German Law of Sterilisation* (London: Catholic Medical Guardian, 1938); my thanks to Dr William E. Seidelman for obtaining copies of these pamphlets for me from the Wiener Library, University of Tel Aviv.
44 For an excellent account of the Catholic position on eugenics, see Hervé Blais, *Les Tendances Eugénistes au Canada* (Montreal: L'Institut Familial, 1942), 133–41.
45 Idem, 150–1.
46 Blacker to Brock, letter d. 25 May 1936, Eugen.Soc. Papers, D50.

47 Charles P. Blacker, ed., *The Chances of Morbid Inheritance* (London: Lewis, 1934).
48 The original statement of this idea was by J. Langdon Down, 'Ethnic classification of idiots', *Clinical Lectures and Reports, London Hospital* 3 (1866):259–62; see obituary for 'Reginald Langdon Down (1866–1955)', *Eugen. Rev.* 47 (1955–56): 149(n).
49 Sir Humphrey Rolleston, 'Eugenics and medicine', in Blacker, *Morbid Inheritance* (1934), n. 47, ix–xi.
50 Aubrey Lewis, 'Inheritance of mental disorders', in Blacker, *Morbid Inheritance* (1934), n. 47, 86–133.
51 Lancelot Hogben, 'The analysis of pedigrees', in Blacker, *Morbid Inheritance* (1934), n. 47, 405–27.
52 Fisher to Blacker, letter d. 8 March 1933, Eugen. Soc. Papers, SA/108.
53 Blacker to Fisher, letter d. 9 March 1933, Eugen. Soc. Papers, SA/108.
54 Lancelot Hogben, *Nature and Nurture, being the William Withering Memorial Lectures on the Methods of Clinical Genetics, delivered at the Faculty of Medicine of the University of Birmingham, 1933* (London: Williams, 1933).
55 R.A. Fisher, review of Hogben, *Genetic Principles in Medicine and Social Science* (London: Williams, 1931), in *Health and Empire* 7 (1932): 147–50.
56 Harry Harris, 'Development of Penrose's ideas in genetics and psychiatry', *Brit. J. Psych.* 125 (1974): 529–36; Harris, 'Lionel Sharples Penrose 1898–1972', *Biog. Mems. of Fellows of Roy. Soc.* (London) 19 (1973): 521–61; Daniel J. Kevles, *In the Name of Eugenics: Genetics and the Uses of Human Heredity* (New York, NY: Knopf, 1985), 148–63; Alexander Shapiro, 'A biographical note', *Brit. J. Psych.* 125 (1974): 517–20.
57 E.O. Lewis, 'Investigation into the incidence of mental deficiency in six areas, 1925–27', *Wood Report* (1929), n. 2, *Part IV*, 44–138; *Part II*, 78–102.
58 Great Britain, Committee of the Privy Council for Medical Research, *Report(s) of Medical Research Council for the Year(s) 1930–31*, to *1938–39* (London: HMSO, 1932–40). Penrose's project is defined in *Report* (1930–31), 89. Subsequent years comment on its progress until the final account was published in 1938: *Report* (1936–37), 25–7.
59 Central Association for Mental Welfare, *Conference on Mental Welfare* (1931–32), Afternoon Session, 137–66: R. Langdon-Down and C.P. Blacker spoke for sterilisation, A.F. Tredgold (146–52), F. Shrubsall, Lord Brackenbury and F.D. Turner spoke against; Blacker regarded the session as a political arrangement by the CAMW designed to give the well-known *contras* the last word: see Blacker to Fisher, letter d. 15 June 1932, Eugen. Soc. Papers, C107.
60 Charles P. Blacker, *A Social Problem Group?* (Oxford: University Press, 1937).
61 Blacker to Penrose, letter d. 1 Oct. 1931, Penrose Papers, 130/9,

includes prospectus of the study; *Eugenics Society Annual Report* (1936–37), 8; the sections offered to Penrose were later to be contributed by A.A.E. Newth and Eliot Slater.

62 Penrose to Blacker, letter d. 2 Oct. 1931, Penrose Papers, 130/9.

63 L.S. Penrose and F. Douglas Turner, 'An investigation into the position in family of mental defectives', *J. Ment. Sci.* 77 (1931): 512–24.

64 Lancelot Hogben, 'The genetic analysis of familial traits I: Single gene substitutions', *J. Genet.* 25 (1931): 97–112; Hogben, 'The genetic analysis of familial traits II: Double gene substitutions with special reference to hereditary dwarfism', *J. Genet.* 25 (1931): 211–39.

65 L.S. Penrose, *The Influence of Heredity on Disease*, Buckston Browne Prize Essay, 1933 (London: Lewis, 1934), 10.

66 Penrose, *Influence of Heredity* (1934), n. 65, 10–15.

67 Idem, 71.

68 Idem, 60.

69 Harris, 'Penrose' (1974), n. 56, 521, 549; Kevles, *In the Name of Eugenics* (1985), n. 56, 151–6; 397–8 (sources).

70 G.P. Wells, 'Lancelot Hogben', *Biographical Memoirs of Fellows of Roy. Soc.* (London) 24 (1978): 183–221.

71 Fenner Brockway, *Inside the Left: Thirty Years of Platform, Press, Prison and Parliament* (London: Allen, 1942), 47.

72 Idem, 53.

73 Horace G. Alexander, *The Growth of the Peace Testimony of the Society of Friends* (1939) (London: Quaker Peace and Service, 1982).

74 John Rae, *Conscience and Politics: the British Government and the Conscientious Objector to Military Service 1916–1919* (London: Oxford University Press, 1970), 72–93.

75 John O. Greenwood, *Quaker Encounters*, vol. I: *Friends and Relief* (York: Sessions, 1975), 182–90; Meaburn Tatham and James E. Miles, *The Friends' Ambulance Unit 1914–1919: a Record* (London: Swarthmore, 1919), 133–65, on the trains.

76 Greenwood, *Friends and Relief* (1975), n. 75, 183–4.

77 Thomas C. Kennedy, *The Hound of Conscience: a History of the No-Conscription Fellowship 1914–1919* (Fayetteville, AR: University of Arkansas Press, 1981), 45–50.

78 Thomas C. Kennedy, 'Fighting about peace: the No-Conscription Fellowship and the British Friends' Service Committee 1915–1919', *Quaker Hist.* 69 (1980): 3–22.

79 Brockway, *Inside the Left* (1942), n. 71, 67.

80 Lancelot Hogben, File at Friends House, London.

81 L.S. Penrose, 'Mental deficiency II; the subcultural group', *Eugen. Rev.* 24 (1933): 289–91.

82 L.S. Penrose, *Mental Defect*, in series, Textbooks of Social Biology, edited by Lancelot Hogben (London: Sidgwick, 1933), 76, 77, 80.

83 Harris, 'Penrose' (1974), n. 56; Penrose had gone up to Cambridge ten years behind the Fisher–Hogben generation, and had read mathematics and psychology. As a postgraduate, he had gone to

Vienna where he had contact with Sigmund Freud and psycho-analysis; his interest in abnormal psychology led him back to Cambridge to read medicine.

84 Penrose, *Mental Defect* (1933), n. 82, 57–8.
85 Idem, 64–5.
86 Idem, 146. E.J. Lidbetter had linked his pauper pedigrees with the *Wood Report*'s social problem group by titling his book *The Social Problem Group*; and see his 'The social problem group as illustrated by a series of East London pedigrees', *Eugen. Rev.* 24 (1932): 7–12.
87 Great Britain, Medical Research Council, Special Report Series No. 229: *A Clinical and Genetic Study of 1280 Cases of Mental Defect* by Lionel S. Penrose (London: HMSO, 1938) [*Colchester Survey*].
88 *Colchester Survey* (1938), n. 87, Preface, i.
89 Idem, 70.
90 Idem.
91 L.S. Penrose, 'Eugenic prognosis with respect to mental deficiency', *Eugen. Rev.* 31 (1939): 35–7. In the *Colchester Survey* he cites Brugger's 'Genealogische Untersuchungen an Schwachsinnigen' (1930), n. 32, though not Luxenburger's paper of 1936 to which he refers here.
92 *Brock Report* (1934), n. 22, 60–74; Appendix IX, 131–4.
93 Joint Committee on Voluntary Sterilisation: Lecturer's Report from Colchester Rotary Club, d. 30 Oct. 1934: 'Discussion stifled by presence of three eminent medical men, Dr Penrose, Dr Turner and Dr Turnbull – who simply laid down the law. ... No resolution was submitted' Eugen. Soc. Papers, D245.
94 *Wood Report* (1929), n. 2, 133–7; E.O. Lewis, 'Types of mental deficiency and their social significance', *J. Mental Sci.* 79 (1933): 298–304.
95 L.S. Penrose, 'Mental deficiency II: the subcultural group', *Eugen. Rev.* 24 (1933): 289–91; he is referring to R.A. Fisher, *The Correlation between Relatives on the Supposition of Mendelian Inheritance* (1918), P.A. Moran and C.A.B. Smith, eds, Eugenics Laboratory Memoirs No. 41 (Cambridge: University Press, 1966).
96 L.S. Penrose, 'On the interaction of heredity and environment in the study of human genetics (with special reference to mongolian imbecility)', *J. Genet.* 25 (1932): 407–22; Penrose, 'The relative effects of paternal and maternal age in mongolism', idem, 27 (1933): 219–24; Penrose, 'A method of separating the relative aetiological effects of birth order and maternal age in mongolism', *Proc. Roy. Soc.* (London) B 115 (1934): 431–50; Penrose, 'A method of separating the relative aetiological effects of birth order and maternal age, with special reference to mongolian imbecility', *Ann. Eugen.* 6 (1934): 108–22.
97 L.S. Penrose, 'The inheritance of phenylpyruvic amentia (phenyl-ketonuria)', *Lancet* ii (1935): 192–4.
98 M. Gunther and L.S. Penrose, 'The genetics of epiloia', *J. Genet.* 31 (1935): 413–30.
99 L.S. Penrose and J.B.S. Haldane, 'Mutation rates in man', *Nature*

135 (1935): 907–8; Penrose, 'Autosomal mutation and modification in man with special reference to mental defect', *Ann. Eugen.* 7 (1936): 1–16.

100 L.S. Penrose, 'The detection of autosomal linkage in data which consist of pairs of brothers and sisters of unspecified parentage', *Ann. Eugen.* 6 (1935): 133–8.

101 L.S. Penrose, 'The blood grouping of mongolian imbeciles', *Lancet* i (1932): 394–5; Margaret Penrose and L.S. Penrose, 'The blood group distribution in the eastern counties of England', *Brit. J. Exper. Path.* 14 (1933): 160–1.

102 J.L. Gray, review of E.J. Lidbetter, *The Social Problem Group*, v. 1 (London: Arnold, 1933), in *Sociol. Rev.* 27 (1935): 236–7.

103 For the Galton–Darwin family see Karl Pearson, *Life, Letters and Labours of Francis Galton* (Cambridge: University Press, 1914), v. 1, 5–61 and pedigree plates A–E in pocket of cover; and also the Frontispiece of this book.

104 Leonard Huxley, *Life and Letters of Thomas Henry Huxley* 2 v (New York, NY: Appleton, 1900), v. 1, 391.

105 Julian Huxley to J.R. Baker, letters d. 5 and 15 Nov. 1940, replying to Baker's invitation to join the Society for Freedom in Science, an anti-Marxist organisation promoting individualism and decrying teamwork in science. Huxley appears to be both for and against both Marxist and the Society's ideals; for Fisher's response to the same invitation, see n. 130.

106 Naomi Mitchison, 'Beginnings', in K.R. Dronamraju, ed., *Haldane and Modern Biology* (Baltimore: Johns Hopkins Press, 1968), 299–305; (302).

107 Eugenics Education Society, *Sixth Ann. Rep.* (1913–14), 50–1, Oxford Branch list of members.

108 J.B.S. Haldane, *Heredity and Politics* (London: Allen, 1938), 126.

109 Lancelot Hogben, 'The experimental analysis of sex – a review', *Eugen. Rev.* 15 (1923–24): 316–29.

110 R.W. Clarke, 'Haldane, John Burdon Sanderson', in C.C. Gillespie, ed., *Dictionary of Scientific Biography* (New York, NY: Scribner's, 1972), v. 6.

111 J.B.S. Haldane, 'Methods for the detection of autosomal linkage in man', *Ann. Eugen.* 6 (1934): 26–65.

112 R.A. Fisher, 'The amount of information supplied by families as a function of linkage in the population sampled', *Ann. Eugen.* 6 (1934): 66–70.

113 R.A. Fisher, 'The detection of linkage with dominant abnormalities', *Ann. Eugen.* 6 (1935): 187–210; Fisher, 'The detection of linkage with recessive abnormalities', *Ann. Eugen.* 6 (1935): 339–51.

114 J.B.S. Haldane, 'A search for incomplete sex linkage in man', *Ann. Eugen.* 7 (1936): 28–57.

115 R.A. Fisher, 'Tests of significance applied to Haldane's data on partial sex linkage', *Ann. Eugen.* 7 (1936): 87–104.

116 Great Britain, Committee of the Priry Council for Medical Research, *Report* (1934–35), 32–4 (*MRC Report*).

117 The change of emphasis first appears in the Rockefeller Foundation's *Annual Report* (1932), 203–12. The fellowships were maintained for a short time by the Medical Research Council, and then restored by the Rockefeller Foundation. See *MRC Report* (1935–36), n. 112, 149 and *MRC Report* (1936–37), n. 116, 171.

118 *MRC Report* (1936–37), n. 113, 171.

119 *MRC Report* (1933–34), n. 113, 12–16, 12.

120 For the terms of the Mental Deficiency Act (1913), their relation to the recommendations of the Royal Commission and the powers of the Board of Control, see R.A. Leach, *The Mental Deficiency Act as amended, etc., with introduction and annotations* . . . R.W. Leach, ed. of 3rd ed. (London: Poor Law Publications, 1924), esp. 33–8.

121 L.S. Penrose, *Mental Defect* (1933), n. 82, 79.

122 W.H. Beveridge, memorandum d. 16 July 1935, 'Origin of social biology in the School of Economics', LSE Archives, 213 E (1935).

123 Rockefeller Foundation, *Annual Report* (1934), n. 117, 77.

124 Penrose, *Mental Defect*, (1933), n. 82, 79–96.

125 Tisdale to Weaver, letter d. 17 Nov. 1934, Rockefeller Archives, 401 A.

126 Fisher to O'Brien, memorandum d. 18 July 1934, 'Research in human genetics', Rockefeller Archives, 401 A.

127 O'Brien to Alan Gregg, memorandum d. 1 March 1935, 'Genetic study of mental defectives through serological approach at Galton Laboratory, University College London', Rockefeller Archives, 401 A.

128 'Resolution RF 35057' d. 17 April 1935, Rockefeller Archives, 401 A.

129 R.A. Fisher, 'Eugenics, academic and practical', *Eugen. Rev.* 27 (1935–36): 95–100; Joan Fisher Box, *R.A. Fisher: the Life of a Scientist* (New York, NY: Wiley, 1978), 344–51.

130 Fisher, 'Eugenics, academic and practical' (1935–36), n. 126, 97.

131 *Brock Report* (1934), n. 22, 26–7.

132 Lancelot Hogben, *Genetic Principles in Medicine and Social Science* (London: Williams, 1931), 89–90.

133 Fisher to J.R. Baker, letter d. 4 Nov. 1940, explaining his reasons for *not* joining the proposed Society for Freedom in Science, an anti-Marxist group which also emphasised individualism and decried teamwork in science; for Julian Huxley's more ambivalent response to the same proposal, see above, n. 105.

134 Robert R. Race, ms notebook on Huntington's chorea families, d. 1938, in the possession of Ruth Sanger (Mrs R.R. Race).

135 A.F. Tredgold, *Mental Deficiency (Amentia)* (London: Ballière, 1908).

136 L. Minski and E. Guttmann, 'Huntington's chorea: a study of thirty-four families', *J. Mental Sci.* 84 (1938): 21–76; Race's own reprint of this paper is marked to show the families he was following up.

137 Race, ms notebook (1938), n. 134.

138 R.R. Race, 'On the inheritance and linkage relations of acholuric jaundice', *Ann. Eugen.* 11 (1942): 365–84.

139 Race, 'Linkage relations of acholuric jaundice.' (1942), n. 138, 366, referring to M. Gänsslen, E. Zipperlen and E. Schütz, 'Die haemolytische Konstitution', *Deutsche Arch. klin. Med.* 146 (1925): 1–46; M. Gänsslen, 'Der haemolytische Ikterus und die haemolytische Konstitution', *Klin. Wschr.* 6(i) (1927): 929–33.

140 For R.A. Fisher's treatment of this method see 'Tests of ... independence and homogeneity', in his *Statistical Methods for Research Workers* (1926) (New York, NY: Hafner, 14th ed, 1970), 85–99.

141 R.A. Fisher, 'Detection of linkage with dominant abnormalities', *Ann. Eugen.* 6 (1935): 187–201.

142 D.J. Finney, 'The detection of linkage I, II, III', *Ann. Eugen.* 10 (1940): 171–214; 11 (1941): 10–30, 115–35; Finney has said that 'The ideas for the whole series of papers' were put before him by Fisher, though the detailed algebra was his own'; see Box, *Fisher* (1978), n. 129, 272.

143 Great Britain, Medical Research Council, *Medical Research in War: Report of the Medical Research Council for the years 1939–1945* Cmd 7335 (London: HMSO, 1947), 183–7; 188–95.

144 Lionel S. Penrose, 'The Galton Laboratory: its work and its aims', *Eugen. Rev.* 41 (1949): 17–27.

145 Lionel S. Penrose, 'Report on the Galton Laboratory, Department of Eugenics, Biometry and Genetics (1945–1946)', Penrose Papers, 159; Penrose, 'Syllabus of proposed course of lectures on human genetics', n.d., Penrose Papers, 53/3.

146 Sir Bernard Mallet, 'The social problem group: the President's account of the Society's next task', *Eugen. Rev.* 23 (1931–32): 203–6; Mallet had become the Society's president in 1929, succeeding Major Leonard Darwin.

147 Idem, 206.

148 Charles P. Blacker, ed., *A Social Problem Group?* (1937) n. 60, Introduction, 6.

149 Eliot Slater, 'Mental disorder and the social problem group', in Blacker, ed., *Social Problem Group?* (1937), n. 60, 37–49.

150 David Caradog Jones, ed., *The Social Survey of Merseyside*, 3 v (Liverpool: University Press, 1934) v. 3, last 8 chapters deal with subnormal types in the population, and their localisation, fertility and heredity; Alexander Carr-Saunders and David Caradog Jones, *Social Structure of England and Wales* (Oxford University Press, 1937), on the increase in numbers of defectives, pp. 202–3.

151 David Caradog Jones, 'Mental deficiency on Merseyside: its connection with the social problem group', *Eugen. Rev.* 24 (1932–33): 97–105; Jones, 'Differential class fertility: a further report of the Merseyside Social Survey', *Eugen. Rev.* 24 (1932–33) 175–90; Jones, 'Eugenic aspects of the Merseyside Survey', *Eugen. Rev.* 28 (1936–37): 103–13.

152 Report of the Committee appointed to consider the Eugenic Aspect of Poor Law Reform. 'Section I. The eugenic principle in

Poor Law administration', *Eugen. Rev.* 2 (1910–11): 167–77; cited in Chapter 2, n. 51.

153 Great Britain, Parliamentary Papers, Committee on Social Insurance and Allied Services, *Report* by Sir William Beveridge, 2 v Cmd 6404 and 6405 (London, HMSO, 1942) (*Beveridge Report*) v. 1, 6, No. 8.

154 Great Britain, Parliamentary Papers, *Royal Commission on the Law Relating to Mental Illness and Mental Deficiency (1954–1957)* 2 v. Cmd 167 (London: HMSO, 1957) (*Percy Report*) v 1, 199–200, No. 585. The later part of the nineteenth century saw the beginning of a tendency to set up various special services, such as those for the blind and for mothers and children, outside the Poor Law. The Local Government Act of 1929 encouraged local authorities to use these powers rather than those of the Poor Law, thus taking a step towards breaking up the Poor Law. During the thirties, there was a growth of hospital and health-related services outside the framework of the Poor Law, but the Board of Control continued to be responsible for lunatics and the mentally defective.

155 See Anthony Giddens, *The Class Structure of Advanced Societies* (London: Hutchinson, 1981) 53–68; T.B. Bottomore, *Sociology as Social Criticism* (London: Allen, 1975), 19–28.

156 Richard M. Titmuss, *The Irresponsible Society*, No. 323 in series, Fabian Tracts (London: The Fabian Society, 1959), 3.

157 Problem Families Committee, 'Problem Families: Proposed Pilot Inquiries', ms d. Nov. 1947. Eugen. Soc. Papers, D 167.

158 Charles P. Blacker and R.C. Wofinden, *Social Problem Families: Two Contributions*, reprinted June 1948 from *Eugen. Rev.* 38 (1946–47): 127; these constituted preliminary statements; Wofinden, *Problem Families in Bristol*, No. 6 in series, Occasional Papers in Eugenics (London: Eugenics Society and Cassell, 1950).

159 Wofinden, *Problem Families* (1950), n. 158, 12.

160 Lewis to Blacker, letter d. 1 Feb. 1952. Eugen. Soc. Papers D 171.

161 *Percy Report* (1957), n. 154, v. 1, 202.

162 Idem, v. 2, Evidence, 1349.

163 [Editor], 'Notes of the Quarter', *Eugen. Rev.* 25 (1933): 6; the Burdon Trust was set up by Mrs R.G. Burdon in 1933 to support research on 'familial genetical and national aspects of mental disease'. R.J.A. Berry, who had been instrumental in securing this benefaction, was Chairman of the Research Committee that administered the Trust.

164 *Percy Report* (1957), n. 154, v. 2, Evidence, 610–11.

165 Lionel S.Penrose, 'From eugenics to human genetics', lunch-hour lecture, d. 4 March ?1963, Penrose Papers, 77/2.

166 N. O'Connor, 'The prevalence of mental defect', in Ann M. Clarke and Alan D.B. Clarke, *Mental Deficiency: the Changing Outlook* (London: Methuen, 1958, 2nd ed., 1965), 23–43.

167 Lionel S. Penrose, 'The supposed threat of declining intelligence', *Am. J. Ment. Deficiency* 53 (1948): 114–18; Penrose, 'Genetical influences on the intelligence level of the population', paper

read to the British Association for the Advancement of Science, Newcastle, 1949. *Brit. J. Psychol.* 40 (1950): 128–36.

168 Lionel S. Penrose, 'Eugenics', lecture to the British Medical Association, ms d. 24 Oct. 1962, Penrose Papers, 77/2.

169 Harris explains that Karl Pearson was the first Galton Professor, with two laboratories, Biometrics and Eugenics. When he retired in 1933, Fisher was appointed to the Galton Chair, with the Eugenics laboratory alone; Pearson's son Egon took over the Statistics Chair. From 1935,Haldane had a separate Chair of Biometry, and when Fisher resigned in 1943, Haldane succeeded him, and the two chairs were again combined into a Department of Eugenics and Biometry. Penrose was appointed in 1945 to Fisher's chair, and when Haldane left for India in 1957, Penrose took over Biometry as well as Eugenics, thus reconstituting the original Pearsonian arrangement; Harris, 'Penrose' (1973), n. 56, 537.

170 Lionel S. Penrose, 'Presidential Address – the influence of the English tradition in human genetics', *Proc. III Intl. Congr. of Human Genetics*, University of Chicago, 5–10 Sept. 1966, Plenary Sessions and Symposia (Baltimore, MD: Johns Hopkins, 1967), 13–25.

171 Charles P. Blacker, 'Foreword', *Eugen. Rev.* 60 (1968): 1.

EPILOGUE AND CONCLUSION

1 Michel Foucault, *L'Archéologie du Savoir* (Paris: Gallimard, 1969), 74, 182.

2 Norman Birnbaum, cited by T.B. Bottomore, *Sociology as Social Criticism* (London: Allen, 1975), 44.

3 Robert R. Race and Ruth Sanger, *Blood Groups in Man* (Oxford: Blackwell, 1st ed. 1950, 6th/last ed. 1975).

4 Sylvia D. Lawler, 'Family studies showing linkage between elliptocytosis and the Rhesus blood group system', *Caryologia*, Supplement 6 (1954): 26–7; Lawler and M. Sandler, 'Data on linkage in man: elliptocytosis and blood groups. III. Family 4', *Ann. Eugen.* 18 (1954): 328–34; J.H. Renwick and Lawler, 'Linkage between the ABO and nail-patella loci,' *Ann. Human Genetics* 19 (1955): 312–31.

5 J.H. Renwick, 'Mapping of human chromosomes', in *Ann. Rev. Genet.* 5 (1971): 81–120 (contains useful bibliography).

6 Victor A. McKusick and Frank H. Ruddle, 'Status of the gene map of the human chromosome', *Science* 196 (1977): 390–405.

7 L.N. Went and W.S. Volkers, 'Genetic linkage', *Advances in Neurology* 23 (1979): 37–42; special issue on Huntington's disease.

8 Ray White and Jean-Marc Lalouel, 'Chromosome mapping with DNA markers', *Scientific American* 258 (1988): 40–8.

9 James F. Gusella, Nancy S. Wexler *et al.*, 'A polymorphic DNA marker genetically linked to Huntington's disease', *Nature* 306 (1983): 234–8; Congress of the United States, Office of Technology Assessment (OTA), *Mapping our Genes. Genome Projects: How Big, How Fast?* (Baltimore, MD: Johns Hopkins University Press, 1988), 134–6 (Box 7–A. The Venezuelan Pedigree Project).

10 Victor A. McKusick, 'The morbid anatomy of the human genome: a review of gene mapping and clinical medicine', *Medicine* 65 (1986): 1–33; OTA, *Mapping our Genes*, (1988), n. 9, 28–44.
11 David Botstein, Ray L. White, M. Skolnick *et al.*, 'Construction of a genetic linkage map using restriction fragment length polymorphisms', *Am. J. Human Genetics* 32 (1980): 314–31.
12 White and Lalouel, 'Chromosome mapping', (1988), n. 8, 40–8.
13 Victor A. McKusick, Testimony and prepared statement, 'Medical applications of mapping and sequencing the human genome (human genomics)', US Congress, OTA, *Report on the Human Genome Project: Hearing before the Subcommittee on Oversight and Investigations of the Committee on Energy and Commerce*, House of Representatives, 100th Congress, Serial No. 100–123 (Washington, DC: US Government Printing Office, 1988), 55–66 (58).
14 OTA, *Mapping our Genes* (1988), n. 9, 146.
15 James B. Wyngaarden, Director of the National Institutes of Health, testimony and prepared statement, in OTA Report on the Human Genome Project, *Hearing* (1988), n. 13, 81–103 (86).
16 Bruce M. Alberts, Chairman, National Research Council Committee on Mapping and Sequencing the Human Genome, testimony and prepared statement, in OTA Report on the Human Genome Project, *Hearing* (1988), n. 13, 3–16 (11).
17 OTA, *Mapping our Genes* (1988), n. 9, 139–59; Peter Newmark, 'Mapping and sequencing the human genome in Europe', OTA, *Mapping our Genes. Federal Genome Projects: How Vast – How Fast?* Contractor Reports, Order No. PB88–162805 (Springfield, VA: US Department of Commerce, National Technical Information Service, 1988) v. 2, 1–56.
18 John Maddox, 'Brenner homes in on the human genome', *Nature* 326 (1987): 119.
19 OTA, *Mapping our Genes* (1988), n. 9, 136–9.
20 Dorothy Nelkin and Laurence Tancredi, *Dangerous Diagnostics: the Social Power of Biological Information* (New York, NY: Basic Books, 1989), 11–13.
21 Nelkin and Tancredi, *Dangerous Diagnostics* (1989), n. 20, 75.
22 Stephanie Yanchinski, 'Genetic screening: employees under a microscope', Toronto *Globe and Mail* (3 Feb. 3 1990), D1; 3.
23 Robin Maranz Henig, 'Body and mind: high-tech fortune-telling', *New York Times Magazine* (24 Dec. 1989), 20–2.
24 Leon Jaroff, with J. Madeleine Nash and Dick Thompson, 'The gene hunt', and Philip Elmer-Dewitt, with Andrea Dorfman and J. Madeleine Nash, 'The perils of treading on heredity', *Time* (20 March 1989), 54–61; 62–3; my thanks to Ms Chantelle Ung, of the University of Toronto, for bringing this article to my attention.
25 Lori Andrews, 'The gene prophets', American *Vogue* (Jan. 1990), 198–9; 241.
26 David Dickson, 'Genome project gets rough ride in Europe', *Science* 243 (2 Feb. 1989), 599.
27 Commission of the European Communities, *Predictive Medicine:*

Human Genome Analysis (1989–1991), COM Documents: COM/88/ 424 – C2-119/88.

28 For an outline of the parties in the European Parliament, see Directorate-General for Research, *Forging Ahead: European Parliament 1952–1988: 36 Years* (Luxembourg: Office of Official Publications of the European Communities, 1989), 5.4.2; for an indication of where they stand in terms of left and right, see *European Community News*, No. 26/89 for 1 Aug. 1989, 3; this displays the membership spectrum after the 1989 election.

29 Benedikt Härlin, 'Predictive Medicine: Human Genome Analysis (1989–1991): Report drawn up on behalf of the Committee on Energy, Research and Technology, on the proposal from the Commission to the Council (COM/88/424 – C2–119/88) for a decision adopting a specific research programme in the field of health', European Communities, European Parliament, *Session Documents* Series A, Document A2–0370/88 SYN 146.

30 Härlin, *Report*, n. 29, 23–4.

31 Härlin, (ARC) rapporteur, Debate on genome analysis, *Official Journal of the European Communities*, No. 2–374: Debates of the European Parliament, 1988–89 Session: Report of Proceedings 13–17 Feb. 1989, Sitting of Tuesday, 14 Feb. 1989, 2–374/69 – 2–374/ 76 (69).

32 Pandolfi, Vice-President of the Commission, idem, 75.

BIBLIOGRAPHY

ARCHIVAL SOURCES

Eugenics Society, now (1989) The Galton Institute, 19 Northfields Prospect, Northfields, London SW18 1PE.

——, Cambridge University Eugenics Society's Minute Book, (May 1911–May 1913); in the Society's possession.

——, Eugenics Education Society, Council Minute Books, 1907–09, 1909–12; in the Society's possession.

——, Eugenics (Education) Society, Research Minute Books, 1923–25, 1925–31; in the Society's possession.

——, Card index for the use of speakers, in the Society's possession.

——, Library Catalogue, examined at the Society's library, then at 69 Eccleston Square, London SW1V 1PJ, courtesy of Eileen Walters, General Secretary; the library was transferred in 1989 to the Wellcome Institute for the History of Medicine.

——, Eugenics Society Papers, Contemporary Medical Archives Centre, Wellcome Institute for the History of Medicine, 183 Euston Road, London, NW1 2BP; courtesy of Julia Sheppard, Archivist, G.M. Prescott, Assistant Curator, Iconographic Collections, and the Wellcome Trustees.

Fisher Papers, see Galton Chair.

Galton Chair of Human Genetics, papers relating to, University College Records, University College, Gower Street, London, WC1E 6BT.

Hogben, Lancelot, 'An unauthorised autobiography of Lancelot Hogben', edited by Adrian and Anne Hogben, in their possession, c/o Dr Adrian Hogben, RFD No. 1, Box 243, Ellesworth, ME 04605, USA.

Penrose Papers, The Library, University College, Gower Street, London, WC1E 6BT; courtesy of the Librarian, F.J. Friend.

Race, Robert R., ms notebook (1938) in possession of Ruth Sanger (Mrs R.R. Race).

Rockefeller Archives, Rockefeller Archives Center, Hillcrest, Pocantico Hills, North Tarrytown, NY 10591, USA, courtesy of the then Director, Joseph W. Ernst.

Social Biology, Chair of, papers relating to, The Archives, London School of Economics, Houghton Street, London WC2A 2AE.

GOVERNMENT DOCUMENTS

European Communities, Commission of the European Communities, 'Predictive medicine: human genome analysis (1989–1991)', *COM Documents*: COM/88/424 – C2–119/88.

——, European Parliament, Benedikt Härlin, rapporteur, 'Predictive medicine: human genome analysis (1989–91)', Report drawn up on behalf of the Committee on Energy, Research and Technology, on the proposal from the Commission to the Council (COM/88/424 – C2–119/88) for a decision adopting a specific research programme in the field of health', *Session Documents* Series A, Document A2–0370/88 SYN 146.

——, Härlin, (ARC) rapporteur, Debate on genome analysis, *Official Journal of the European Communities*, No. 2–374: Debates of the European Parliament, 1988–89 Session: Report of Proceedings 13–17 Feb., Sitting of Tuesday, 14 Feb. 1989, 2–374/69 – 2–374/76.

——, Directorate-General for Research, *Forging Ahead: European Parliament 1952–1988: 36 Years* (Luxembourg: Office of Official Publications of the European Communities, 1989), 5.4.2.

——, *European Community News* No. 26/89 (1 Aug. 1989)

Great Britain, Poor Law Commissioners, *Report to Her Majesty's Principal Secretary of State from the Poor Law Commissioners, on an Inquiry into the Sanitary Condition of the Labouring Population of Great Britain, with Appendices* (London: HMSO, 1842) (*Chadwick Report*). See also M.W. Flinn, edition with introduction (1965).

——, Commissioners for Inquiring into the State of Large Towns and Populous Districts (Health of Towns Commission), *First Report* (London: HMSO, 1844).

——, Commissioners for Inquiring into the State of Large Towns and Populous Districts (Health of Towns Commission), *Second Report* (London: HMSO, 1845).

——, Royal Commission on the Aged Poor, appointed to consider whether any Alterations in the System of Poor Law Relief are Desirable in the Case of Persons whose Destitution is Occasioned by Incapacity for Work Resulting from Old Age, or whether Assistance could Otherwise be Afforded in these Cases, *Report and Minutes of Evidence* (London: HMSO, 1895).

——, Interdepartmental Committee on Physical Deterioration, *Report* Cmd 2175, 2210, 2186 (London: HMSO, 1904) (*Fitzroy Report*).

——, Royal Commission on the Care and Control of the Feeble-Minded, *Minutes of Evidence and Reports*, Cmd 4215–4221; 4202 (London: HMSO, 1908) (*Bath-Radnor Report*).

——, Royal Commission on the Poor Laws and the Relief of Distress, *Volume I, being Parts I to VI of the Majority Report* Cmd 4499 (London: HMSO, 1909) (*Majority Report*).

——, *The Break Up of the Poor Law, being part 1 of the Minority Report of the Poor Law Commission*, edited with an introduction by Sidney and Beatrice Webb (London: Longmans, 1909) (*Minority Report*).

——, Royal Commission on Venereal Disease, *Reports and Minutes of*

Evidence Cmd 7474, 7475; 8189, 8190 (London: HMSO, 1916) (*Sydenham Report*).

———, Royal Commission on Lunacy and Mental Disorder, Report Cmd 2700 (London: HMSO, 1926) (*Macmillan Report*).

———, Joint Committee of the Board of Education and the Board of Control, *Report of the Mental Deficiency Committee* (London: HMSO, 1929) (*Wood Report*).

———, Ministry of Health, Departmental Committee on the Casual Poor, *Report* Cmd 3640 (London: HMSO, 1930) (*Phelps Report*).

———, Committee of the Privy Council for Medical Research, *Report(s) of the Medical Research Council for the Year(s) 1930–1931 to 1938–1939* (London: HMSO, 1932–40).

———, Medical Research Council, *Vitamins: a Survey of Present Knowledge*, No. 167 in Special Report series (London: HMSO, 1932).

———, Medical Research Council, *A Clinical and Genetic Study of 1280 Cases of Mental Defect* by L.S. Penrose, No. 229 in Special Report series (London: HMSO, 1938) (*Colchester Survey*).

———, Board of Control, Committee on Sterilisation, *Report* Cmd 4485 (London: HMSO, 1934) (*Brock Report*).

———, Committee on Social Insurance and Allied Services, *Report* by Sir William Beveridge, 2 v, Cmd 6404 and 6405 (London: HMSO, 1942) (*Beveridge Report*).

———, Medical Research Council, *Medical Research in War: Report of the Medical Research Council for the Years 1939–1945* Cmd 7335 (London: HMSO, 1947).

———, Royal Commission on the Law Relating to Mental Illness and Mental Deficiency 1954–1957, *Report* Cmd 169 (London: HMSO, 1957) (*Percy Report*).

United States of America, Congress, Office of Technology Assessment, *Mapping our Genes. Federal Genome Projects: How Vast – How Fast?* in series, Contractor Reports, Order No. PB88–162805 (Springfield, VA: US Department of Commerce, National Technical Information Service, 1988) v. 2, 1–56.

———, Congress, Office of Technology Assessment, *Mapping our Genes. Genome Projects: How Big, How Fast?* (Baltimore, MD: Johns Hopkins University Press, 1988).

———, Congress, Office of Technology Assessment, Report on the Human Genome Project, *Hearing before the Subcommittee on Oversight and Investigations of the Committee on Energy and Commerce*, House of Representatives, 100th Congress Serial No. 100–123 (Washington, DC: US Government Printing Office, 1988).

PRIMARY SOURCES

Alexander, Horace G., *The Growth of the Peace Testimony of the Society of Friends* (1939) (London: Quaker Peace and Service, reprinted 1982).

Allaun, F.J., Letter to the Editor, 'Eugenics and capitalism', *Eugen. Rev.* 19 (1927–28): 98.

Andrews, Lori, 'The gene prophets', *Vogue* American Ed., (Jan. 1990) 198–9; 241.

Anon., 'Article I. Meliora', *Meliora, a Quarterly Review of Social Science in its Ethical, Economical and Ameliorative Aspects* 1 (1858): 1–16.

Anon., 'The foundation of the Society for the Study of Inebriety', *Brit. J. Inebriety* 1 (1903): i–iv.

——, 'Origin and work of the Society', Eugenics Education Society, *First Annual Report* (1907–8): 16–18.

——, 'Worst family in the world: interesting and curious exhibition: pedigrees of the great', *Pall Mall Gazette* 29, 29 July 1912.

——, 'The Commission of Inquiry into the National Birth Rate', *The Times*, (13 Oct. 1913).

——, 'Editorial', *Moral Education Q.* 35 (1914): 1.

——, 'Population studies in Edinburgh', *Eugen. Rev.* 18 (1926–27): 227–30.

——, (leading article), 'The dwindling family: a case for enquiry', *The Times* (19 Sept. 1936).

——, (Special Correspondent), 'A menace to the future: I. Britain and Europe', *The Times*, 28 Sept. 1936.

——, (Special Correspondent), 'A menace to the future: II. Planning for population: Germany and Italy', *The Times*, (29 Sept. 1936).

'Ardent Mendelian', 'The present position of the Mendelians and the biometricians', *Mendel J.* 1 (1909): 159–63.

Babak, E. *et al.*, see Winterstein, H. (1910–14).

Bateson, William, *Mendel's Principles of Heredity* (Cambridge: University Press, 1909).

Baur, Erwin, Eugen Fischer and Fritz Lenz, *Grundriss der menschliche Erblichkeitsforschung* 2 v (Munich: Lehmann, 1921) translated 1931 by Eden and Cedar Paul, from the 3rd ed., 1927.

Bell, Julia, see Pearson, K. *et al.* (1912).

Bernal, J. Desmond, *The Social Function of Science* (London: Macmillan, 1939).

Bernstein, Felix, 'Ergebnisse einer biostatistischen zusammenfassenden Betrachtung über die erblichen Blutstrukturen des Menschen', *Klin. Wschr.* 3 (1924): 1495–97; and translated by the F.C. Farnham Co. for F.R. Camp, Jr, F.R. Ellis and C.E. Shields (eds), in series Selected Contributions to the Literature of Blood Groups and Immunology: Dunsford Memorial v. 1 The ABO System (Fort Knox, KY: Blood Transfusion Division, US Army Medical Research Laboratory, 1966), 83–90.

——, 'Zusammenfassenden Betrachtungen über die erblichen Blutstrukturen des Menschen', *Z.f. indukt. Abstammungs- u.Vererbungslehre* 37 (1925): 237–70.

——, 'Über mendelistische Anthropologie', Verhandlungen des V Internationalen Kongresses für Vererbungswissenschaft, Berlin, 1927, 2 v (Leipzig: Bornträger, 1928) v. 1 431–8.

——, 'Über die Ermittlung und Prüfung von Genhypothesen aus Vererbungsbeobachtungen am Menschen und über die Unzulässigkeit der Weinbergschen Geschwistermethode als Korrektur der Auslesewirkung', *Arch. f. Rassen- u. Gesellsch. biol.* 22 (1929): 241–4.

BIBLIOGRAPHY

——, 'Zur Grundlegung der Chromosomentheorie der Vererbung beim Menschen, mit besonderer Berücksichtigung der Blutgruppen', *Z.f. indukt. Abstammungs- u. Vererbungslehre* 57 (1931): 113–38.

[? Blacker, Charles P.], Editorial, 'The sterilisation proposals: a history of their development', *Eugen. Rev.* 22 (1930): 239–47.

Blacker, Charles P., see *Brock Report* (1934), Appendix IX, 131–4.

——, *A Social Problem Group?* (Oxford: University Press, 1937).

——, 'Eugenics in retrospect and prospect (Galton Lecture)', *Eugen. Rev.* 37 (1945–46): 184 (N).

—— and R.C. Wofinden, *Social Problem Families: Two Contributions*, reprinted as a pamphlet (June 1948) from Blacker, 'Social problem families in the limelight', *Eugen. Rev.* 38 (1946–47): 117–27; Wofinden, 'Social problem families', *idem*, 127–32.

——, 'Voluntary sterilisation: the last sixty years. introduction and summary', *Eugen. Rev.* 53 (1961–62): 145–7.

——, 'Voluntary sterilisation: the last sixty years', *Eugen. Rev.* 54 (1962–63): 9–23.

——, 'Voluntary sterilisation: transitions throughout the world', *Eugen. Rev.* 54 (1962–63): 143–62.

——, 'Voluntary sterilisation: its role in human betterment', *Eugen. Rev.* 56 (1964–65): 77–80.

——, *Voluntary Sterilisation* reprints from the *Eugenics Review*, with an Appendix by the Legal Correspondent, *British Medical Journal*, reprinted from *Brit. Med. J.* (19 Nov. 1960) (London: Eugenics Society, 1961).

——, *Eugenics: Galton and After* (London: Duckworth, 1972).

Blais, Hervé, *Les Tendances Eugénistes au Canada* (Montreal: L'Institut Familial, 1942).

Booth, Charles, 'The inhabitants of Tower Hamlets (School Board Division), their conditions and occupations', *J. Roy. Stats. Soc.* 50 (1887): 326–401.

——, *The Aged Poor in England and Wales: Condition* (London: Macmillan, 1894).

——, 'Poor Law statistics', *Econ. J.* 6 (1896): 70–4.

——, *Life and Labour of the People in London* 17 v (London: Macmillan, 1902–3).

Bosanquet, Bernard, ed., *Aspects of the Social Problem by various Writers* (London: Macmillan, 1895).

Bosanquet, Helen, (Mrs Bernard), see Dendy, Helen.

Botstein, David, Ray L. White, M. Skolnick *et al.*, 'Construction of a genetic linkage map using restriction fragment length polymorphisms', *Am. J. Human Genetics* 32 (1980): 314–31.

Brackenbury, Henry, Lord, 'Sterilisation of the unfit', *Brit. Med. J.* i (1933): Supplement, 11 Feb., 42–3.

Bridges, Calvin B., 'The chromosome hypothesis of linkage applied to cases of sweet peas and primula', *American Naturalist* 40 (1914): 524–34.

——, 'Direct proof through non-disjunction that the sex-linked genes of *Drosophila* are borne by the X-chromosome', *Science* 40 (1914): 107–9.

——, see Morgan, T.H., and —— (1920).

British Medical Association, 'Report of the Mental Deficiency Committee', *Brit. Med. J.* i (1932): Supplement, 25 June, 322–44.

British Population Society, aims, members and rules, in *Bulletin of the International Union for the Scientific Investigation of Population Problems* 1 (1930): 23–5.

British Social Hygiene Council, Inc., founded 1925 by amalgamation of National Council for the Prevention of Venereal Disease, and the Society for the Prevention of Venereal Disease (*q.v.*).

——, *Foundations of Social Hygiene* (London: British Social Hygiene Council Inc., 1926).

Brockway, Fenner, *Inside the Left: Thirty Years of Platform, Press, Prison and Parliament* (London: Allen, 1942).

Brugger, Carl, 'Genealogische Untersuchungen an Schwachsinnigen', *Z.f.d. ges. Neurol. u. Psychiatrie* 130 (1930): 66–103.

Bukharin, Nikolai Ivanovich, Boris Hessen, B.M. Zavadovskii *et al.*, *Science at the Crossroads: Papers Presented to the International Congress of the History of Science and Technology, London, 1931, by the Delegates of the USSR*, edited and introduced by Gary Werskey (London: Cass, 1971).

Burt, Sir Cyril, see Hearnshaw, L.S. (1979); Kamin, L.J. (1974); Gillie, O. (1976).

——, 'The inheritance of mental characters', *Eugen. Rev.* 4 (1912–13): 168–200.

——, *Mental and Scholastic Tests: Report by the Education Officer* ... (London: County Council, 1921).

Carpenter, Mary, *Reformatory Schools for the Children of the Perishing and Dangerous Classes, and for Juvenile Offenders* (1851) (Montclair, NJ: Patterson Reprints, 1970).

——, 'Juvenile delinquency in its relation to the educational movement', in A. Hill, ed., *Essays on Educational Subjects* (1857), 320–33.

Carpenter, William B., *Principles of Human Physiology* (Philadelphia, PA: Blanchard, from 4th London ed., 1852).

——, *Principles of Mental Physiology, with their Applications to the Training and Discipline of the Mind and the Study of its Morbid Conditions* (1874) (London: Kegan Paul, 6th ed., 1881).

Carr-Saunders, Alexander M., Major Greenwood, Ernest J. Lidbetter and Alfred F. Tredgold, 'The standardisation of pedigrees: a recommendation', *Eugen. Rev.* 4 (1912–13): 383–90.

—— and P.A. Wilson, *The Professions* (Oxford: University Press, 1933).

——, *World Population* (Oxford: Clarendon, 1936).

—— and David Caradog Jones, *A Survey of the Social Structure of England and Wales, as Illustrated by Statistics* (Oxford: Clarendon, 2nd ed., 1937).

Cattell, Raymond B., 'Is national intelligence declining?' *Eugen. Rev.* 28 (1936): 181–203.

Chatterton-Hill, Georges, *The Philosophy of Nietzsche: an Exposition and an Appreciation* (London: Ousely, 1912); for review, see Lindsay, J.A. (1913).

Clark, F. LeGros, 'Food prices and poverty', *Labour Monthly* 20 (1938): 231–6.

Clarke, Ann M., and Alan D.B. Clarke, eds, *Mental Deficiency: the Changing Outlook* (London: Methuen, 1st ed., 1958, 2nd ed., 1965).

Clarke, R.W., 'Haldane, John Burdon Sanderson', in C.C. Gillespie, ed., *Dictionary of Scientific Biography* (New York, NY: Scribner's, 1972).

Coit, Stanton, Report of a talk, 'Moral education', Eugenics Education Society, *First Annual Report* (1907–8): 17.

Collins, S. Hare, *Chemical Fertilizers and Parasiticides* (London: Ballière, 1920).

[Crackanthorpe, Montague] 'Presidential address, 5 May 1910', Eugenics Education Society, *Second Annual Report* (1909–10): 1–16.

Crew, Frank A.E., *Animal Genetics: the Science of Animal Breeding*, in series Biological Monographs and Manuals, edited by F.A.E. Crew and D. Ward Cutler (Edinburgh: Oliver, 1925).

——, and E. Moore, 'Outline of problems to be investigated by Commission II, on differential fertility, fecundity and sterility', *Bulletin of the International Union for the Scientific Investigation of Population Problems* 1 (1930): 17–22.

Crowther, J.G., *British Scientists of the Nineteenth Century* (London: Kegan Paul, 1935).

——, *Fifty Years of Science* (London: Barrie, 1970).

Cutler, D. Ward, *Evolution, Heredity and Variation* (London: Christopher, 1925).

Darwin, Leonard, Major, 'First steps towards eugenic reform', *Eugen. Rev.* 4 (1912–13): 26–38; lecture, Cambridge University, 8 Feb. 1912, under the auspices of Cambridge University Eugenics Society; reported in *Cambridge Daily News*, 12 Feb. 1912.

——, *Quality not Quantity* (London: The Eugenics Education Society, n.d.) reprinted from *Eugen. Rev.* 8 (1916–17): 297–321.

——, 'Memorandum on the evidence proposed to be given before the Royal Commission on Income Tax', *Eugen. Rev.* 11 (1919–20): 213–18.

——, 'The aims and methods of eugenics societies', *Eugenics and the Family: Scientific Papers Presented at the Second International Eugenics Congress, New York, 1922* (Baltimore, MD: Williams, 1923), 5–19.

——, 'Letter to the Chancellor of the Exchequer [from the President of the Eugenics Society]', Pamphlet d. Jan. 1927, reprinted from *Eugen. Rev.* 19 (1927–28): 96–7.

——, Introduction to E.J. Lidbetter, *Heredity and the Social Problem Group* v. 1 (London: Arnold, 1933).

——, 'E.J. Lidbetter, 1878–1962', *Eugen. Rev.* 54 (1962–63): 191.

Davenport, Charles, see Heron, D. (1913); Rosenberg, C. (1976); Allen, G.E. (1986); Kimmelman, B. (1983).

——, *Heredity in Relation to Eugenics* (New York, NY: Holt, 1911).

Dendy, Helen, 'The industrial residuum', in Bosanquet, B., ed. (1895) 82–102.

Dickson, David, 'Genome project gets rough ride in Europe', *Science* 243 (2 Feb. 1989): 599.

Diem, Otto, Exhibit C16, 'Distribution of particular taints in every hundred of tainted members among nearest relations, &c.', First

327

International Eugenics Exhibition, *Catalogue of the Exhibition* (London: Knight, 1912).

——, 'Die psychoneurotische erbliche Belastung der Geistegesunden und Geisteskranken: eine statische-kritische Untersuchung auf Grund eigener Beobachtungen', *Arch. f. Rassen- u. Gesellsch. biol.* 2 (1905): 215–52; 336–68.

Dobell, Clifford, *Anthony van Leeuwenhoek and his Little Animals* (London: Ball, 1932).

—— and F.W. O'Connor, *Intestinal Protozoa of Man* (London: Ball, 1921).

Doncaster, L., 'Sex limited inheritance', read to Cambridge University Eugenics Society, 14 Feb. 1912; report in Cambridge Minute Book.

Down, J. Langdon, 'Ethnic classification of idiots', *Clinical Lectures and Reports, London Hospital* 3 (1866): 259–62.

Down, Reginald Langdon, see obituary, 'Reginald Langdon Down, 1866–1955', *Eugen. Rev.* 47 (1947–48): 149 (N).

Elderton, Ethel M., A. Barrington, H.G. Jones, E.M. de G. Lamotte, Harold J. Laski and Karl Pearson, *On the Correlation of Fertility with Social Value: a Cooperative Study Series*. Eugenics Laboratory Memoirs XVIII (London: Dulau, 1913).

——, *Report on the English Birth Rate, Part I* (London: Dulau, 1914).

Elmer-Dewitt, Philip, 'The perils of treading on heredity', *Time* (20 March 1989) 62–3.

Engels, Friedrich, *The Condition of the Working Class in England* (1845) translated by W.O. Henderson and W.H. Chaloner (Stanford, CA: Stanford University Press, 1968).

Eugenics Congress, First International, *Problems in Eugenics: Papers Communicated to the First International Eugenics Congress, &c., London, 1912* (London: Knight, 1912).

——, First International, *Catalogue of the Exhibition* (London: Knight, 1912).

——, Second International, *Eugenics and the Family: Scientific Papers Presented at the Second International Eugenics Congress, &c., New York, 1921* (Baltimore, MD: Williams, 1923).

——, Second International, *The Second International Exhibition of Eugenics, &c., New York 1932* (Baltimore, MD: Williams, 1923).

——, Third International, *A Decade of Progress in Eugenics: Scientific Papers of the Third International Congress of Eugenics, &c., New York, 1932* (Baltimore, MD: Williams, 1934).

Eugenics Society, since 1989 known as Galton Institute.

Eugenics (Education) Society, *Annual Reports*, 1907–89.

——, Poor Law Committee, 'Report of the Committee appointed to Consider Poor Law Reform, Section I. "The eugenic principle in Poor Law administration", *Eugen. Rev.* 2 (1910–11): 167–77.

——, *Record and Programme 1908–1914* n.d., n.p.

——, *Outline of a Practical Eugenic Policy, approved by the Council of the Eugenics Education Society* (London: Eugenics Education Society, n.d.).

——, Committee for Legalising Eugenic Sterilisation (1930–34), see also Joint Committee on Voluntary Sterilisation (1934–).

——, Committee for Legalising Eugenic Sterilisation, *Eugenic Sterilisation* (London: The Eugenics Society, 1930).

——, Committee for Legalising Eugenic Sterilisation, (physician members of), 'Sterilisation of mental defectives', Letter to the Editor, *Brit. Med. J.* i (1933): 18 March 483.

——, Committee for Legalising Sterilisation, *The Elimination of Mental Defect* by R.A. Fisher (London: Eugenics Society, n.d.); reprint with update of Fisher, 'Elimination of mental defect,' *Eugen. Rev.* 16 (1924–25): 114–16.

—— and Central Association for Mental Welfare, Mental Hospitals Association and National Council for Mental Hygiene, forming the Joint Committee on Voluntary Sterilisation, *Eugen. Rev.* 26 (1934–35): 100; 178; 251.

——, ——, —— and ——, Joint Committee on Voluntary Sterilisation, Activities of, *Eugen. Rev.* 26 (1936–37): 61; 291.

——, 'The aims and objects of the Eugenics Society', Eugenics Society, *Annual Report* (1936–37).

Falk, S., see Jordan, E.O. and ——, eds (1928).

Fairfield, Letitia, *The Case against Sterilisation* (London: Catholic Truth Society, 2nd ed., 1935).

——, *Catholics and the German Law of Sterilisation* (London: Catholic Medical Guardian, 1938).

Finney, D.J., 'The detection of linkage, I. II. III'. *Ann. Eugen.* 10 (1940): 171–214; 11 (1941): 10–30, 115–35.

Fisher, Ronald Aylmer, see Joan Fisher Box (1978); Hacking, I. (1988); Norton, B.J., and E.S. Pearson (1976); Yates, F. (1964); Yates, F. and K. Mather (1963).

——, 'Heredity: paper given in Mr C.E. Shelley's rooms on Friday November 10, 1911', in Norton, B.J. and E.S. Pearson (1976).

——, 'Some hopes of a eugenist', *Eugen. Rev.* 5 (1913–14): 309–15; read at the Second Annual Meeting of the Cambridge University Eugenics Society, 12 Oct. 1913.

—— and C.S. Stock, 'Cuenot on preadaptation', *Eugen. Rev.* 7 (1915–16): 184–92.

——, 'The evolution of sexual preference', *Eugen. Rev.* 7 (1915–16): 184–92.

——, 'Positive eugenics', *Eugen. Rev.* 9 (1917–18): 206–12.

——, 'The correlation between relatives on the supposition of Mendelian inheritance', *Trans. Roy. Soc.* (Edinburgh) 52 (1918): 399–433; reprinted with introduction and commentary by P.A. Moran and C.A.B. Smith, No. 41 in series, Eugenics Laboratory Memoirs (Cambridge: University Press, 1966).

——, 'Studies in crop variation, I. An examination of the yield of dressed grain from Broadbalk', *J. Agric. Sci.* 11 (1921): 107–35.

—— and W.A. Mackenzie, 'Studies in crop variation, II. The manurial response of different potato varieties', *J. Agric. Sci.* 13 (1923): 311–20.

——, 'The elimination of mental defect', *Eugen. Rev.* 16 (1924–25): 114–16; reprinted as a pamphlet by the Eugenics Society, Committee for Legalising Sterilisation.

——, 'The biometrical study of heredity', two lectures given at the London School of Economics, 6 and 11 June 1924, *Eugen. Rev.* 16 (1924–25): 198–210.

——, *Statistical Methods for Research Workers* (London: Oliver, 1925).

——, 'The arrangement of field experiments', *J. Min. Ag.* (1926): 503–13.

——, see Eden, T. and R.A. Fisher (1929).

——, 'Family allowances in the contemporary economic situation', *Eugen. Rev.* 24 (1932–33): 87–95, reprinted in *Eugen. Rev.* 60 (1968): 109–17.

——, 'The amount of information supplied by families as a function of linkage in the population sampled', *Ann. Eugen.* 6 (1934): 66–70.

——, 'Report of an enquiry into children of mental defectives', *Brock Report* (1934), 60–74.

——, 'The detection of linkage with dominant abnormalities', *Ann. Eugen.* 6 (1935): 187–201.

——, 'The detection of linkage with recessive abnormalities', *Ann. Eugen.* 6 (1935): 339–51.

——, *The Design of Experiments* (Edinburgh: Oliver, 1935).

——, 'Eugenics, academic and practical', *Eugen. Rev.* 27 (1935–36): 95–100.

——, 'Tests of significance applied to Haldane's data on partial sex linkage', *Ann. Eugen.* 7 (1936): 87–104.

——, 'Heterogeneity of linkage data for Friedreich's ataxia and the spontaneous antigens', *Ann. Eugen.* 7 (1936–37): 17–21.

——, 'Statistical methods in genetics', Bateson Lecture, 1951 *Heredity* 6 (1952): 1–12.

Fison, Margaret, *Handbook of the National Association for the Promotion of Social Science* (London: Longmans, 1859).

Forel, Auguste-Henri, 'Alkohol und Keimzellen (blastophthorische Entartung)', *Münch. med. Wschr.* 58 (1911): 2596–601.

Galton, Francis, Sir, see Pearson, K. (1914–30); Cowan, R.S. (1969, 1970).

——, 'Hereditary talent and character', *Macmillan's Mag.* 12 (1865): 157–5; 318–27.

——, *Hereditary Genius: an Inquiry into its Laws and Consequences* (London: Macmillan, 1869).

——, *English Men of Science: their Nature and Nurture* (1874) edited and introduced by Ruth Schwarz Cowan (London: Cass, 1970).

——, 'Presidential address', *Transactions of the International Congress of Hygiene and Demography, London August 1891* (London: Ballantyne, 1892), Section on Demography, 7–12.

——, 'Eugenics, its definition, scope and aims', *Sociological Papers* 1 (1904): 43–99.

——, 'Eugenics', *Sociological Papers* 2 (1905): 1–54.

—— and Edgar Schuster, *Noteworthy Families (Modern Science): An Index to Kinships in Near Degrees between Persons whose Achievements are Honorable and have been Publicly Recorded* v. 1 in series, Publications of the Eugenics Record Office of the University of London (London: Murray, 1906).

BIBLIOGRAPHY

——, *Memories of my Life* (London: Methuen, 1908).

——, *Essays in Eugenics* (London: The Eugenics Education Society, 1909).

Gänsslen, M., 'Der haemolytische Ikterus und die haemolytische Konstitution', *Klin. Wschr.* 6 (i) (1927): 929–33.

——, E. Zipperlen and E. Schütz, 'Die haemolytische Konstitution', *Deutsche Arch. klin. Med.* 146 (1925): 1–46.

Garrod, Archibald, *Inborn Errors of Metabolism: the Croonian Lectures* (1909); edited and introduced by Harry Harris, in series, Oxford Monographs on Medical Genetics (London: Oxford University Press, 1963).

Gibson, George, 'Sterilisation of the unfit', *Report of Proceedings at the 66th Annual Trades Union Congress, September 3–7, 1934* (London: Cooperative Printing Society, 1934).

Goddard, H.H., 'The heredity of feeblemindedness', *Bull. Eugen. Record Office* 1 (1911): 1–14.

Gotschlich, Emil, ed., unter Mitwirkung namhafter Fachgelehrter, *Handbuch der hygienische Untersuchungsmethoden*, 3 v (Jena: Fischer, 1926–29)

Gotto, Sybil, see Rolfe, Sybil Neville.

Gray, J.L., review of Lidbetter (1933) in *Sociol. Rev.* 27 (1935): 236–7

—— and Pearl Moshinsky, 'Ability and opportunity in English education', *Sociol. Rev.* 27 (1935): 113–62; and in Hogben, L., ed., (1938), 334–76.

Greenwood, Major, see Carr-Saunders *et al.* (1912–13).

Grotjahn, Alfred, see Kantorovitz, M. (1940).

—— and J. Kaup, eds, *Handwörterbuch der sozialen Hygiene*, 2 v (Leipzig: Vogel, 1912).

——, 'Der Unterricht der Studierenden und der Ärzte', in Gottstein A., A. Schlossman and L. Telecky, eds, *Handbuch der sozialen Hygiene und Gesundheitsfürsorge*, 8 v (Berlin: Springer, 1925), v. 1, 21–47.

——, *Erlebtes und Erstrebtes: Erinnerung eines sozialistischen Ärztes* (Berlin: Herbig, 1932).

Gruber, Max von, and Ernst Rüdin, eds, *Fortpflanzung, Vererbung, Rassenhygiene: Illustrierte Führer durch die Gruppe Rassenhygiene der Internationalen Hygiene-Ausstellung 1911 in Dresden* (Munich: Lehmann, 1911).

——, 'Hygienische Aufgaben der Gegenwart', in R. Eucken and Max von Gruber, *Ethische und hygienische Aufgaben der Gegenwart: Vorträge gehalten den 8 Januar 1916 in der neuen Aula der Berliner Universität* (Berlin: Massigkeits-Verlag der Deutschen Vereins gegen den Missbrauch geistiger Getränke, 1916).

Gunther, M. and Penrose, L.S., 'The genetics of epiloia', *J. Genet.* 31 (1935): 413–30.

Gusella, James F., Nancy S. Wexler *et al.*, 'A polymorphic DNA marker genetically linked to Huntington's disease', *Nature* 306 (1983): 234–8.

Haldane, Charlotte Franken, (Mrs J.B.S.), *Truth will Out* (London: Vanguard, 1951).

Haldane, John Burdon Sanderson, for bio-ergographical materials, see Anon. (1964); Clark, R.W. (1972); Dronamraju, K.R. (1968); Mitchison, N. (1968); Paul, D. (1984); [Penrose, L.S.] (1964); Penrose, L.S. (1966); Pirie, N.W. (1966); Smith, C.A.B. (1965); Wurmser, R. (1968); Wersky, P.G. (1978).

—— and A.E. Gairdner, 'A case of balanced lethal factors in *Antirrhinum majus*', *J. Genet.* 21 (1929): 315–25.

——, *Enzymes* (London: Longmans, 1930).

——, *The Inequality of Man and Other Essays* (London: Chatto, 1932).

——, *The Causes of Evolution* (1932) (Ithaca, NY: Cornell University Press, 1966).

——, 'A method for investigating recessive characters in man', *J. Genet.* 25 (1932): 251–5.

—— and D. DeWinton, 'The genetics of *Primula sinensis*, II. Segregation and interaction of factors in the diploid', *J. Genet.* 27 (1933): 1–44.

——, *Science and Human Life* (New York, NY: Harper, 1933).

——, 'Methods for the detection of autosomal linkage in man', *Ann. Eugen.* 6 (1934): 26–65.

——, *Human Biology and Politics: Tenth Annual Norman Lockyer Lecture to the British Science Guild* (London: British Science Guild, 1935).

——, 'A search for incomplete sex linkage in man', *Ann. Eugen.* 7 (1936): 28–57.

——, 'A provisional map of a human chromosome', *Nature* 137 (1936): 398–400.

——, *The Chemistry of the Individual* (Oxford: University Press, 1936).

——, *Heredity and Politics* (London: Allen, 1938; New York, NY: Norton, 1938).

——, *New Paths in Human Genetics* (London: Allen, 1941); for reviews, see *Times Lit. Suppl.* (27 Jan. 1942) 28; Waddington, C.H., *New Statesman and Nation* 23 n.s. (1942): 246.

——, 'A defense of bean-bag genetics', *Persp. Biol. Med.* 7 (1964) 343–59.

Haldane, Naomi, see Mitchison, Naomi.

Hall, Sir A. Daniel, *The Book of the Rothamsted Experiments* (London: Murray, 1905).

——, *Fertilizers and Manures* (London: Murray, 1909; 2nd ed., 1913; 3rd ed., 1920).

Hall, Stanley, *Adolescence* 2 v (New York, NY: Appleton, 1904).

——, *Youth* (New York, NY: Appleton, 1907).

——, *The Physical and Mental Life of Schoolchildren* (London: Longmans, 1913).

Hardy, G.H., 'Mendelian proportions in a mixed population', *Science* 28 (1908): 49.

Henig, Robin Maranz, 'Body and mind: high-tech fortune-telling', *New York Times Magazine* (24 Dec. 1989) 20–2.

Heron, David, *On the Relation of Fertility in Man to Social Status and on the Changes in this Relation that have taken Place during the Last Fifty Years*,

No. 1 in series, Drapers' Company Research Memoirs: Studies in National Degeneration (London: Dulau, 1906).

———, *Mendelism and the Problem of Mental Defect: a Criticism of Recent American Work*, No. 7 in series, Questions of the Day and of the Fray (London: Dulau, 1913).

Hill, A., ed., *Essays on Educational Subjects, read at the Educational Conference of June 1857, with a Short Account of the Objects and Proceedings of the Meeting* (London: Longmans, 1857).

Hogben, Lancelot T., see Anon. (1975) for obituary; Wersky, G. (1978) 60–7; 101–15.

———, 'Modern heredity and social science', *Socialist Rev.* 16 (1919): 147–56.

———, 'The pigmentary effector system, IV. A further contribution to the role of pituitary secretion in amphibian colour response', *Brit. J. Exper. Biol.* 1 (1923): 249–70.

———, 'The experimental analysis of sex – a review', *Eugen. Rev.* 15 (1923–24): 316–29.

———, *The Pigmentary Effector System*, No. 1 in series, Biological Monographs and Manuals, edited by Frank A.E. Crew and D. Ward Cutler (Edinburgh: Oliver, 1924).

———, *Comparative Physiology*, in series, Textbooks of Animal Biology, edited by Julian S. Huxley (London: Sidgewick, 1926).

———, *Principles of Evolutionary Biology* (Cape Town: Juta, 1927).

———, *Principles of Animal Biology* (London: Christophers, 1930).

———, *The Nature of Living Matter* (London: Kegan Paul, 1930).

———, 'Contemporary philosophy in Soviet Russia', *Psyche* 12 (1931): 2–18.

———, *Genetic Principles in Medicine and Social Science* (London: Williams, 1931); for reviews, see *The Medical Officer* 47 (1932): 59; *Brit. Med. J.* i (1932): 293–4; *The Times*, 1 July 1932; *Times Lit. Suppl.* (7 July 1932): 492; *New Statesman and Nation* (n.s.) 2 (26 Dec. 1931); 816–17; Haldane, J.B.S., *Nature* 129 (5 March 1932): 345–6; Zuckerman, Solly, *Spectator* 148 (13 Feb. 1932): 221.

———, 'The genetic analysis of family traits, I. Single gene substitution; II. Double gene substitution, with especial reference to hereditary dwarfism; III. Mating involving one parent exhibiting a trait determined by a single recessive gene substitution with special reference to sex-linked conditions', *J. Genet.* 25 (1931): 97–112; 211–40; 293–314.

———, R.L. Worrall and I. Zieve, 'The genetic basis of alcaptonuria', *Proc. Roy. Soc.* (Edinburgh) 52 (1932): 264–95.

———, 'Factorial analysis of small families', *J. Genet.* 26 (1932): 75–9.

———, *Nature and Nurture: being the William Withering Memorial Lectures on the Method of Clinical Genetics, Delivered at the Faculty of Medicine of the University of Birmingham, 1933* (London: Williams, 1933).

———, 'The limits of applicability of the correlation technique in human genetics', *J. Genet.* 27 (1933): 379–406.

———, 'The analysis of pedigrees', in Blacker, C.P. (1934), 405–27.

——— and Ray Pollack, 'A contribution to the relation of the gene loci involved in the iso-agglutinin reaction, taste blindness and major brachydactyly of man', *J. Genet.* 31 (1935): 353–61.

——, 'Our social heritage', *Science & Society* 1 (1936): 137–51.

——, *Mathematics for the Million: a Popular Self-Educator*, No. 1 in series, Primers for an Age of Plenty (London: Allen, 1936).

——, *Science for the Citizen: a Self-Educator based on the Social Background of Scientific Discovery*, No. 2 in series, Primers for the Age of Plenty (London: Allen, 1938).

——, *Political Arithmetic: a Symposium of Population Studies* (London: Allen, 1938).

——, *Lancelot Hogben's Dangerous Thoughts* (London: Allen, 1939).

——, *Author in Transit* (New York, NY: Norton, 1940).

——, 'Origins of the Society', in M. Sleigh and J. Sutcliffe, *The Society for Experimental Biology: Origins and History* (Cambridge: Company of Biologists, 1974).

——, 'An unauthorised autobiography of Lionel Hogben', ms. edited by Adrian and Anne Hogben, in their possession.

Huxley, Leonard, *Life and Letters of Thomas Henry Huxley*, 2 v (New York, NY: Appleton, 1900).

Huxley, Thomas Henry, 'Autobiography', (1989) in Gavin de Beer, ed., *Charles Darwin, Thomas Henry Huxley, Autobiographies* (London: Oxford University Press, 1974).

Inebriety, Society for the Study of, see Berridge, Virginia (1984).

——, see Anon., 'Foundation of the Society' (1903).

——, Membership Lists, *Brit. J. Inebriety* 1 (1903): v–xv.

Inge, William R., 'Some moral aspects of eugenics', *Eugen. Rev.* 1 (1909–10): 26–36.

Jaroff, Leon, 'The gene hunt', *Time* (20 March 1989): 54–61.

Jones, David Caradog, see Trend, Rt. Hon. Lord (1984).

——, 'Mental deficiency on Merseyside: its connection with the social problem group', *Eugen. Rev.* 24 (1932–33): 97–105.

——, 'Differential class fertility: a further report of the Merseyside Social Survey', *Eugen. Rev.* 24 (1932–33): 175–90.

——, David Caradog Jones, ed., *The Social Survey of Merseyside* 3 v (Liverpool: University Press, 1934).

——, 'Eugenic aspects of the Merseyside Survey', *Eugen. Rev.* 28 (1936–37): 103–13.

——, Review of Glass, *Struggle for Population* (1936) and Carr-Saunders, *World Population* (1936), 'Eugenics and the decline in population', *Eugen. Rev.* 28 (1936–37): 213–15.

——, see Carr-Saunders, A., and —— (1937).

——, *The Social Problem Group: Poverty and Subnormality of Intelligence* in series English Studies in Criminal Science, from the Department of Criminal Science. Faculty of Law, University of Cambridge, edited by L. Radzinowicz and J.W. Cecil Turner (Toronto: Canadian Bar Association, 1945).

Jones, Robert, Report of talk, 'Mental integrity and how to attain it', *Eugen. Ed. Soc., First Annual Report* (1907–8): 17.

Jordan, Edwin O., and Sidney Falk, *The Newer Knowledge of Bacteriology and Immunology* (Chicago, IL: Chicago University Press, 1928).

Kantorovitz, Myron, 'Alfred Grotjahn as a eugenist', *Eugen. News* 15 (1940): 15–19.

Karn, Mary N., 'Comparison of the mean physique in the schools of the three suburban boroughs, and of the variance of physique within the schools', *Ann. Eugen.* 7 (1936): 226–39.

Kay-Shuttleworth, James, Sir, see Tholfsen, Trygve.

Kidd, F., 'Natural selection and Mendelism', read to Cambridge University Eugenics Society, 13 Feb. 1912; Cambridge Minute Book.

Kraepelin, Emil, *Clinical Psychiatry: a Textbook for Students and Physicians*, abstracted and adapted from 7th German ed. by Ross Diefendorf (New York, NY: Macmillan, 1907). Facsimile with introduction by Eric T. Carlson; see section on *Dementia praecox* and Paraphrenia, from v. 3, part ii.

Landsteiner, Karl, and Philip Levine, 'A new agglutinable factor differentiating human bloods', *Proc. Soc. Exper. Biol. Med* 24 (1926–27): 600–2.

Laughlin, Harry H., see Ludmerer, K. (1972) 90–5.

——, *Eugenical Sterilisation in the United States* (Chicago, IL: Municipal Court, 1922).

——, 'Historical background of the Third International Congress of Eugenics', in Third International Congress of Eugenics, *A Decade of Progress in Eugenics: Scientific Papers of the Third International Congress of Eugenics, &c., New York, 1932* (Baltimore, MD: Wilkins, 1934).

Lawes, Sir John Bennett, and Sir Henry Gilbert, 'On agricultural chemistry', *J. Roy. Agric. Soc.* 8 (1847): 226–60.

—— and ——, 'On agricultural chemistry, especially in relation to the mineral theory of Baron Liebig', *J. Roy. Agric. Soc.* (1851): 1–40.

Lawler, Sylvia D., 'Family studies showing linkage between elliptocytosis and the Rhesus blood group system', *Caryologia*, (Supplement) 6 (1954): 27–7.

—— and M. Sandler, 'Data on linkage in man: elliptocytosis and blood groups. III. Family 4', *Ann. Eugen.* 18 (1954): 328–34.

——, see Renwick, J.H.

Lenz, Fritz, 'Die Bedeutung der statistisch ermittleten Belastung mit Blutverwandschaft der Eltern', *Münch. med. Wschr.* 66 ii (1919): 1340–2; translated in Boyer, S.H. (1963), 16–25.

——, *Menschliche Auslese und Rassenhygiene* v. 2 of Baur, E., E. Fischer and —— (1921).

——, 'Methoden der menschliche Erblichkeitsforschung', in Gotschlich, E., ed. (1929), v.3, 689–739.

Levien, Max, 'Stimmen aus dem deutschen Urwald (Zwei neue Apostel des Rassenhasses)', *Unter dem Banner des Marxismus* 2 (1928): 150–95.

Levine, Philip, see Landsteiner, K. (1926–27).

Lewis, Aubrey, 'The inheritance of mental disorders', in Blacker, C.P. (1934), 86–133.

Lewis, E.O., see *Wood Report* (1929): Part II, 78–102; Part IV, 44–138.

——, 'Types of mental deficiency and their social significance', *J. Mental Sci.* 79 (1933): 298–304

Lidbetter, Ernest J., Obituary, 'E.J. Lidbetter, 1878–1962', *Eugen. Rev.* 54 (1962–63): 191; and see Darwin, L., Introduction to Lidbetter (1933).

——, 'Eugenics and the prevention of destitution: a paper read at the Conference on the Prevention of Destitution', *Eugen. Rev.* 3 (1911–12): 170–3.

——, 'Nature and nurture: a study in conditions', *Eugen. Rev.* 4 (1912–13): 54–73.

——, see Carr-Saunders *et al.* (1912–13).

——, *Heredity and the Social Problem Group* v. 1 (London: Arnold, 1933) [No more appeared.].

——, 'The social problem group as illustrated by a series of East London pedigrees', *Eugen. Rev.* 24 (1932): 7–12.

Lindsay, J.A., review of Chatterton-Hill, G., *The Philosophy of Nietzsche* (1912) in *Eugen. Rev.* 5 (1913–14): 72.

Loch, Charles S., 'Mr Charles Booth on the aged poor', *Econ. J.* 4 (1894): 468–87.

——, 'Some recent investigations as to the number of "poor" in the community', *Fitzroy Report* (1904) 1: 104–11 (Appendix III).

——, 'Eugenics and the Poor Law: the *Majority Report*', *Eugen. Rev.* 2 (1910–11): 229–32.

Lokay, Alfons, 'Über die heriditäre Beziehungen der Imbezillität', *Z. f. d. ges. Neurologie u. Psychiatrie* 122 (1929): 90–143.

Lord, J.R., ed., *Contributions to Psychiatry, Neurology and Sociology, Dedicated to the Late Sir Frederick Mott, K.B.E.* (London: Lewis, 1929); includes biographical articles and bibliography.

Luxenburger, Hans, 'Wilhelm Weinberg', *Allgem. Z. f. Psych. u. ihre Grenzgebiet* 108 (1938): 378–81.

MacBride, Ernest William, see Calman, W.T. (1940) for obituary; Bowler, P.J. (1984).

——, *Zoology: the Study of Animal Life* (London: Jack, 1913).

——, 'Do we inherit our habits?' *Radio Times* (12 Oct. 1923).

——, *An Introduction to the Study of Heredity* (London: Williams, 1924).

——, 'Biological memory, a new theory of life', *Scientia* (Bologna) 38 (1925): 153–64.

McCollum, E.V., Elsa Orent-Keiles and H.G. Day, *The Newer Knowledge of Nutrition* (New York, NY: Macmillan, 4th ed., 1929).

MacKenzie, J.S., 'Moral education and social progress', *Moral Education Q.* 29 (1912): 1–3.

McKusick, Victor A., 'The morbid anatomy of the human genome: a review of gene mapping and clinical medicine', *Medicine* 65 (1986): 1–33.

——, Testimony and prepared statement, 'Medical applications of mapping and sequencing the human genome (human genomics)', U States Congress, Office of Technology Assessment, Report on the Human Genome Project: *Hearing before the Subcommittee on Oversight and Investigations of the Committee on Energy and Commerce*, House of

Representatatives, 100th Congress, Serial No. 100–123 (Washington, DC: US Government Printing Office, 1988), 55–66.

——, and Frank H. Ruddle, 'Status of the gene map of the human chromosome', *Science* 196 (1977): 390–405.

Maddox, John, 'Brenner homes in on the human genome', *Nature* 326 (1987): 119.

Mallet, Sir Bernard, 'The social problem group: the President's account of the Society's next ta̧sk', *Eugen. Rev.* 23 (1931–32): 203–6.

Malthus, Thomas Robert, *An Essay on the Principle of Population, or, a View of its Past and Present Effects on Human Happiness, with an Inquiry into our Prospects Respecting Future Removal of the Evils which it Occasions* (1798) 2 v (London: Johnson, 3rd ed., 1806)

——, *A Letter to Samuel Whitbread, Esq., M.P., on his Proposed Bill for the Amendment of the Poor Laws* (London: Hatchard's, 1807), reprinted in Glass, *Introduction to Malthus* (1953), 183–285.

——, *Summary of the Principle of Population* (London: Murray, 1830) reprinted in Glass, *Introduction to Malthus* (1953), 115–81.

Mannheim, Karl, *Ideologie und Utopie*, in series, Schriften zur Philosophie und Soziologie, K. Mannheim, ed. (Bonn: Lohen, 1929).

Marrack, John R., 'A national food policy', *Labour Monthly* 20 (1938): 502–7.

Martius, Friedrich, 'Die Vererbbarkeit des konstitutionellen Factors bei Tuberculose', *Berl. klin. Wschr.* 38 (1901): 1125–30.

Mayr, Ernst, 'Where are we?' *Cold Spring Harbor Symposia on Quantitative Biology* 24 (1959): 1–14.

Mearns, Andrew, (pseudonym) *The Bitter Cry of Outcast London* (London: Congregational Union, 1883).

Mental Welfare, Central Association for, (CAMW) *Annual Reports* (previously National Association for the Care and Protection of the Feeble-Minded (1896).

——, Central Association for, see Eugenics Society, Joint Committee on Voluntary Sterilisation.

——, Central Association for, *Mental Welfare*, 1 (1920): (previously *Studies in Mental Inefficiency*).

Minski, L., and E. Guttmann, 'Huntington's chorea: a study of thirty-four families', *J. Mental Sci.* 84 (1938): 21–76.

Mitchison, Naomi, 'Beginnings', in Dronamraju, K.R. (1968).

'Moral Education Congress, Close of the', *Manchester Guardian* (30 Sept. 1908).

Moral Education Congress, *Record of Proceedings of the First International, &c., London, 1908* (London: Nutt, 1908).

——, see Muirhead, J.H. (1909); Sadler, M.E. (1909).

Moral Education League, see [Spiller, G.A.], (1914); *Moral Education League Q.* 35 (1914): 1.

Moral Education League Quarterly 1 (1898).

Morgan, Thomas H., and Calvin B. Bridges, *The Third Chromosome Group of the Mutant Characters of* Drosophila melanogaster (Washington, DC: Carnegie Institution, 1920).

Mott, Sir Frederick, see Lord, J.R., ed., (1929) for biography and bibliography.

Mott, Frederick W., 'Heredity and insanity', *Lancet* i (1911): 1251–9.
——, 'Heredity and eugenics in relation to insanity', *Problems in Eugenics: Papers Communicated to the First International Eugenics Congress, &c., London, 1912* (London: Knight, 1912), 400–28.
——, 'Alcohol and insanity', *Brit. J. Inebriety* 9 (1911–12): 5–27.
Mügge, Maximilian, 'Eugenics and the superman: a racial science and a racial religion', *Eugen. Rev.* 1 (1909–10): 184–93.
——, *Friedrich Nietzsche, his Life and Work* (London: Unwin, 1909).
Muirhead, J.H., 'The central problem of the International Congress on Moral Education', *Hibbert J.* 6 (1909): 346–51.
Murphy, Sir Shirley, 'Sanitary science and preventive medicine: presidential address to the Congress of the Royal Sanitary Institute, on "Some points in the decline of birth and death rates"', *J. Roy. Sanitary Inst.* 33 (1912): 345–9.
——, Evidence on effects of overcrowding on infant mortality, *Fitzroy Report* (1904) 3: 50–5 (Appendix XIII).
National Council of Public Morals, see National Birth Rate Commission.
National Birth Rate Commission, *The Declining Birth Rate: its Causes and Effects. Being the Report and Chief Evidence Taken by the National Birth Rate Commission, Instituted with Official Recognition by National Council of Public Morals, for the Promotion of Race Regeneration, Spiritual, Moral and Physical* (London: Chapman, 1916).
National Birth Rate Commission, see Anon., *The Times*, 13 Oct. 1913.
Needham, Joseph, *Time, the Refreshing River: Essays and Addresses* (London: Allen, 1943).
Needham, Joseph, *Order and Life* (Cambridge, MA: Massachussetts Institute of Technology Press, 1968).
——, ed., *The Chemistry of Life: Lectures on the History of Biochemistry* (Cambridge: University Press, 1971).
——, *Moulds of Understanding: a Pattern of Natural Philosophy*, edited by Gary Werskey (London: Unwin, 1976).
Nelkin, Dorothy, and Laurence Tancredi, *Dangerous Diagnostics: the Social Power of Biological Information* (New York, NY: Basic Books, 1989).
Newman, Sir George, *The Building of a Nation's Health* (London: Macmillan, 1939).
Nietzsche, Friedrich, see Mügge, M. (1909); Chatterton-Hill, G. (1912); and review by Lindsay, J.A. (1913); Jaspers, K. (1965); Thatcher, D.S. (1970).
——, *The Case of Wagner*, translated by Thomas Common, introduced by Alexander Tille (London: Henry, 1896).
——, *Thus Spake Zarathustra*, translated by Alexander Tille (1896) (London: Henry, 1908).
O'Brien, T., Speech seconding anti-sterilisation resolution proposed by George Gibson, *Report of Proceedings at the 66th Annual Trades Union Congress, 3–7 September 1934* (London: Cooperative Printing Society, 1934): 400.
O'Connor, Nicholas, 'The prevalence of mental defect', in Clarke, Ann M., and Alan D.B. Clarke, *Mental Deficiency: the Changing Outlook* (London: Methuen, 1958, 2nd ed., 1965).

Orr, Sir John Boyd, *Food, Health and Income: Report on a Survey of Adequacy of Diet in Relation to Income* (London: Macmillan, 1936).

——, *As I Recall* (New York, NY: Doubleday, 1967).

Ottenberg, Reuben, and David Beres, 'The heredity of the blood groups', in Jordan, E.O., and S. Falk, eds (1928), 909–20.

Paul, Eden, and Cedar Paul, *Population and Birth Control: a Symposium* (New York, NY: Critic and Guide, 1917).

—— and ——, translation of Baur, E., E. Fischer and F. Lenz, *Human Heredity*, from 3rd German ed., 1927 (London: Allen, 1931).

Pearson, Karl, see Yule, G.U., and L.N.C. Filon (1936) obituary; Froggatt, P., and N.C. Nevin (1971) a and b; Norton, B.J. (1975, 1978, 1983).

——, 'Contributions on the mathematical theory of evolution', *Phil. Trans., Roy. Soc.* (London), A 185 (1894): 70–110.

——, 'Mathematical contributions to the theory of evolution. On the law of ancestral heredity', *Proc. Roy. Soc.* (London) 62 (1898): 386–412.

——, 'On the inheritance of the mental and moral characters in man and its comparison with the inheritance of physical characters', Huxley Lecture, 1903, *J. Anthropol. Inst. Brit. and Ireland* 33 (1903): 179–237.

——, 'On a generalised theory of alternative inheritance with special reference to Mendel's laws', *Phil. Trans., Roy. Soc.* (London) 203 (1904): 53–86.

——, *On the Theory of Contingency and its Relation to Association and Normal Correlation*, Drapers' Company Research Memoirs, Biometric Series T (London: Dulau, 1904).

——, Letter to the editor, *Brit. Med. J.* ii (1908): 1720; i (1909): 184; 372; 568; 694.

——, 'The law of ancestral heredity', *Biometrika* 2 (1909): 211–36.

——, 'On a new method of determining correlation when one variable is given by alternative and the other by multiple categories', *Biometrika* 7 (1910): 248–57.

——, Preface to Julia Bell, *Treasury of Human Inheritance*, v. 1, name and subject index. No. 16 in series, Eugenics Laboratory Memoirs (London: Dulau, 1912).

——, *A First Study of the Statistics of Pulmonary Tuberculosis (Inheritance)*, No. 2 in series, Studies in National Deterioration. Drapers' Company Research Memoirs (London: Dulau, 1910).

——, see Elderton *et al.* (1913).

——, *On the Handicapping of the First-Born*, No. 10 in Eugenics Lecture series, Galton Laboratory Publications (London: Dulau, 1914).

—— and G.A. Jaederholm, *Mendelism and the Problem of Mental Defect, II. On the Continuity of Mental Defect*, No. 8 in series, Questions of the Day and of the Fray (London: Dulau, 1914).

——, *Mendelism and the Problem of Mental Defect, III. On the Graded Character of Mental Defect and on the Need for Standardising Judgements as to the Grade of Social Inefficiency that shall Involve Segregation*, No. 9 in series, Questions of the Day and of the Fray (London: Dulau, 1914).

——, *Francis Galton: A Centenary Appreciation* (London: Cambridge University Press, 1922).

——, *Life, Letters and Labours of Francis Galton*, 3 v in 4 (Cambridge: University Press, 1914–30).

Peddie, Alexander, 'Dipsomania, a proper subject for legal decision', *Trans. Nat. Assoc. for the Promotion of Social Sci.* (1860): 538–46.

Penrose, Lionel S., see Harris, H. (1973, 1974); Kevles, D.J. (1985), 148–63; Shapiro, A. (1974).

——, and F. Douglas Turner, 'An investigation into the position in family of mental defectives', *J. Mental Sci.* 77 (1931): 512–24.

——, 'On the interaction of heredity and environment in the study of human genetics (with special reference to mongolian imbecility)', *J. Genet.* 25 (1932): 407–22.

——, 'The blood grouping of mongolian imbeciles', *Lancet* i (1932): 394–5.

——, 'The relative effects of paternal and maternal age in mongolism', *J. Genet.* 27 (1933): 219–24.

——, *Mental Defect*, in series, Textbooks of Social Biology, edited by Lancelot Hogben (London: Sidgewick, 1933).

——, 'Mental deficiency, II. The subcultural group', *Eugen. Rev.* 24 (1933): 289–91.

——, see Penrose, M., and —— (1933).

——, *The Influence of Heredity on Disease*, Buckston Browne Prize Essay, 1933 (London: Lewis, 1934).

——, 'A method of separating the relative aetiological effects of birth order and maternal age in mongolism', *Proc. Roy. Soc.* (London), B 115 (1934): 431–50.

——, 'A method of separating the relative aetiological effects of birth order and maternal age, with special reference to mongolian imbecility', *Ann. Eugen.* 6 (1934): 108–22.

——, 'The inheritance of phenylpyruvic amentia (phenylketonuria)', *Lancet* ii (1935): 192–4.

—— and J.B.S. Haldane, 'Mutation rates in man', *Nature* 135 (1935): 907–8.

——, 'The detection of autosomal linkage in data which consist of pairs of brothers and sisters of unspecified parentage', *Ann. Eugen.* 6 (1935): 133–8.

——, see Gunther, M., and —— (1935).

——, 'Autosomal mutation and modification in man with special reference to mental defect', *Ann. Eugen.* 7 (1936): 1–16.

——, see Great Britain, Medical Research Council (1938).

——, 'Eugenic prognosis with respect to mental deficiency', *Eugen. Rev.* 31 (1939): 35–7.

——, 'The supposed threat of declining intelligence', *Am. J. Ment. Deficiency* 53 (1948): 114–18.

——, 'The Galton Laboratory: its work and its aims', *Eugen. Rev.* 41 (1949): 17–27.

——, 'Genetical influences on the intelligence level of the population', paper read to the British Association for the Advancement of Science, Newcastle, 1949; *Brit. J. Psychol.* 40 (1950): 128–36.

——, Obituary, J.B.S. Haldane, *Brit. Med. J.* ii (1964): 1936.

——, 'Presidential Address: the influence of the English tradition in human genetics', *Proc. III Internat. Congress of Human Genetics, University of Chicago, September 5–10, 1966: Plenary Sessions and Symposia,* (Baltimore, MD: Johns Hopkins, 1967).

Penrose, Margaret, and Lionel S. Penrose, 'The blood group distribution in the eastern counties of England', *Brit. J. Exper. Path.* 14 (1933): 160–1.

Pigou, Arthur C., 'The economic aspect of the problem', in [Slater] *Problem of the Feeble-Minded* (1909), 97–101.

Pirie, N.W., 'John Burdon Sanderson Haldane', *Biog. Mems of Fellows of Roy. Soc.* (London) 12 (1966): 212–49.

Pleger, Werner, 'Erblichkeits-untersuchungen an schwachsinnigen Kindern', *Z. f. d. ges. Neurol. u. Psych.* 135 (1931): 225–52.

Punnett, Reginald C., *Mendelism* (London: Macmillan, 1905, 1907, 1911).

——, 'Genetics and eugenics', read before public meeting of Cambridge University Eugenics Society, Friday, 5 December 1911, ms, Cambridge Minute Book; reported in *Cambridge Daily News,* 6 Dec. 1911.

——, 'Eliminating feeblemindedness', *J. Heredity* 8 (1917): 464–5.

Race, Robert R., ms notebook (1938).

——, 'On the inheritance and linkage relations of acholuric jaundice', *Ann. Eugen.* 11 (1942): 365–84.

—— and Ruth Sanger, *Blood Groups in Man* (Oxford: Blackwell, 1st ed. 1950, 6th/last ed., 1975).

Rathbone, Eleanor, *The Disinherited Family,* introduction by S. Fleming (London: Falling Wall Press, 1986).

Reid, G. Archdall, *Alcoholism, a Study in Heredity* (London: Unwin, 1901).

——, 'Human evolution and alcohol', *Brit. J. Inebriety* 1 (1903–4): 186–201.

——, 'The biological foundation of society', *Sociological Papers* 3 (1906): 3–52.

Renwick, J.H., and Sylvia D. Lawler, 'Linkage between the ABO and nail-patella loci', *Ann. Human Genet.* 19 (1955): 312–31.

——, 'Mapping of human chromosomes', *Ann. Rev. Genet.* 5 (1971): 81–120.

Roberts, J.A. Frazer, 'Reginald Ruggles-Gates, 1882–1962', *Biographical Memoirs of Fellows of Roy. Soc.* (London) 10 (1964): 83–106.

Rockefeller Foundation, *Annual Reports.*

——, *Archives.*

Rolfe, Sybil, (Mrs Neville), (a.k.a. Sybil Gotto), see obituary, 'Sybil Neville Rolfe, O.B.E., 1886–1955', *Eugen. Rev.* 47 (1955–56): 149 (N); 214(N).

——, 'The relation between venereal disease and the regulation of prostitution', *Proceedings of the Imperial Social Hygiene Congress, British Empire Exhibition, Wembley, 12–16 May, 1924* (London: National Council for Combatting Venereal Disease, 1924).

Rolleston, Sir Humphrey, 'Eugenics and medicine', in Blacker, C.P. (1934), ix–xi.

Rothamsted Experimental Station, *Guide to the Experimental Farms* (Harpenden, Hertfordshire: Lawes Agricultural Trust, 1962).

——, *Guide to the Classical Field Experiments* (Harpenden, Hertfordshire: Lawes Agricultural Trust, 1984).

Rüdin, Ernst, see Gruber, M. von, and —— (1911).

——, 'Veröffentlichung aus der genealogischen Abteilung', Bibliography, prepared 1932; ms, Eugen. Soc. Papers, C301.

——, 'Einige Wege und Ziele der Familienforschung, mit Rücksicht auf die Psychiatrie', *Z. f. d. ges. Neurol. u. Psychiatrie* 7 (1911): 487–585.

——, *Studien über Vererbung und Entstehung geistiger Störungen, I. Zur Vererbung und Neuentstehung der* Dementia praecox, No. 12 in series Monographien aus dem Gesamtgebiete der Neurologie und Psychiatrie (Berlin: Springer, 1916).

——, 'Psychiatrische Indikation zur Sterilisierung', *Das kommende Geschlecht* 5 (1929): 1–19; reprinted by the Eugenics Society of London as a pamphlet.

——, 'Praktische Ergebnisse der psychiatrischen Erblichkeitsforschung', *Arch. f. Rassen- u. Gesellsch. biol.* 24 (1930): 228–37.

——, 'Empirische Erbprognose', *Arch. f. Rassen- u. Gesellsch. biol.* 27 (1933): 271–83.

——, ed., *Erblehre und Rassenhygiene im volkischen Staat* (Munich: Lehmann, 1934).

Russell, Sir Edward John, *Soil Conditions and Plant Growth* (1912) (London: Longmans, 4th ed., 1921).

——, *Plant Nutrition and Crop Production* (Berkeley, CA: University of California Press, 1926).

——, 'Field experiments: how they are made and what they are', *J. Min. Ag.* 32 (1926): 989–1001.

——, *History of Agricultural Science in Great Britain*, 1620–1954 (London: Allen, 1966).

——, *The Land Called Me: an Autobiography* (London: Allen, 1956).

Russell, A.S., 'Ability and educational opportunity', *The Listener* (2 Oct. 1935), 554.

Sadler, M.E., 'The International Congress on Moral Education', *Int. J. Ethics* 7 (1909): 158–73.

Sayer, Ettie, Report of speech to Moral Education Congress, 'A woman doctor's remedies', *Daily Mail* (30 Sept. 1908).

Schenk, Faith, and A.S. Parkes, 'The activities of the Eugenics Society', *Eugen. Rev.* 60 (1968): 142–61.

Schuster, Edgar, see Galton, F., and —— (1906).

——, *The Promise of Youth and the Performance of Manhood: Being a Statistical Examination into the Relation Existing between Success in the Examinations for the B.A. Degree at Oxford and Subsequent Success in Professional Life. (The Professions Considered are the Bar and the Church)*, No. 3 in series, Eugenics Laboratory Memoirs (London: Dulau, 1907).

—— and Ethel M. Elderton, *The Inheritance of Ability: Being a Statistical*

Examination of the Oxford Class Lists from the Year 1800 Onwards, and of the School Lists of Harrow and Charterhouse, No. 1 in series, Eugenics Laboratory Memoirs (London: Dulau, 1907).

Sjögren, Torsten, 'Die juvenile amaurotische Idiotie: klinische und erblichkeitsmedizinische Untersuchungen', *Hereditas* (Lund) 14 (1931): 197–425.

Slater, Eliot, 'Mental disorder and the social problem group', in Blacker, C.P. (1937), 37–49.

[Slater, (Mrs Walter)], *The Problem of the Feeble-Minded: an Abstract of the Royal Commission on the Care and Control of the Feeble-Minded, with an Introduction by the Rt. Hon. Sir Francis Galton, F.R.S., &c.* (London: King, 1909).

Slaughter, James W., Report of talk on eugenics, 'Biology and moral education', *Moral Education Congress, Record of Proceedings of the First International, &c., London, 1908*, (London: Nutt, 1908), 67.

——, The Adolescent (London: Allen, 1912).

Slome, David, 'The genetic basis of amaurotic family idiocy', *J. Genet.* 25 (1931): 363–78.

Smith, C.A.B., 'Professor J.B.S. Haldane', *Ass. Scientific Workers J.* 2 (1965): 3–4.

'Social biology and population improvement', *Nature* (16 Sept. 1939): 521–2; signed by F.A.E. Crew, J.B.S. Haldane, L. Hogben, J.S. Huxley *et al.*

Social Hygiene, see British Social Hygiene Council, Inc., also Venereal Disease, National Council for Combatting, also Venereal Disease, Society for the Prevention of.

Spearman, Charles, see Norton, B.J. (1979); Fancher, R.E., (1985); Gould, S.J. (1981).

——, 'General intelligence, objectively determined and measured', *Am. J. Psychol.* 15 (1904): 201–93.

——, The heredity of abilities', *Eugen. Rev.* 6 (1914–15): 219–37.

——, *The Abilities of Man* (New York, NY: Macmillan, 1927).

Spielmeyer, Walther, 'Die Eröffnung des Neubaues der Deutschen Forschungsanstalt für Psychiatrie (Kaiser Wilhelm Institut) in München', *Z. f. d. ges. Neurol. u. Psychiatrie* 113 (1928): 117–84.

[Spiller, G.A.], 'The growth of an idea', *Moral Education League Q.* 35 (1 Jan. 1914): 2–4.

Stewart, Alan, and Maurice J. Kendall, *Statistical Papers of George Udny Yule* (London: Griffith, 1971).

Stock, C.S., 'Eugenics', read to Cambridge University Eugenics Society (29 Oct. 1911); ms in Cambridge Minute Book.

——, Secretary's Report, 1911–12, ms in Cambridge Minute Book.

——, 'The principles of eugenics', *Cambridge Mag.* (18 May 1912).

——, see Fisher, R.A., and —— (1915–16).

Sydenham, Lord, [George Sydenham Clarke], 'The work of the National Council', *National Council for Combatting Venereal Disease, First Annual Report.* (1916), 12–17.

Tandler, J., 'Konstitution und Rassenhygiene', *Z. f. angewandte Anat. u. Konstitutionslehre* 1 (1914): 11–26.

Taylor, E.C., 'The pauper inebriate: a note on the aetiology of poverty', *Brit. J. Inebriety* 2 (1904–5): 112–16.

Taylor, Sir William, 'Memorandum', *Fitzroy Report* (1904), 1: 95–7 (Appendix I).

Thomson, Sir Godfrey H., *The Factorial Analysis of Human Ability* (London: London University Press, 1939).

Thomson, J. Arthur, 'The sociological appeal to biology', *Sociological Papers* 3 (1906): 157–96.

——, *Heredity* (London: Murray, 1909).

Tjio, Joe-Hin, and Albert Levan, 'Chromosome number in man', *Hereditas* (Lund) 42 (1956): 1–6.

Tredgold, Alfred F., *Mental Deficiency (Amentia)* (London: Ballière, 1st ed., 1908; New York, NY: Wood, 1912).

——, see Carr-Saunders *et al.* (1912–13).

Trend, Rt. Hon. Lord, 'The Caradog Jones Lecture: the self and society', *Biology & Society* 1 (1984): 14–28.

Turner, F. Douglas, 'Mental deficiency: the Presidential Address at the 92nd Annual Meeting of the Royal Medico-Psychological Association, Colchester, July 5, 1933', *J. Mental Sci.* 79 (1933): 563–77.

——, see Penrose, L.S. and —— (1931).

Venereal Disease, National Council for the Combatting of, *Annual Reports* 1916–; see Sydenham (1916).

——, Society for the Prevention of, see British Social Hygiene Council.

Webb, Beatrice, *My Apprenticeship* (London: Longman, 1926).

——, *Our Partnership*, B. Drake and M.I. Cole, eds (London: Longman, 1948).

[——], *Break up the Poor Law and Abolish the Workhouse: being Part I of the Minority Report of the Poor Law Commission* (London: Fabian Society, 1909).

——, *The Case for the National Minimum* (London: National Committee for the Prevention of Destitution, 1913).

Webb, Sidney, 'Eugenics and the Poor Law: the Minority Report', *Eugen. Rev.* 2 (1910–11): 233–7; reprinted in *Eugen. Rev.* 60 (1968): 71–5.

—— and Beatrice Webb, *The Decay of Capitalist Civilisation* (London: Fabian Society, 1923).

Weinberg, Wilhelm, see Boyer, S.H. (1963); Luxenburger, H. (1938); Stern, C. (1943).

——, 'Über Nachweis der Vererbung beim Menschen', *Jahrbuch d. vaterl. Naturkunde in Württemberg* 64 (1908): 368–82; reprinted in Boyer, S.H. (1963), 3–15.

——, 'Mathematischen Grundlagen der Probandenmethode', *Z. f. indukt. Abstammungs- u. Vererbungslehre*, 48 (1927): 179–228.

Went, L.N., and W.S. Volkers, 'Genetic linkage', *Advances in Neurology* 23 (1979): 37–42.

Wexler, Nancy, see Gusella, J.F.

White, Ray L., and Jean-Marc Lalouel, 'Chromosome mapping with DNA markers', *Scientific American* 258 (1988): 40–8.

Wiener, Alexander S., M. Lederer and S.H. Polayes, 'Studies in isohemagglutination III. On the heredity of the Landsteiner blood groups', *J. Immunol.* 18 (1930): 201–21.

——, I. Zieve and J.H. Fries, 'The inheritance of allergic disease', *Ann. Eugen.* 7 (1936): 141–62.

Winterstein, Hans, and E. Babak *et al.*, *Handbuch der vergleichende Physiologie*, 4 v in (Jena: Fischer, 1910–14).

Wofinden, R.C., *Problem Families in Bristol*, No. 6 in series Occasional Papers in Eugenics (London: Eugenics Society and Cassell, 1950).

——, see Blacker, C.P., and —— (1946–47).

Yanchinski, Stephanie, 'Genetic screening: employees under a microscope', Toronto *Globe and Mail* (3 Feb. 1990), D1; 3.

Yates, Frank, *The Design and Analysis of Factorial Experiments* (London: Commonwealth Bureau of Soil Science, 1937).

Yule, George Udny, see Stewart, A. and Kendall, M.G., eds (1971).

——, 'On the correlation of total pauperism with the proportion of out-relief, I. All ages; II. Males over 65', *Econ. J.* 5 (1895): 603–11; 6 (1896): 613–23.

——, 'Notes on the history of pauperism in England and Wales from 1850, treated by the method of frequency curves, with a note on the method', *J. Roy. Stats. Soc.* 59 (1896): 318–49.

——, 'Note on the teaching of the theory of statistics at University College', *J. Roy. Stats. Soc.* 60 (1897): 456–8.

——, 'On the theory of correlation', *J. Roy. Stats. Soc.* 60 (1897): 812–54.

——, 'Investigation into the causes of changes in pauperism in England, chiefly during the last two intercensal decades', *J. Roy. Stats. Soc.* 62 (1899): 249–56.

——, 'On the association of attributes in statistics', (1900) in Stewart, A., and Kendall, M.G. (1971).

——, 'Mendel's laws and their probable relation to interracial heredity', *New Phytologist* 1 (1902): 226–7.

——, 'On the theory of inheritance of quantitative compound characters on the basis of Mendel's laws – a preliminary note', *Report of the Third International Conference on Genetics* (London: Spottiswoode, 1907), 140–2.

——, *Introduction to the Theory of Statistics* (London: Griffin, 1911, 14th ed. 1950); subsequent editions were revised by Maurice G. Kendall.

——, 'On the method of measuring association between two attributes', (1912); reprinted in Stewart, A., and M.G. Kendall, eds (1971), 107–70.

——, 'Statistical methods in relation to eugenics: syllabus of a course given in the autumn of 1913 at the offices of the Society', Eugenics Education Society, *Sixth Annual Report* (1913–14).

——, *Introduction to the Theory of Statistics* (London: Griffin, 1911; last edition 1932).

—— and L.N.C. Filon, 'Karl Pearson', *Obituary Notices of Fellows of Roy. Soc.* (London) 2 (1936): 73–110.

——, *Statistical Papers of*, Stewart, A., and M.G. Kendall, eds (1971).

Zieve, I., Alexander S. Wiener and J.H. Fries, 'On the linkage relations of the genes of allergic disease and the genes determining blood groups, MN groups and eye colour in man', *Ann. Eugen.* 7 (1936): 163–78.

SECONDARY SOURCES

Abrams, Philip, 'History, sociology, historical sociology', *Past and Present* 87 (1980): 3–16.
Allen, Garland E., 'The introduction of *Drosophila* into the study of heredity and evolution', *Isis* 66 (1975): 322–33.
——, 'The Eugenics Record Office at Cold Spring Harbor, 1910–1940: an essay in institutional history', *Osiris* 2 (1986): 225–64.
Aly, Götz, ed., *Totgeschweigen 1933–1944: Die Geschichte der Karl-Bonhoeffer-Nervenklinik*, Arbeitsgruppe zur Erforschung der Geschichte der Karl-Bonhoeffer-Nervenklinik (Berlin: Hentrich, 1988).
Anon., 'John Burdon Sanderson Haldane', *New York Times*, (1 Dec. 1964): 1, 45.
Anon., 'Lancelot Hogben', *The Times*, (23 Aug. 1975): 14.
Baader, Gerhard and Ulrich Schulz, eds, *Medizin und Nationalsozialismus: tabuisierte Vergangenheit – ungebrochene Tradition?* (Berlin: Verlag Gesundheit, 2nd ed., 1983).
Banks, J.A., and David V. Glass, 'A list of books and articles on the population question, published in Britain in the period 1793–1880', in Glass, D.V. (1953), 79–112.
Beales, H.L., 'The historical context of the *Essay on Population*, in Glass, D.V. (1953), 1–24.
Berridge, Virginia, 'Editorial', *Brit. J. Addiction (Inebriety)* 79 (1984): 1–6.
Birnbaum, Norman, in Hans P. Dreitzel, ed., *Recent Sociology*, No. 1 (a yearbook) (New York, NY: Macmillan, 1969); cited by Bottomore, T.B. (1975).
Bottomore, Thomas B., *Sociology as Social Criticism* (London: Allen, 1975).
Bowler, Peter J., 'E.W. MacBride's Lamarckian eugenics and its implications for the social construction of scientific knowledge', *Ann. Sci.* 41 (1984): 245–60.
Box, Joan Fisher, *R.A. Fisher: the Life of a Scientist* (New York, NY: Wiley, 1978).
Boyer, S.H., *Papers on Human Genetics* (Englewood Cliffs, NJ: Prentice Hall, 1963).
Briggs, Asa, and Anne Macartney, *Toynbee Hall: the First Hundred Years* (London: Routledge, 1985).
Burrow, J.W., *Evolution and Society: a Study in Victorian Social Theory* (Cambridge: University Press, 1966).
Bynum, William P., 'Alcohol and degeneration in twentieth century European medicine and psychiatry', *Brit. J. Addiction (Inebriety)* 79 (1984): 59–70.
Calman, W.T., Obituary, 'Ernest William MacBride', *Biographical Memoirs of Fellows of Roy. Soc.* (London) 3 (1940): 747–59.
Carlson, E.A., *The Gene: a Critical History* (Philadelphia, PA: Saunders, 1966).

Carlson, Eric T., 'Medicine and degeneration: theory and praxis', in Chamberlin, J.E., and S.L. Gilman, eds (1985) 121–144.

Carpenter, James Estlin, *The Life and Work of Mary Carpenter* (London: Macmillan, 1881).

Clark, Ronald W., 'Haldane, John Burdon Sanderson', in C.C. Gillespie, ed., *Dictionary of Scientific Biography* (New York, NY: Scribner's, 1972).

Coale, Ansley K., 'The decline of fertility in Europe from the French revolution to World War II', in S.J. Behrman, L. Corsa and R. Freeman, eds, *Fertility and Family Planning: a World View* (Ann Arbor, MI: University of Michigan Press, 1970), 3–24.

Coleman, William, *Death is a Social Disease: Public Health and Political Economy in Early Industrial France*, (Madison, WI: University Press, 1892).

Cowan, Ruth Schwarz, 'Sir Francis Galton and the study of heredity in the nineteenth century', Dissertation, Johns Hopkins University, 1969 (Ann Arbor, MI: University Microfilms, 1969).

——, Introduction to Galton (1874/1970).

Cullen, M.J., *The Statistical Movement in Early Victorian Britain: the Foundations of Empirical Social Research*, (Hassocks, Sussex: Harvester, 1975).

Dahlberg, Kenneth A., *Beyond the Green Revolution: the Ecology and Politics of Global Agricultural Development* (New York, NY: Plenum, 1979).

Dalrymple, D.G., *Development and Spread of High Yielding Varieties of Wheat and Rice in the Less Developed Nations*, No. 95 in series, Foreign Agriculture Reports (Washington, DC: US Department of Agriculture, 6th ed., 1978).

Dronamraju, K.R., ed., *Haldane and Modern Biology* (Baltimore, MD: Johns Hopkins, 1968).

Dunn, L.C., *A Short History of Genetics: the Development of some of the Main Lines of Thought 1864–1939* (New York, NY: McGraw-Hill, 1965).

Eversley, D.E.C., *Social Theories of Fertility and the Malthusian Debate* (Oxford: Clarendon, 1959).

Fancher, Raymond E., *The Intelligence Men: Makers of the IQ Controversy* (New York, NY: Norton, 1985).

Farrall, Lyndsay A., 'The origin and growth of the British eugenics movement 1865–1925', dissertation, University of Indiana, 1970 (Ann Arbor, MI: University Microfilms, 1970).

——, 'The role of controversy and conflict in science – a case study: the English biometric school and Mendel's laws', *Social Stud. Sci.* 5 (1975): 269–301.

Flinn, Michael W., Editor's introduction to *Report on the Sanitary Condition of the Labouring Population of Great Britain, by Edwin Chadwick (1842)* (Edinburgh: University Press, 1965), 1–75.

Foucault, Michel, *L'Archéologie du Savoir* (Paris: Gallimard, 1969).

Frazer, Derek, *The Evolution of the British Welfare State: a History of Social Policy since the Industrial Revolution* (London: Macmillan, 1973).

Freeden, Michael, 'Eugenics and progressive thought', *Historical J.* 22 (1979): 645–71.

Froggatt, Peter, and N.C. Nevin, 'Galton's law of ancestral heredity: its influence on the early development of human genetics', *Hist. Sci.* 21 (1971): 1–27.
—— and ——, 'The "law of ancestral heredity" and the Mendelian-ancestrian controversy in England, 1899–1906', *J. Med. Genet.* 8 (1971): 1–36.
Giddens, Anthony, *The Class Structure of Advanced Societies* (London: Hutchinson, 1981).
Gilbert, B.B., *British Social Policy 1914–1939* (London: Batsford, 1970).
Gillie, Oliver, 'Crucial data was faked by eminent psychologist', *The Sunday Times* (24 Oct. 1976).
Glass, David V., *The Struggle for Population* (Oxford: Clarendon, 1936).
——, 'The Berlin Population Congress and recent population movements in Germany', *Eugen. Rev.* 27 (1935–36): 207–12.
——, 'Changes in fertility in England and Wales, 1851–1931', in Hogben, L. (1938), 161–212.
——, *Population: Policies and Movements in Europe* (1940), reprinted with a new introduction (London: Cass, 1967).
——, *Introduction to Malthus* (London: Watts, 1953).
—— and D.E.C. Eversley, eds, *Population in History* (London: Arnold, 1964).
—— and R. Revelle, eds, *Population and Social Change* (London: Arnold, 1972).
Gould, Stephen Jay, *The Mismeasure of Man* (New York, NY: Norton, 1981).
Graham, Loren R., 'Science and values: the eugenics movement in Germany and Russia in the 1920s', *Am. Historical Rev.* 82 (1977): 1133–64.
——, *Between Science and Values* (New York, NY: Columbia University Press, 1981).
——, 'The socio-political roots of Boris Hessen: Soviet Marxism and the history of science', *Soc. Stud. Sci.* 15 (1985): 705–22.
Greenwood, John O., *Quaker Encounters*, v. I: *Friends and Relief* (York: Sessions, 1975).
Günther, Maria, 'Die Institutionalizierung der Rassenhygiene an den deutschen Hochschulen vor 1933', Dissertation, Johann Gutenberg Universität, Mainz, 1982.
Hacking, Ian, 'Telepathy: origins of randomisation in experimental design', *Isis* 79 (1988): 427–51.
Hajnal, John, 'European marriage patterns in perspective', in David V. Glass and D.E.C. Eversley, eds, *Population in History* (1964), 101–43.
Harman, H.H., *Modern Factor Analysis* (Chicago, IL: University of Chicago Press, 3rd ed., 1976).
Harris, Harry, Obituary, 'Lionel Sharples Penrose, 1898–1972', *Biographical Memoirs of Fellows of Roy. Soc.* (London) 19 (1973): 521–61.
——, 'Development of Penrose's ideas in genetics and psychiatry', *Brit. J. Psychiatry* 125 (1974): 529–36.
Harris, Jose, *William Beveridge: a Biography* (Oxford: Clarendon, 1977).

Harrison, Brian, *Drink and the Victorians: the Temperance Question in England, 1815–1872* (London: Faber, 1971).

Hearnshaw, L.S., *Cyril Burt, Psychologist* (London: Hodder, 1979).

Heer, David M., 'Economic development and the fertility transition', in Glass, D.V., and R. Revelle, eds (1972), 99–113.

Hobsbawm, Eric J., *Labour's Turning Point, 1880–1900* (London: Lawrence, 1948).

——, *Labouring Men: Studies in the History of Labour* (London: Weidenfeld, 1968).

Holmes, C., 'Bukharin in England', *Soviet Stud.* (July 1972): 86–90.

Hogben, Lancelot, ed., *Political Arithmetic: a Symposium of Population Studies* (London: Allen, 1938).

James, Patricia, *Population Malthus, his Life and Times* (London: Routledge, 1979).

Jaspers, Karl, *Nietzsche: an Introduction to his Philosophical Activity* (1935), trans. C.F. Wallraff and F.J. Schmitz (Flagstaff, AR: University of Arizona Press, 1965).

Johnson, Richard, 'Three problematics: elements of a theory of working-class culture', in John C. Clarke, Charles Critcher and Richard Johnson, eds, *Working-Class Culture: Studies in History and Theory* (London: Hutchinson, 1979), 201–37.

Jones, Gareth Stedman, *Outcast London: a Study in the Relationship between Classes in Victorian Society* (1971) (Harmondsworth, Middlesex: Penguin, 1976).

——, 'Class expression vs. social control? A critique of recent trends in the history of leisure', Jones, G. Stedman (1983), 76–89.

——, *Languages of Class: Studies in English Working Class History* (Cambridge: University Press, 1983).

Jones, Greta, *Social Hygiene in Twentieth Century Britain* (London: Croom Helm, 1986).

Jones, Kathleen, *Mental Health and Social Policy, 1845–1959* (London: Routledge, 1972).

Joravsky, David, 'Soviet views on the history of science', *Isis* 46 (1955): 3–13.

Joshi, Heather, and Vijay Joshi, *Surplus Labour and the City: a Study of Bombay* (Delhi: Oxford University Press, 1976).

Kamin, Leon J., *The Science and Politics of IQ* (1974) (Harmondsworth, Middlesex: Penguin, 1977).

Kennedy, Thomas C., 'Fighting about peace: the No-Conscription Fellowship and the British Friends' Service Committee, 1915–1919', *Quaker Hist.* 69 (1980): 3–22.

——, *The Hound of Conscience: a History of the No-Conscription Fellowship and the British Friends' Service Committee 1915–1919* (Fayetteville, AR: University of Arkansas Press, 1981).

Kevles, Daniel J., 'Genetics in the United States and Britain, 1890–1930: a review with speculations', *Isis* 71 (1980): 441–55.

——, *In the Name of Eugenics: Genetics and the Uses of Human Heredity* (New York, NY: Knopf, 1985).

Kimmelman, Barbara, 'The American Breeders' Association: genetics and eugenics in an agricultural context, 1903–1913', *Social Stud. Sci.* 13 (1983): 163–204.

Knodel, J., 'Law, marriage and illegitimacy in nineteenth century Germany', *Population Studies* (March 1967): 279–94.

Koestler, Arthur, *The Case of the Midwife Toad* (London: Hutchinson, 1971).

Kuczynski, Robert René, 'British demographers' opinions on fertility and the Malthusian debate', in Hogben, L., ed., (1938), 283–327.

Lawson, J., and Harold Silver, *A Social History of Education in England* (London: Methuen, 1973).

Leach, R.A., *The Mental Deficiency Act as Amended, &c., with Introduction and Annotatations* ... 3rd ed., edited by R.W. Leach (London: Poor Law Publications, 1924).

Ludmerer, Kenneth, *Genetics and American Society: a Historical Appraisal* (Baltimore, MD: Johns Hopkins, 1972).

McCandless, Peter, 'Curses of civilisation: insanity and drunkenness in Victorian Britain', *Brit. J. Addiction* 79 (1984): 49–58.

MacKenzie, Donald A., 'Eugenics in Britain', *Social Studies of Science* 6 (1976): 499–532.

——, *Statistics in Britain, 1865–1930: the Social Construction of Scientific Knowledge* (Edinburgh: University Press, 1981).

——, 'Sociobiologies in competition: the biometrician–Mendelian debate', in Charles Webster, ed. *Biology, Medicine and Society* (1981), 243–88.

McLaren, Angus, *Birth Control in Nineteenth Century England* (New York, NY: Holmes & Meier, 1978).

MacLeod, Roy M., 'The edge of hope: social policy and alcoholism, 1870–1900', *J. Hist. Med.* 22 (1967): 215–45.

McOuat, Gordon, 'Was Haldane a eugenist?' (in preparation).

Mayr, Ernst, and William B. Provine, *The Evolutionary Synthesis: Perspectives on the Unification of Biology,* (Cambridge, MA: Harvard University Press, 1980).

Mazumdar, Dipak, 'Labour supply in early industrialisation: the case of the Bombay textile industry', *Econ. Hist. Rev.* 26 (1973): 477–96.

——, 'The urban informal sector', *World Development* (Oxford) 5 (1976): 655–80.

Mazumdar, Pauline M.H., 'Karl Landsteiner and the problem of species, 1838–1968', dissertation, Johns Hopkins University, 1976 (Ann Arbor, MI: University Microfilms, 1981).

——, 'The eugenists and the residuum: the problem of the urban poor', *Bull. Hist. Med.* 54 (1980): 204–15.

——, 'Anatomical physiology and the reform of medical education 1825–1835', *Bull. Hist. Med.* 57 (1983): 230–46.

——, 'Blood and soil: the serology of the Aryan racial state', *Bull. Hist. Med.* 64 (1990): 187–219.

——, 'Two models for human genetics: blood grouping and psychiatry in Germany between the wars', (in preparation).

Meek, Ronald L., ed., *Marx and Engels on Malthus: Selections from the Writings of Marx and Engels dealing with the Theories of Thomas Robert Malthus* (New York, NY: International, 1954).

Mowat, C.L., *The Charity Organisation Society 1869–1913, its Ideas and Work* (London: Methuen, 1961).

Nathan, H., 'Bernstein, Felix', in C.C. Gillespie, ed., *Dictionary of Scientific Biography* (New York, NY: Scribner's, 1970), v 2, 58–79.

Norton, Bernard J., 'Biology and philosophy: the methodological foundation of biometry', *J. Hist. Biol.* 6 (1975): 85–93.

—— and Egon S. Pearson, 'A note on the background to, and refereeing of, R.A. Fisher's 1918 paper, "On the correlation between relatives on the supposition of Mendelian inheritance"', *Notes and Records of Roy. Soc.* (London) 31 (1976): 151–62.

——, 'Karl Pearson and statistics: the social origin of scientific innovation', *Social Stud. Sci.* 8 (1978): 3–34.

——, 'Charles Spearman and the general factor in intelligence: genesis and interpretation in the light of socio-personal considerations', *J. Hist. Behav. Sci.* 15 (1979): 142–54.

——, 'The biometric defense of Darwinism', *J. Hist. Biol.* 13 (1983): 283–316.

Nowak, Kurt, *'Euthanasie' und Sterilisierung im 'Dritten Reich': die Konfrontation der evangelischen und katholischen Kirche mit dem 'Gesetz zur Verhütung-erbkranken Nachwuchses', und der 'Euthanasie'-Aktion* (Göttingen: Vandenhoek, 1984).

Olby, Robert C., *The Origins of Mendelism* (New York, NY: Schlocken, 1966).

Parkin, Frank, *Middle Class Radicalism: the Social Bases of the British Campaign for Nuclear Disarmament* (Manchester: University Press, 1968).

Paul, Diane, 'Eugenics and the left', *J. Hist. Ideas* 45 (1984): 576–90.

Petty, C., 'The MRC's interwar dietary surveys', *Soc. Social Hist. Med. Bull.* (London) 37 (1985): 76–8.

Provine, William B., see Mayr, E., and —— (1980).

——, *The Origins of Theoretical Population Genetics* (Chicago, IL: University Press, 1971).

——, 'The role of mathematical models in the evolutionary synthesis of the 1930s and 1940s', *Stud. Hist. Biol.* 2 (1978): 167–92.

Rae, John, *Conscience and Politics: the British Government and the Conscientious Objector to Military Service, 1916–1919* (London: Oxford University Press, 1970).

Ritt, Lawrence, 'The Victorian conscience in action: the National Association for the Promotion of Social Science, 1857–1886', dissertation, Columbia University, 1959 (Ann Arbor, MI: University Microfilms, 1959).

Rosen, George, 'Cameralism and the concept of medical police', *Bull. Hist. Med.* 27 (1952): 21–42; reprinted in Rosen (1974), 120–41.

——, *From Medical Police to Social Medicine: Essays on the History of Health Care* (New York, NY: Science History, 1974).

Rosenberg, Charles, *No Other Gods: Science and American Social Thought* (Baltimore, MD: Johns Hopkins Press, 1976).

Sandbrook, Richard, and J. Arn, *The Labouring Poor and Urban Class Formation*, No.12 in Monograph Series, Centre for Developing-Area Studies (Montreal: McGill University Press, 1977).

Searle, G.R., 'Eugenics and class', in Webster, C., ed., (1981), 212–42.

Shapiro, Alexander, 'A biographical note', [on L.S. Penrose] *Brit. J. Psychiatry* 125 (1974): 517–20.

Silver, Harold, *English Education and the Radicals, 1780–1850* (London: Routledge, 1971).

Spengler, J.J., 'French population theory since 1800. I.', *J. Econ.* 44 (1926): 577–611; 743–66.

Stern, Curt, 'The Hardy-Weinberg Law', *Science* 97 (1943): 137–8.

Sutherland, Gillian, 'Measuring intelligence: English Local Education Authorities and mental testing, 1919–1939', in Webster, C., ed. (1981), 315–35.

Tatham, Meaburn, and James E. Miles, eds, *The Friends' Ambulance Unit 1914–1919: a Record* (London: Swarthmore, 1919).

Tholfsen, Trygve, ed., *Sir James Kay-Shuttleworth on Popular Education* (New York, NY: Teachers' College Press, 1974).

Thompson, Edward P., *The Making of the English Working Class* (New York, NY: Vintage, 1963).

——, *William Morris: Romantic to Revolutionary* (London: Merlin, 2nd ed., 1977).

Thompson, F.M.L., 'Social control in Victorian Britain', *Econ. Hist. Rev.* 34 (1981): 189–208.

Titmuss, Richard M., *The Irresponsible Society*, No. 323 in series, Fabian Tracts (London: Fabian Society, 1959).

Walker, Helen M., *Studies in the History of Statistical Method* (Baltimore, MD: Williams, 1929).

Waterman, Lawrence S., 'The Eugenics Movement in Britain in the nineteen-thirties', Dissertation, University of Sussex, 1975.

Webb, R.K., *Harriet Martineau: a Radical Victorian* (London: Heinemann, 1960).

Webster, Charles, ed., *Biology, Medicine and Society, 1840–1940* (Cambridge: University Press, 1981).

——, 'Health, welfare and unemployment during the depression', *Past & Present* 109 (1985): 204–30.

Wells, G.P., Obituary, 'Lancelot Hogben', *Biographical Memoirs of Fellows of Roy. Soc.* (London) 24 (1978): 183–221.

Werskey, P. Gary, see Bukharin, N.I. (1931/1971).

——, *The Visible College* (London: Lane, 1978).

——, 'Haldane and Huxley: the first appraisals', *J. Hist. Biol.* 4 (1971): 171–83.

Wurmser, R., 'Haldane as I knew him', in Dronamraju, K.R., (1968): 313–17.

Yates, Frank, and K. Mather, Obituary, 'Ronald Aylmer Fisher', *Biographical Memoirs of Fellows of Roy. Soc.* (London) 9 (1963): 91–120.

——, 'Sir Ronald Fisher and the design of experiments', *Biometrics* 20 (1964): 307–21.

INDEX

acholuric jaundice (haemolytic anaemia) 240–1, 316 n.139
Adams, Mrs Bridges 26
alcaptonuria 175, 181–2, 304 n.89
alcoholism, 13, 20, 80, 85, 207; *British Journal of Inebriety*, 31; cause of pauperism 20, 56, 198, 276 n.97; social problem group and 198; Society for Promoting Legislation for the Control and Cure of Habitual Drunkards 30; Society for the Study of Inebriety 9, 25, 30; Tredgold, A.F. on 80, Fig.2.4
Alexander, Horace G. 312 n.73
Allaun, Frank 50, 282 n.174
Allbut, Sir Clifford 102
Allen, Clifford 223
Allen, Garland E. 287 n.47
Aly, Götz 301 n.28
Alzheimer's disease 261, 318 nn.8, 12
amaurotic family idiocy 175, 229, 301 n.59, 304 n.90
amentia *see also* feeblemindedness, mental deficiency, primary and secondary 198, 215; Tredgold, A.F. on 80, Fig. 2.4, 107; *Mental Deficiency (Amentia)* 79; *Wood Report* 198–200, 215
American Breeder's Association 82, 89, 287 n.47, 288 n.77

Annals of Eugenics becomes *Annals of Human Genetics* 253, 257
ante-dating (anticipation) 140, 218
Anthropological Institute, Royal 126
Anthropology, Department of, Oxford 126–7
'Ardent Mendelian' 70, 82, 95, 287 n.48
Arn, J. 272 n.42
Association for the Education of Women 25
Association of Headmistresses 25
asthma 213

Baader, Gerhard 278 n.127
Babak, E. 152, 299 n.25
Bateson, William 232, 286 n.31; eugenics and 232; MacBride, E.W. and 67; Mendelism and 60, 98, 283 n.5; presence and absence theory 60, 67, 82; Provine, W.B. on 60, 283 n.2; Punnett, R.C. and 61, 98–9, 177
Beales, H.L. 37, 277 n.19
Baur, Erwin 178, 305 n.99
Bell, Daniel 258
Bell, Julia 283 n.1
Bernal, J. Desmond 190, 307 n.130
Bernstein, Felix 149, 162; ABO blood groups, inheritance of 164–5, 166–9, 184, 253;

Printed in Great Britain
by Amazon